INFECTIOUS DISEASES IN THE ELDERLY

Edited by
Burke A. Cunha

PSG Publishing Company, Inc.
Littleton, Massachusetts

Library of Congress Cataloging-in-Publication Data

Infectious diseases in the elderly.

    Includes bibliographies and index.
    1. Communicable diseases—Age factors. 2. Aged—
Diseases—Treatment.   I. Cunha, Burke A. [DNLM:
1. Communicable Diseases—in old age. WC 100 I4184]
RC112.I46 1988   618.97'69   88-17915
ISBN 0-88416-475-6

Published by
PSG Publishing Company, Inc.
545 Great Road
Littleton, Massachusetts 01460

Copyright © 1988 by PSG Publishing Company, Inc.

All rights reserved. No part of this publication may be reproduced or transmitted in any form or by any means, electronic or mechanical, including photocopy, recording, or information storage or retrieval system, without permission in writing from the publisher.

Printed in United States of America.

International Standard Book Number: 0-88416-475-6

Library of Congress Catalog Card Number: 88-17915

92 91 90 89 88 9 8 7 6 5 4 3 2 1

This book is dedicated to:

Marie, just Marie!*

For her unfailing love, inspiration, support, encouragement, and the faith to keep going against all odds.

                                                  With love and appreciation,

                                                             BAC

*And to all those in medicine providing competent and loving care to those patients in their twilight years.

CONTRIBUTORS

Robert C. Aber, MD
Vice Chairman Department of
 Medicine
Milton S. Hershey Medical Center
Pennsylvania State University
Hershey, Pennsylvania

John G. Bartlett, MD
Head, Division of Infectious Diseases
Johns Hopkins University School
 of Medicine
Baltimore, Maryland

Constance A. Benson, MD
Assistant Professor of Medicine
Infectious Disease
Rush-Presbyterian-St. Luke's
 Medical Center
Chicago, Illinois

Jerome A. Boscia, MD
Associate Professor of Medicine
Department of Medicine
Medical College of Pennsylvannia
Philadelphia, Pennsylvannia

Burke A. Cunha, MD
Chief, Infectious Disease Division
Winthrop-University Hospital
Mineola, New York

Carlos E. Donayre, MD
Surgical Research Fellow
Department of Surgery
Harbor / UCLA Medical Center
Torrance, California

Robert Fekety, MD
Professor, Internal Medicine
Chief, Division of Medical Infectious
 Diseases
University of Michigan Medical
 School and Hospitals
Ann Arbor, Michigan

Paul N. Gobbo, MD
Infectious Disease Division
Interfaith Medical Center
St. John's Episcopal Hospital Division
Brooklyn, New York

Peter A. Gross, MD
Director of Internal Medicine
Hackensack Medical Center
Professor of Medicine
New Jersey Medical School
Newark, New Jersey

Inge Gurevich, RN, MA
Coordinator, Infection Control
Infectious Disease Division
Winthrop-University Hospital
Mineola, New York

William J. Holloway, MD
Director, Infectious Disease Research
 Laboratory
Wilmington Medical Center
Wilmington, Delaware

Donald Kaye, MD
Chairman and Professor of Medicine
Department of Medicine
Medical College of Pennsylvania
Philadelphia, Pennsylvania

Carol A. Kauffman, MD
Professor, of Internal Medicine
Chief, Infectious Disease Medical
 Service
Veterans Administration Hospital
Ann Arbor, Michigan

Stuart Levin, MD
Director, Infectious Disease
Rush-Presbyterian-St Luke's Medical
 Center
Chicago, Illinois

Donald B. Louria, MD, FACP
Chairman and Professor
Department of Preventive Medicine
and Community Health
UMDNJ-NJ Medical School
Newark, New Jersey

Martin C. McHenry, MD, MS
Chairman, Department of
Infectious Diseases
The Cleveland Clinic Foundation
Cleveland, Ohio

Aksel G. Nordestgaard, MD
Research Fellow, Department of
Surgery
Harbor / UCLA Medical Center
Torrance, California

Dean C. Norman, MD
Associate Chief
Clinical Section GRECC
Veterans Administration
Wadsworth Medical Center
Los Angeles, California

George A. Pankey, MD
Head, Section of Infectious Diseases
Ochsner Clinic
New Orleans, Louisiana

Richard H. Parker, MD
Director, Education and Research
Section of Infectious Diseases
Providence Hospital
Associate Professor of Medicine and
Pharmacy
Howard University
Washington, DC

John P. Phair, MD
Section of Infectious Disease and
Hypersensitivity
Department of Medicine
North Western University Medical
School
Chicago, Illinois

Anne Sacks-Berg, MD
Infectious Disease Division
Winthrop-University Hospital
Mineola, New York

Purnendu Sen, MD, FACP
Division of Infectious Diseases
Department of Internal Medicine
Raritan Bay Medical Center
Perth Amboy, New Jersey

John W. Sensakovic, MD, PhD
Director of Medical Education and
Nosocomial Disease Laboratory
St Michael's Medical Center
Newark, New Jersey

Leon G. Smith, MD, FACP
Director of Medicine
Chief of Infectious Diseases
St Michael's Medical Center
Newark, New Jersey

Michael J. Strampher, MD
Associate Director, Infectious Disease
Division
Winthrop-University Hospital
Mineola, New York

Dennis H. Sullivan, MD
Clinical Assistant Professor
Department of Medicine
University of Arkansas Medical
Science
Little Rock, Arkansas

Reisa F. Ullman, MD
Infectious Disease Division
Winthrop-University Hospital
Mineola, New York

Gregory T. Valainis, MD
Section on Infectious Diseases
Ochsner Clinic
New Orleans, Louisiana

Louis Weinstein, MD, PhD
Senior Consultant in Medicine
Brigham and Women's Hospital
Lecturer in Medicine
Harvard Medical School
Boston, Massachusetts

Michael R. Weitkamp, MD
Director, Department of Medicine
 Polyclinic Medical Center
Harrisburg, Pennsylvania

Richard P. Wenzel, MD, MSc
Professor and Director
Division of Clinical Epidemiology
Department of Internal Medicine
Iowa City, Iowa

Russell A. Williams, MD
Associate Chairman, Department of
 Surgery
Harbor / UCLA Medical Center
Torrance, California

Samuel E. Wilson, MD
Professor and Chairman,
Department of Surgery
Harbor/UCLA Medical Center
Torrance, California

Thomas T. Yoshikawa, MD
Chief, Division of Infectious Diseases
Veterans Administration
Wadsworth Medical Center
Los Angeles, California

CONTENTS

Preface   xi

SECTION I: GENERAL CONCEPTS

1   Infectious Diseases in the Elderly — An Overview   1
Louis Weinstein

2   Host Defenses in the Elderly   6
John P. Phair

3   Infection and Fever in the Elderly   18
Dean C. Norman and Thomas T. Yoshikawa

SECTION II: CLINICAL SYNDROMES

4   Central Nervous System Infections   25
Purnendu Sen and Donald B. Louria

5   Encephalitis   44
Reisa F. Ullman and Burke A. Cunha

6   Upper Respiratory Tract Infections in the Elderly   61
Constance A. Benson and Stuart Levin

7   Atypical Pneumonias   93
Paul N. Gobbo and Burke A. Cunha

8   Community-Acquired Pneumonias   116
Martin C. McHenry

9   Nosocomial Pnenumonias   144
Michael R. Weitekamp and Robert C. Aber

10   Endocarditis   159
Carol A. Kauffman and Robert Fekety

11   Infections of the Biliary Tract   173
Aksel G. Nordestgaard and Russell A. Williams

12 **Bacterial Infections of the Liver** 185
    Carlos E. Donayre and Samuel E. Wilson

13 **Viral Hepatitis** 194
    Inge Gurevich and Anne Sacks-Berg

14 **Intra-Abdominal Infections** 205
    John G. Bartlett

15 **Urinary Tract Infections** 216
    Jerome A. Boscia and Donald Kaye

16 **Prostatitis** 235
    William J. Holloway

17 **Skin and Soft Tissue Infections** 243
    Leon G. Smith and John W. Sensakovic

18 **Bone and Joint Infections** 254
    Richard H. Parker

SECTION III: SPECIAL PROBLEMS

19 **Fever of Unknown Origin** 271
    Michael J. Strampfer and Burke A. Cunha

20 **Infections in the Nursing Home Patient** 285
    Dennis H. Sullivan and Richard P. Wenzel

21 **Tuberculosis** 303
    George A. Pankey and Gregory T. Valainis

22 **Infections in the Diabetic Patient** 312
    Thomas T. Yoshikawa

23 **Immunizations** 324
    Peter A. Gross

24 **Antimicrobial Therapy** 330
    Burke A. Cunha

Index 345

PREFACE

The study of infectious diseases of the elderly has almost become a discipline in itself by the late 1980s. With each passing decade, a larger portion of the population becomes older with a resultant increase in multisystem diseases that accompany the aging process. The host defenses wane with advancing years and are further diminished by diseases or medications making the elderly person a special kind of compromised host. Infectious diseases in the older population warrant a special attention because infections in the aged differ in kind, severity, and presentation from younger adults. Many infectious diseases in the elderly individual are not unlike those in younger adults, but they tend to be more severe or prolonged and may have varied or atypical manifestations. Therapy is a special challenge in the elderly because host defenses are suboptimal. Special attention should be given to antibiotic dosing in the elderly because the majority of these patients will have some degree of hepatic renal insufficiency.

The rationale for a book like this is to make the clinician who cares for geriatric patients with infections more aware of their special problems. The aim of this book is to provide the clinician with a practical guide to the most important infectious disease problems in the elderly.

Burke A. Cunha, MD
Mineola, NY
1988

SECTION I
GENERAL CONCEPTS

1

Infectious Diseases in the Elderly — An Overview

Louis Weinstein

That the elderly have an increased susceptibility to infections appears to be well established. This is primarily a quantitative phenomenon that reflects the augmented risk of the development of a variety of infectious disorders and the increased fatality rates associated with them. There is, however, another aspect of the problem in older individuals that has received much less attention than the matter of a general increase in susceptibility. This involves the remarkable changes that have occurred in the natural history and clinical features of some infectious diseases, especially subacute infective endocarditis, pulmonary tuberculosis, and pneumonia caused by *Mycoplasma pneumoniae*, in older individuals. In addition to these qualitative differences, there is also ample evidence to support the fact that these diseases have increased in frequency in the elderly.

The prevalence of bacteremia is higher in elderly than in young persons, and is associated with a decrease in longevity.[1,2] Ten percent of older men and 20% of aging women experience episodes of bacteremia. Comparative figures in young persons are 0.1% and 5%, respectively. The attack rate of herpes zoster has been reported to range from 2.3 per 1000 patients 30 to 39 years of age, to 6.8 per 1000 in those 60 to 69 years old and 10 per 1000 in persons between the ages of 60 and 79 years.[3] Elderly patients are particularly susceptible to the development of pneumococcal pneumonia, and are at much higher risk of complications such as meningitis and endocarditis, when compared to young persons.[4,5] Pneumococcal bacteremia has been observed in 30% of the elderly and in 10% to 20% of the young; the associated fatality rates are 40% to 60%

and 10% to 20%, respectively.[4,5] Infection produced by gram-negative organisms such as *Escherichia coli, Enterobacter* and *Klebsiella pneumoniae* are involved in the pathogenesis of pneumonia much more commonly in the older age group than in the younger one. An important factor that predisposes the elderly to invasion by these organisms is the risk of aspiration of oropharyngeal contents associated with an altered state of consciousness, diminished gag and cough reflexes, esophageal dysfunction, and the presence of nasogastric or tracheostomy tubes.

A number of studies designed to examine the role of abnormalities of immune mechanisms that might be responsible for the increased susceptibility of the elderly to infection have not yielded promising results. Although it has been shown that the function of T cells is impaired in older individuals,[6-10] the data are open to question because they were derived from hospitalized and chronically institutionalized patients in whom the influence of factors such as underlying major illness and the nutritional status were not taken into consideration. Studies of the chemotactic and phagocytic activity of polymorphonuclear leukocytes, and the activity of the classic and alternate complement pathways have demonstrated no age differences.[11,12-14] It is clear that, at this moment, observation of immune mechanisms has not indicated that they play a critical role in altering the susceptibility of the elderly to infection.

A very important aspect of the problem of infection in the elderly is essentially qualitative in nature, and is related to changes in the clinical presentation and natural history of some infectious diseases in which increasing age appears to play a major role. Most striking, in this regard, are subacute infective endocarditis, pulmonary tuberculosis, and pneumonia caused by *M pneumoniae*. In addition to the qualitative changes, it is clear that there are also some quantitative ones.

There is no question that the incidence of subacute infective endocarditis is increasing in older individuals. It has become apparent that, among the patients with this disease, the mean age in the 1960s had already risen to 50 to 54 years. It is presently occurring commonly in those 60 to 80 years old. The ratio of men to women is now 9:1.[15] The most common type of underlying cardiac disorder is atherosclerotic valvular or annular disease; the aortic valve is most often involved. Because of the progressive decrease in the temperature of the body with increasing age, older patients are often considered to be afebrile when their oral temperature does not exceed 98.6°F when, in fact, this represents fever. Cultures of the blood appear to be sterile more often in older than in young patients. This may be related to delay in obtaining these because the patient has no "fever."

Although pulmonary tuberculosis is considered to be decreasing in incidence, a serious question may be raised as to whether, in fact, this is true. The writer's experience with this disease over the past 40 years has made it clear that a number of changes in the clinical behavior of this disease have confused the diagnosis when it is based on old descriptions of its presentation. One striking feature is a remarkable change in the age and sex distribution. In the past, tuberculosis of the lung was most common in women between the ages of 16 to 30 years. Presently, it occurs most often in men over 50 years old; its presence has been detected in not a small number of patients in their seventies and eighties. Two other features of pulmonary tuberculosis appear to be more frequent in elderly than in young persons. One involves the location of the lesion in the lung. Although the classic presentation in the posterior basilar segment of an upper lobe is still the most common, the writer has been impressed by the increasing frequency with which the lower lobes or even the right middle lobe are involved. Very striking has been his experience with an increasing incidence of negative tuberculin reactions in elderly patients from whose gastric aspirates *Mycobacterium tuberculosis* was recovered. These patients fell into two groups. Most were tuberculin-negative, but responded positively to intradermal injection of *Candida*, streptokinase-streptodornase (SK-SD), and mumps. A small number failed to react to all antigens. The fact that the suppression of reactivity to tuberculin was related to active infection was proved by demonstration of a strongly positive reaction 3 to 4 months after specific therapy was instituted.

An infection that has undergone most remarkable changes in its natural history that appear to be associated with aging is the pneumonia produced by *M pneumoniae*. As first described in the early 1940s when it was called "atypical viral pneumonia," the disease was reported to have the following characteristic clinical features. It occurred primarily in young persons and involved older ones very infrequently. The classic pulmonary lesion was present in the right middle lobe ("right middle lobe syndrome"). The temperature was only moderately elevated in most cases. There were no complications or recurrences, and no deaths. Treatment was not recommended unless the temperature was 102°F or higher; antimicrobial agents were given primarily to make patients "feel better," and not to alter the course of what was considered a benign disorder.

Over the years since it was first recognized, the changes in the clinical behavior of this common pulmonary disease have been most striking. First, and probably most important, has been the rapidly increasing incidence of this pneumonia in the elderly in whom it now appears to be very common. The clinical picture in older persons is, for the most part, very different from that which characterizes the disease in young persons. The level of fever is usually higher. There is no preferred site of the lesion in the lungs; it may be present in the upper or lower lobes or in the left lingula, and be nodular or diffuse. Complications involving the nervous system — mononeuritis, polyneuritis, Guillain-Barré syndrome, meningitis and encephalitis — although rare, occur most often in the elderly, and are not due to active infection, but are probably the result of presently undefined immunologic reactions. The writer has noted recurrence of pneumonia only in old people. One patient studied by him had four such episodes over a period of about 8 months. Each was characterized by a single "coin" lesion located in different areas of the lungs. The diagnosis was established during the last three infections by isolation of *M pneumoniae* from sputum and by serial serologic studies. Although rare, death has occurred in older persons. It is now clear that all older individuals with infection of the lung by *M pneumoniae* must be treated with an appropriate antimicrobial agent.

That aging is associated with an overall increase in susceptibility to a number of bacterial infections, many of which have a fatal outcome, is well established. Although a number of investigations directed to evaluation of the relation of immunologic competency to this have been carried out, none of the data obtained from these studies explain the basis for the increase in susceptibility. The results of some of these have been confused by failure to take into consideration the role played by extraneous factors such as the presence of illness other than infection and the nutritional status of patients.

It is interesting that, in most instances, immunologic studies in the elderly have been performed when the subjects are relatively well and not infected. An important question can be raised concerning the time at which such studies need to be carried out. In my opinion, an ideal approach to this problem involves examination of the level of immunocompetence of older individuals when they are well and again when they develop an infection. Such studies may disclose that while immunologic function is relatively normal during a healthy period, the stress of an acute infectious process decreases its effectiveness. Such investigations require the establishment of a cohort of elderly individuals who are studied longitudinally. A base of data concerning the adequacy of immunologic activity prior to infection will serve to define any important aberrations that may be induced after it develops.

The reasons for the striking changes in the natural history of tuberculosis, subacute infective endocarditis, and pneumonia caused by *M pneumoniae*, as indicated not only by an increase in their incidence but also in their clinical presentation, cannot be explained at this time. That this may also be the case in other infections in older persons is a possibility that needs to be examined. Ideal studies of this phenomenon would involve evaluation of specific factors such as the level of immunocompetence from youth to old age.[16] This is obviously not feasible. However, the first step in investigation of this phenomenon involves careful clinical study of patients throughout their lifetimes, an approach available to all internists and family physicians who often care for patients over extended periods. While this may not identify the reasons for the unusual behavior of some infections in the elderly, it would be most helpful in determining whether or not such changes in clinical behavior are peculiar to the infections listed above or whether they represent a general response to aging. Such information would be very valuable because it would prevent major diagnostic errors. The experience of the writer underscores the importance of this. He has learned that, were he to use the criteria on which diagnosis of subacute infective endocarditis was made 40 years ago, when the vast majority of patients were relatively young, the presence of the disease would be overlooked in over 90% of patients seen today.

REFERENCES

1. Nordenstam GR, Brandberg CA, Oden AS, et al: Bacteriuria and mortality in an elderly population. *N Engl J Med* 1986; 314:1152–1156.
2. Stamey TA, Fair WR, Timothy MM, et al: Antibacterial nature of prostate fluid. *Nature* 1968;218:444.
3. Hope-Simpson RE: The nature of herpes zoster: A long-term study and a new hypothesis. *Proc R Soc Med* 1965;58:9.
4. Austrian R, Gold J: Pneumococcal bacteremia with special reference to bacteremic pneumococcal pneumonia. *Ann Intern Med* 1964;60:759.
5. Mufson MA, Kruss DM, Wasil RE, et al: Capsular types and outcome of bacteremic pneumococcal disease in the antibiotic era. *Arch Intern Med* 1974;134:505.
6. Diaz-Jouanen E, Strickland RG, Williams RC: Studies of human lymphocytes in the newborn and aged. *Am J Med* 1975;58:620.
7. Hallgren HM, Buckley CE, Gilbertsen VA, et al: Lymphocyte phytohemagglutinin responsiveness, immunoglobins and auto-antibodies in aging humans. *J Immunol* 1973; 111:1101.
8. Weksler ME, Hutteroth TH: Impaired lymphocyte function in aged humans. *J Clin Invest* 1974;53:99.
9. Antel JP, Weinrich M, Aranson BG: Circulating suppressor cells in man as a function of age. *Clin Immunol Immunopathol* 1978;9:131.
10. Hallgren HM, Kersey JH, Dubey DP, et al: Lymphocyte subsets and integrated immune function in aging humans. *Clin Immunol Immunopathol* 1978;10:65.
11. Phair JP, Kauffman A, Bjornson A, et al: Host defenses in the aged: Evaluation of components of the inflammatory and immune responses. *J Infect Dis* 1978;188:67.
12. Jernigan JA, Gudat JC, Blake JL, et al: Reference values for blood findings in relatively fit elderly persons. *J Am Geriatr Soc* 1980;28:308.
13. MacKinney SA: Effect of age on the peripheral blood lymphocyte count. *J Gerontol* 1978;33:213.
14. Polednak AP: Age changes in differential leukocyte counts among female adults. *Hum Biol* 1978;50:301.
15. Weinstein L: Infective endocarditis, in Braunwald E (ed): *Heart Disease, A Text Book of Cardiovascular Medicine*. Philadelphia, WB Saunders Co, 1984, pp 1136–1182.
16. Murasko DM, Nelson BJ, Silver R, et al: Immunologic response in an elderly population with a mean age of 85. *Am J Med* 1986;81:612–618.

2

Host Defenses in the Elderly

John P. Phair

Clinicians have long accepted that infections in the elderly occur with increased frequency, often present obscurely, and cause high mortality and morbidity.[1] The scientific basis for these assumptions is not firm, partially because of a lack of a suitable definition of senescence. There are no physiologic and metabolic parameters analogous to the changes that delineate childhood from puberty. Cross-sectional investigations of host defenses in the elderly have used chronologic age to define the study population, a technique which can result in a survey of survivors, potentially a physiologically younger population. In addition, these investigations have excluded individuals with age-associated diseases such as cancer or diabetes, conditions known to alter host defenses and often complicated by infection.

The evidence that infections impose a risk for the elderly individual is based upon clinical and epidemiologic studies. An increased frequency of nosocomial infections, tuberculosis, herpes zoster, and an augmented morbidity and mortality in acute endocarditis in aged patients has been reported. Nosocomial urinary tract infections and bacteremia are 5 times more common in patients over 60 as compared to those 20 to 40 years of age. Hospital-acquired pneumonia occurs 3 times and wound infections 2 times as frequently in this older population.[2] These increases may reflect failure of resistance in the aged, or the increased time in hospitals of the elderly for complicated diseases. Invasive techniques of diagnosis and management including urinary instrumentation, intravascular devices, surgery plus the use of antibiotics, corticosteroids, and cytotoxic agents all may contribute to hospital-acquired infections in such patients.[3] The increasing frequency and mortality of infective endocarditis in the elderly contrast with results in younger patients; survival among the latter group is improved with penicillinase-resistant penicillin when compared to the pre- and early antibiotic era.[4] In the elderly with acute endocarditis the cause of the increased prevalence of metastatic infection which contributes to morbidity and mortality is not understood but may relate to ill-defined alterations in host resistance. Currently tuberculosis is a disease of the elderly.[5] This may represent a clinical manifestation of the well-studied changes in cell-mediated immunity in this age group. However, an alternative explanation is possible. Individuals 60 years of age and over are the major population exposed as children to this infection. Therefore they represent the major group who develop reactivation disease and who are exposed to infected patients. The localization of tuberculosis to this age group therefore may reflect successful public health measures introduced 50 to 70 years ago, not alteration in resistance of older individuals. In contrast, reactivation of herpes zoster infection is associated with waning of virus-specific immunity.[6] Shingles, however, is not limited to the old or very old. It is seen in young or middle-aged adults in the absence of an obvious immunologic defect.

HOST DEFENSES

Clinical infection implies that the skin or mucosal barriers have been breached by sufficient numbers of virulent microorganisms to overwhelm local defenses and must be differentiated from colonization. Colonization requires adherence of bacteria to body surfaces such as mucosa and is dependent on the interaction of cellular receptors, bacterial adhesions, and local barriers such as fibronectin and secretory IgA.[7-9] In addition, mechanical factors such as filtering of air by the nasal passages, the mucociliary elevator of the bronchial mucosa, cough reflexes, or urinary flow act to limit colonization and subsequent infection.

Once invasion has occurred the ability to resist infection is based on a complex set of cellular interactions which constitute the immune and inflammatory response. For clarity of presentation, cell-mediated immunity, antibody-dependent responses, and nonspecific resistance based on polymorphonuclear leukocytes (PMNs) and serum opsonins are discussed separately. It should be kept in mind, however, that the immune and inflammatory systems respond concurrently and are interrelated. Table 2-1 lists components of host defense and the common infections associated with specific deficiencies.

The immune response, both cell-mediated and antibody-dependent, requires processing and presentation of antigen by macrophages to responsive lymphocytes.[10] Macrophage processing of microorganisms, probably by enzymatic degradation, results in presentation of antigen in association with the class II major histocompatible complex (MHC) to responsive lymphocytes which have differentiated under the influence of

Table 2-1
Host Defense-Defects and Susceptibility to Infection

Deficiency	Type of Infection
PMN-complement	Staphylococcal
	Gram-negative bacillary
	Fungal
Antibody	Encapsulated pyogenic bacterial
Cell-mediated	Mycobacterial
	Protozoal
	Viral
	Fungal

the thymus gland (T cells).[11] Cell-mediated immune responses generally require this initial step. Protein antigens in high concentration and antigens such as polysaccharides can react directly with bone marrow–derived lymphocytes (B cells) and result in IgM antibody production. The macrophage signal to thymic-derived lymphocytes (T cells) appears to involve antigen presentation plus the elaboration and release of soluble factors by the phagocytic cell. One macrophage factor, interleukin-1 lymphocyte-activating factor, endogenous pyrogen, etc. plays a key role in activating T cells.[12] The activated T cells in turn produce lymphokines which augment cellular immunity. The T cells which produce these augmenting factors are termed T helper/inducer cells (TH). Their soluble products include macrophage-activating factor(s), including interferon-γ, which are important in enabling macrophages to kill ingested organisms such as *Mycobacterium tuberculosis*, *Toxoplasma gondii*, and *Listeria monocytogenes*. Other lymphokines produced by TH cells include interleukin-2 (lymphocyte-activating factor), which augments T cell and B cell responses; interferon, which has antiviral and macrophage-activating effects; and chemotactic factors, which attract macrophages and granulocytes to the site of infection.[13] The TH cells are recognizable by surface membrane antigens identified by the use of tagged monoclonal antibodies. Using this technique they can be distinguished from T suppressor (Ts) cells which act to dampen the immune response. The ratio of TH to Ts cells approximates 1.5:1 in healthy individuals. It should be noted that TH cells in specific circumstances can induce suppressor cell activity.

In addition to thymic cells with helper and suppressor function, other lymphocytes participate in cellular immune responses. Cytotoxic T cells lyse virus-infected cells which express foreign antigen on their surface. Such lysis is restricted. The cytotoxic cell must interact with a class I MHC which is present on the majority of mammalian cells.[11] Killer cells are unsensitized lymphocytes which are capable of lysing infected cells coated with antiviral antibody. Such antibody-dependent cellular cytotoxicity (ADCC) is also mediated by monocytes and PMNs. Natural killer (NK) cells are large granular lymphocytes derived from the bone marrow, are stimulated following exposure to interferon, interferon-inducing agents, and interleukin-2 (IL-2). These cells kill virally transformed cells and appear to play an important role in resistance to herpes infections.

A second major class of lymphocytes, derived from bone marrow, differentiate independently of the thymus and are termed B cells. Surface immunoglobulin serves as an antigen receptor. Antigen alone in collaboration with a second signal from activated T_H cells serves to stimulate B cell proliferation and differentiation of daughter cells, the plasma cells which produce antibody-immunoglobulins.[14] T suppressor cells modulate differentiation of B cells, and therefore antibody production.

Defects in cellular immunity result in infections due to intracellular pathogens, such as *Mycobacterium* sp and *Herpesvirus*, as is seen in patients with acquired immunodeficiency syndrome (AIDS). Defects in the complex cellular interactions leading to antibody production are associated with recurrent infections due to encapsulated pyogenic bacteria such as *Streptococcus pneumoniae*, *Haemophilus influenzae*, and *Neisseria meningitidis*. The polysaccharide capsule of these organisms is a virulence-enhancing factor which inhibits phagocytes by PMNs unless coated with antibody or complement components.[15]

The phagocytic PMN is the central cell involved in nonspecific resistance against the majority of bacterial and certain fungal infections. Polymorphonuclear leukocytes have membrane receptors for the Fc fragment of IgG and IgM immunoglobulins and C3b, the activated third component of complement.[16] The receptors interacting with these proteins facilitate cellular adherence and ingestion of the opsonized microorganisms. Neutropenic patients or individuals with dysfunctional PMNs are at increased risk of infection due to endogenous flora such as the enteric bacilli, *Pseudomonas aeruginosa*, *Staphylococcus aureus*, and fungi such as *Candida* and *Aspergillus* spp.[15]

The complement system mediates much of the inflammatory process. The classic pathway requires the activation of the first component of the cascade by interaction with the Fc fragment of IgG or IgM which is altered following the antigen-antibody reaction. The alternative pathway bypasses this requirement. The third component (C3) of complement can be activated and attach to microbial surfaces by interaction with teichoic acid of the *S aureus* cell wall or lipopolysaccharide of gram-negative bacilli. The fifth component of the cascade, C5, when activated releases chemotactic factors which attract phagocytic cells to the site of infection. The later components of the cascade can lyse specific bacteria, thus providing a serum bactericidal effect which is important for limiting invasiveness of certain bacteria. Deficiencies, either primary or acquired, of C3b can result in infections due to the same microorganisms noted in patients with neutropenia because of diminished phagocytosis. Absence of the later components results in disseminated infections due to *Neisseria* organisms.[15]

The ingestion and intracellular killing of bacteria by PMNs in concert with antibody and complement is the end result of a series of events which define the inflammatory response. Polymorphonuclear leukocytes must be produced in adequate numbers by the bone marrow and released following appropriate stimuli including interleukin-1 (IL-1).[12] Circulating PMNs recognize a poorly defined signal, possibly a complement product, marginate in the postcapillary venules, and adhere to the endothelial cells near a site of infection. Following adherence the PMNs emigrate between endothelial cells into the extravascular tissue.[17] Chemoattractants produced either by bacteria or as a consequence of activation of the complement sequence result in directed migration of the cells to the invading microorganisms.[18] Phagocytosis and intracellular killing then follow. Defects in any step or component of this sequence results in lowered resistance and infection with the organisms cited above.

ALTERATIONS IN HOST DEFENSES WITH AGE

Are there defects in this complex host defense system due to aging alone? As is clear from the description of the immune response, the thymus gland plays a central role in this system. The thymus "educates" lymphocytes derived from the bone marrow to undergo differentiation required for the helper/inducer suppressor/cytotoxic activity involved in both cellular and antibody-mediated responses. It has been known since the 1930s that the thymus begins an involutionary process with puberty. Not only does the gland lose cellular mass[19] but the capacity to induce lymphocyte differentiation declines.

In parallel with these changes there are alterations in thymic-dependent immune mechanisms. Anergy, the inability to respond with delayed-type skin reactions or to be contact-sensitized, is more prevalent in aged than in younger individuals.[20] This manifestation of an alteration in cellular immunity is associated with changes in T cell function. There are normal numbers of circulating thymic cells but a decreased percentage are T suppressor cells (as defined by monoclonal antibodies) in older individuals.[21] The number of T cells which will respond to mitogens or antigens is decreased and the response is altered. The cell cycle of the proliferating clone of cells is prolonged.[22,23] In addition there is altered suppressor cell activity,[24] and recent evidence indicates that production of the key lymphokine, IL-2, is decreased.[25]

Recently, Weksler has reviewed the evidence that the age-associated changes in immunity may be due to mechanisms other than thymic evolution.[26] A thymic deficiency should result in an increase in T lymphocyte precursors as a consequence of the failure of differentiation of precursors. An increase in the number of inducible precursors is found in the marrow of athymic nude mice. In contrast, normal aged mice and humans demonstrate a deficiency of such precursors in the bone marrow. However, this may be due to failure of these cells to respond to appropriate signals. Moreover, the interrelation of the bone marrow and thymus is extremely complex. Not only do thymic hormones induce maturation of bone marrow lymphocytes but apparently bone marrow elements can influence thymic hormone production.

There is evidence of hyperactivity of the suppressor arm of the complex cellular interaction responsible for immune homeostasis. Suppressor activity of either T cells or monocytes may be responsible for the dampened response of lymphocytes to mitogens or antigens and this effect may be mediated through the prostaglandins. T cells of aged individuals are hyperresponsive to effects of these arachidonic acid metabolites.[24] Finally, membrane changes in human T cells with age correlate with a decreased responsiveness to mitogens. The fluidity of the membrane thus may be partly responsible for functional changes in lymphocyte responsiveness.[27]

In addition to alterations in cellular immunity, other manifestations of dysfunction include a decreased ability to respond to new antigens when immunized.[28,29] Although the serum concentrations of immunoglobulins generally are stable or rise with age, a subpopulation of individuals with decreasing IgG levels has been noted in one longitudinal study.[30] This group had an increased early mortality, a finding analogous to the observation that anergy in persons over 80 years old was linked to early death.[31] In contrast, retention of skin test responsiveness and normal immunoglobulin levels in a 24-month study was associated with general good health.[23]

Studies of B cells of aged individuals in vitro indicate depression of function. Plaque-forming cells in one study were not decreased; however, the number of elderly subjects whose cells failed to produce any immunoglobulin was increased.[32] Other authors have reported a deficiency of lymphocytes in men aged over 75 capable of producing immunoglobulin following stimulation by pokeweed mitogen.[33] Cells from older persons fail to respond with specific antibody production in vitro following exposure either to trinitrophenol linked to polyacylamide beads or sheep erythrocytes.[34,35] Coculture with T lymphocytes obtained from younger persons restored the ability to respond; T cells from older subjects did not. Thus there is evidence that primary antibody responses are depressed both in vitro as well as in vivo. These changes may be due to T cell changes as well as inherent B cell defects. Finally, anti-idiotype autoantibody, which regulates B cell responses, may be increased during the immune response of aged animals.[36]

The frequency of nosocomial infections due to gram-negative bacilli and the high morbidity and mortality associated with staphylococcal endocarditis in the elderly suggest a defect in PMN function or serum opsonins. However, complement function as measured by the classic, antibody-associated pathway and the alternative pathway is normal in healthy elderly individuals as is serum opsonic activity for *Escherichia coli* and *S aureus*.[23] Aged individuals are not usually neutropenic and leukocytosis generally occurs with infection implying that myelopoiesis is normal. The ability of PMNs to adhere to nylon, an in vitro correlate of adherence to endothelial cells,[37] is enhanced, not inhibited, in aged persons.[38,39] Thus the early manifestations of the inflammatory response are intact in elderly individuals. Furthermore, there is evidence that production of endogenous pyrogen or IL-1, which mediates the marrow release of PMNs, and induces PMN aggregation and fever, is normal in the majority of aged persons.[40] The PMNs of the elderly are capable of normal movement but there are conflicting reports regarding responses to chemotactic stimuli.[23,39] Ingestion of bacteria occurs normally[23] but some investigators have noted a lower capacity to reduce the dye, nitro blue tetrazolium, indicating change in oxidative metabolism[39] which is activated by phagocytosis. Killing of *S aureus* is normal[23] but decreased fungicidal activity has been reported.[39] Thus studies of healthy older persons have failed to demonstrate a major defect in the inflammatory response underlying an increase in frequency or morbidity due to bacterial infections.

DISEASES OF AGING AND EFFECTS ON HOST DEFENSE

The evidence cited above, however, may not be relevant to the problem of older patients with common diseases of aging that are associated with altered host defenses. Two examples include diabetes and neoplastic disease. Diabetes is prevalent among the older population. Investigators have documented dampened chemotactic responses of PMNs[41] and deficient phagocytosis and intracellular killing,[42] especially in association with hyperglycemia.[43] These alterations may underlie the increased morbidity associated with bacterial and fungal infections in diabetes and therefore contribute to the problems with infection in the elderly.

Malignant disease is associated with an increased frequency of infection.[44] This is true for solid tumors as well as malignant hematologic disease. Solid tumors produce obstruction and secondary infection but neutropenia, either due to therapy or the disease process, is the most important deficit that occurs in patients with malignant disease.[15] In addition, corticosteroid therapy and malnutrition inhibit cell-mediated responses as well as PMN function.[45-48] Hodgkin's disease is associated with infection due to intracellular pathogens as a result of the associated depressed cellular immunity. Finally, hypogammaglobulinemia is frequently found in patients with chronic lymphatic leukemia and multiple myeloma. Recurrent infection due to encapsulated pyogenic organisms are the result. Thus the entire spectrum of host resistance can be altered in such patients[15] and infection remains a major hazard for old as well as young patients with neoplastic disease.

In addition to causing changes in defense mechanisms the diseases common to the older population result in placement of these patients in high-risk environments: hospitals and nursing homes. In the former, invasive diagnostic techniques and therapeutic maneuvers compromise the patient and enhance the risk of infection. Illness and being bedridden apparently favors colonization with pathogenic organisms that are commonly antibiotic-resistant.[49] In the nursing home, the elderly individual is vulnerable to tuberculosis and colonization with antibiotic-resistant bacteria.[50,51] Thus the association of age and frequent illness potentiates the problem of infection.

FUTURE STUDIES

Full understanding of the problem of infections in the elderly will require further study. Factors such as nutrition, bacterial adherence, mucosal barriers such as fibronectin and secretory IgA, and macrophage function have not been adequately investigated in this age group. In addition, the evidence that the response to immunization is inhibited requires that strategies be designed to overcome this problem. This is obviously relevant to the use of influenza vaccine in the elderly. Furthermore, it is important to determine if the relatively normal inflammatory responses in the healthy ambulatory aged person persists during periods of stress. Preliminary evidence indicates that the frequency

Table 2-2
Age-Related Polymorphonuclear Leukocyte Function in Bacteremic Patients With *Staphylococcus aureus*

Age	No of Patients	Abnormal (%)*
<50	14	3 (21.4)
51-60	5	1 (20.0)
61-71	7	2 (28.6)
>71	8	6 (75.0)

* Killed less than 1 log of 10⁶ *S aureus*.

of abnormal PMN function in older individuals increased with serious illness (Table 2-2).[52] These results require confirmation and determination of relevance. Finally, strategies for reconstitution of the thymic-dependent immune response must be carefully thought out. The administration of thymic hormones may not alter the "suppressor state" which appears to be involved in the dampened response in aged individuals. Also, it is possible that the enhanced suppression may be a protective reaction to increasing recognition of self-antigens associated with aging. Evidence suggestive of this possibility is found in the association of anergy and an increased prevalence of autoantibodies. Reversal of this inhibition could have untoward health effects, even if it would improve responses to specific infection.

In summary, there is evidence that infection represents a major problem in the aged. It is not clear if this is due to aging alone or the diseases common to this age group. The alterations of the immune and inflammatory response which have been documented in the healthy elderly do not fully explain the vulnerability of these individuals to infections.

REFERENCES

1. Fox RA (ed): *The Clinical Response to Infection in Immunology and Infection in the Elderly.* Edinburgh, Churchill Livingstone, 1984.
2. Haley RW, Hooton TM, Culver DH, et al: Nosocomial infection in U.S. hospitals 1975–1976. Estimated frequency by selected characteristics of patients. *Am J Med* 1981;70:947–959.
3. Stamm WE: Infections related to medical devices. *Ann Intern Med* 1978;89:764–769.
4. Watanakunakorn C, Tan JS, Phair JP: Some salient features of S aureus endocarditis. *Am J Med* 1973;54:473–481.
5. *Tuberculosis in the United States — 1980.* US Dept of Health and Human Services publication No. (CDC) 83-8322. Atlanta, Centers for Disease Control; 1983.
6. Miller AE: Selective decline in cellular immune response to varicella zoster in the elderly. *Neurology* 1980;30:582–587.
7. Toews GB: Determinants of bacterial clearance from the lower respiratory tract. *Semin Respir Infect* 1986;1:68–78.
8. Tomasi TB, Greg HM: Structure and function of immunoglobulin A. *Prog Allergy* 1972;16:81–213.
9. Woods DE, Strauss DC, Johanson WG, et al: Role of salivary protease activity in adherence of gram negative bacilli to mammalian buccal endothelial cells. *J Clin Invest* 1981;68:1435–1440.
10. Golub ES: The role of the macrophage, in Golub ES (ed): *The Cellular Basis of the Immune Response,* ed 2. Sunderland, Mass, Sinauer Associates, 1981, p 103.
11. McDevitt HO: *Cellular Interaction in the Immune System.* In Fortner JG, Rhonos JE (eds): Accomplishments in Cancer Research. Philadelphia, JB Lippincott Co, 1984.

12. Dinarello CA: Interleukin-1. *Rev Infect Dis* 1984;6:51–95.
13. Rocklin RE: Mediators of cellular immunity, in Fudenberg HH, Stikes DP, Caldwell JL, et al (eds): *Basic and Clinical Immunology*, ed 2. Los Altos, Calif, Lange Medical Publishers, 1978.
14. Levitt D, Cooper MD: B-cells, in Stites DP, Stobo JD, Fudenberg HH, et al (eds): *Basic and Clinical Immunology*, Los Altos, Calif, Appleton and Lange, 1987, pp 72-81.
15. Armstrong D: Infections in patients with neoplastic disease, in Verhoef J, Peterson PK, Quie PG (eds): *Infections in the Immunocompromised Host. Pathogenesis, Prevention and Therapy*. Elsevier, Amsterdam, North Holland Biomedical Press, 1980.
16. Stossel TP: Phagocytosis: Recognition and ingestion. *Semin Hematol* 1975;12:83–116.
17. Grant L: The sticking and emigration of white blood cells in inflammation, in Zweifach BW, Grant L, McCluskey RT (eds): *The Inflammatory Process*, ed 2. New York, Academic Press, 1973, vol 2.
18. Zigmond SH: Chemotaxis by polymorphonuclear leukocytes. *J Cell Biol* 1978;77:267–287.
19. Tosi P, Kraft R, Luzi P, et al: Involution patterns of the human thymus. Size of the cortical area as a function of age. *Clin Exp Immunol* 1982;47:497–504.
20. Waldorf DS, Wilkeas RF, Decker JI: Impaired delayed hypersensitivity in an aging population. *JAMA* 1968;203:831–834.
21. Nagel JE, Chrest FJ, Adler WGH: Enumeration of T-lymphocyte subsets by monoclonal antibodies in young and aged humans. *J Immunol* 1981;127:2086–2088.
22. Tice RR, Schneider EL, Kram D, et al: Cytokinetic analysis of the impaired proliferative responses of peripheral blood lymphocytes from aged human to phytohemagglutinin. *J Exp Med* 1979;149:1029.
23. Phair JP, Kauffman CA, Bjornson A, et al: Host defenses in the aged: Evaluation of components of the inflammatory and immune response. *J Infect Dis* 1978;138:67–73.
24. Goodwin JS, Messner RP: Sensitivity of lymphocytes to prostaglandin E_2 increases in subjects over age 70. *J Clin Invest* 1979;64:434–439.
25. Gilles S, Kozak R, Durante M, et al: Immunological studies of aging. Decreased production of and response to T-cell growth factor by lymphocytes from aged humans. *J Clin Invest* 1981;67:937–942.
26. Weksler ME: The thymus gland and aging. *Ann Intern Med* 1983;98:105–107.
27. Rivnay B, Bergman S, Skinitzky M, et al: Correlations between membrane viscosity, serum cholesterol, lymphocyte activation and aging in man. *Mech Ageing Dev* 1980;12:119–126.
28. Sabin AB, Grinder DR, Matomoto M, et al: Serological response of Japanese children and old people to Japanese B encephalitis mouse brain vaccine. *Proc Soc Exp Biol Med* 1947; 65:135–140.
29. Phair JP, Kauffman CA, Bjornson A, et al: Failure to respond to influenza vaccine in the aged. Correlation with B-cell number and function. *J Lab Clin Med* 1978;92:822–828.
30. Murasko DM, Nelson BJ, Silver R, et al: Immunologic response in an elderly population with a mean age of 85. *Am J Med* 1986;81:612-618.
31. Roberts-Thomson IC, Whittingham S, Younchai YV, et al: Aging, immune response and mortality. *Lancet* 1974;2:368–370.

32. Nagel JE, Chrest FJ, Adler WH: Human B-cell function in normal individuals of various ages: *In vitro* enumeration of pokeweed-induced peripheral blood lymphocyte immunoglobulin synthesizing cells and the comparison of the results with numbers of peripheral B and T-cells, mitogen responses, and levels of serum immunoglobulins. *Clin Exp Immunol* 1981;44: 646–653.
33. Hollingsworth JW, Otte RG: B-lymphocyte maturation in cultures from blood of elderly men: A comparison of plaque forming cells, cells containing intracytoplasmic immunoglobulin and cell proliferation. *Mech Ageing Dev* 1981;15:9–18.
34. Delfraissey JF, Galanaud P, Dormont J, et al: Age-related impairment of the in vitro antibody response in the human. *Clin Exp Immunol* 1980;39: 208–214.
35. Pahwa SG, Pahwa RN, Good RA: Decreased in vitro humoral immune responses in aged humans. *J Clin Invest* 1981;67: 1094–1102.
36. Szewczuk MR, Campbell RJ: Loss of immune competence with age may be due to auto-anti-idiotype antibody regulation. *Nature* 1980;285:164–166.
37. MacGregor RR, Macaraks EJ, Kefalides N: Comparative adherence of granulocytes to endothelial monolayers and nylon fiber. *J Clin Invest* 1978;61:697–702.
38. Silverman EM, Silverman AG: Granulocyte adherence in the elderly. *Am J Clin Pathol* 1977;67:49–52.
39. Corberand J, Nguyen F, Laharrague P, et al: Polymorpho-nuclear functions and aging in humans. *J Am Geriatr Soc* 1981;29:391–397.
40. Jones PG, Kauffman CA, Bergman AG, et al: Fever in the elderly: Production of leukocyte pyrogen by monocytes in elderly persons. *Gerontology* 1984;30:182–187.
41. Molenar DM, Palumbo PJ, Wilson WR, et al: Leukocyte chemotaxis in diabetic patients and their non-diabetic first degree relatives. *Diabetes* 1976;25:880–883.
42. Tan JS, Anderson JL, Watanakunakorn C, et al: Neutrophil dysfunction in diabetes mellitus. *J Lab Clin Med* 1975;85:25–33.
43. Bagdade JD, Root RK, Bulger RJ: Impaired leukocyte function in patients with poorly controlled diabetes. *Diabetes* 1974;23:9–14.
44. Inagaki J, Rodriguez V, Bodey GP: Cause of death in cancer patients. *Cancer* 1974;33:568–573.
45. McMurray DM: Cell-mediated immunity in nutritional deficiency. *Prog Food Nutr Sci* 1984;8:193–228.
46. Dale DC, Fauci AS, Wolff SM: Alternate day prednisone: leukocyte kinetics and susceptibility to infections. *N Engl J Med* 1974;291:1154–1158.
47. Schreiber AD: Clinical immunology of corticosteroids, in Schwartz RS (ed): *Progress in Immunology*. New York, Grune & Stratton, 1977, p 103.
48. Law DK, Dudrick SJ, Abdoub NL: Immunocompetence of patients with protein calorie malnutrition: The effects of nutritional repletion. *Ann Intern Med* 1973;79:545–550.
49. Valenti WM, Trudell RG, Bentley DW: Factors predisposing to oropharyngeal colonization with gram-negative bacilli in the aged. *N Engl J Med* 1978;298:1108–1111.
50. Garibaldi RA, Brodine S, Matsumija S: Infections among patients in nursing homes: policies, prevalence and problems. *N Engl J Med* 1981;305: 731–735.

51. Weir MR, Thornton GF: Extrapulmonary tuberculosis: Experience of a community hospital and review of the literature. *Am J Med* 1986;79:467–478.
52. Phair JP, Riesing KS, Metzger E: Bacteremic infection and malnutrition in patients with solid tumors: investigation of host defense mechanisms. *Cancer* 1980;45:2702–2706.

3

Infection and Fever in the Elderly

Dean C. Norman
Thomas T. Yoshikawa

Infections have a major impact on the geriatric population.[1,2] Diminished physiologic reserve secondary to both biologic changes of aging and coexisting chronic diseases contributes to the higher mortality and morbidity rates observed for serious infection in older compared with younger persons. Aside from preventive measures (eg, immunoprophylaxis), reductions in morbidity and deaths from infection can only be achieved by early diagnosis and institution of effective therapy.

FACTORS INFLUENCING CLINICAL PRESENTATION OF INFECTIONS IN THE ELDERLY

Although many elderly individuals will demonstrate clinical manifestations consistent with a particular disease or disorder, a significant number of geriatric patients will come to the clinician with atypical clinical features. This is especially true in aged persons with infectious diseases, in whom clinical features may be nonspecific, blunted, or even absent. Three factors influence the presentation of disease in geriatric patients: (1) underreporting of illnesses, (2) different patterns of illnesses, and (3) altered response to illnesses.[3]

Underreporting of illnesses by older persons may occur for many reasons, some of which include varied cultural, ethnic, and educational backgrounds, depression, cognitive impairment, and denial. The problem of appendicitis in the elderly is an example of this because geriatric patients may delay seeking medical attention for abdominal pain because of both the failure to appreciate that appendicitis may occur in old age and the fear of economic and other consequences of hospitalization.[4,5]

Changing patterns of illness with age influence presentation of infectious diseases because the etiologic pathogens for a particular infectious disease may also change with age. Thus aerobic gram-negative bacilli are more likely to cause community-acquired pneumonia[6] or septic arthritis in the older age groups.[7] Also, viral meningitis is unusual in the elderly, while bacterial meningitis is more likely to be caused by not only *Streptococcus pneumoniae* and *Neisseria meningitidis* but other unusual pathogens.[8,9] Moreover, these changes in microbial pathogens with age for certain infections, besides influencing presentation and clinical course, have obvious implications for therapeutic decision making, particularly in deciding which antibiotics to use for empiric antimicrobial therapy.

Altered clinical responses to illness by aged individuals occur in part because of underreporting and different patterns of disease. Also, both biologic changes with age (eg, changes in chest wall and pulmonary physiology may result in diminished cough with pneumonia) and coexisting chronic disease (particularly cardiovascular disease) may produce multiple somatic or psychiatric complaints which may mask, confound, or alter the clinical responses to illness. Acute illness may also elicit only nonspecific symptoms in these patients. There are several examples of altered responses to clinical infection in the elderly. Elderly patients with worsening congestive heart failure, or malignancy, or urinary tract infection may all present in a similar fashion with only mental status changes and incontinence.[10] Similarly, fever may be absent in one third of elderly patients with infective endocarditis, and nonspecific symptoms such as weakness, malaise, confusion, and myalgia may be the only clinical manifestations of this disease.[11] Bacterial pneumonia in older persons may present insidiously without high fever or cough.[6] Finally, fever or nuchal rigidity may be lacking in some cases of bacterial meningitis in the older population,[8] and even if present, nuchal rigidity may be wrongly ascribed to cervical osteoarthritis.

FEVER

Fever may be blunted or absent in elderly persons with serious infectious disorders. Since the presence of fever is one of the characteristic factors of infection, its absence may seriously delay or dissuade clinicians from considering this diagnosis. Besides making early diagnosis of infection difficult, the absence of fever has other clinical implications. A febrile response to infection has prognostic significance in that low or normal temperature in patients with bacteremia or other serious infection is associated with diminished chance of survival.[12-15] Furthermore, recent evidence suggests that the explanation for the prognostic significance of fever is that fever in and of itself is an important host defense mechanism against infection.[16] Several animal models, particularly those employing poikilotherms (ie, thermoregulation is achieved only by behavioral mechanisms), have provided the best evidence for a beneficial effect of fever. Kluger et al,[17] in a now classic study, used lizards, which had been shown previously to seek higher environmental temperatures when infected, to investigate the impact of fever on survival. Groups of lizards were maintained at fixed body temperatures by placing them in cages kept at a fixed temperature. Each group was then infected with *Aeromonas hydrophila*. Those groups housed in cages at higher temperatures had dramatically increased survival compared to groups kept at lower temperatures. This same experiment was repeated with infected goldfish kept in tanks at different temperatures, and similar results were obtained.[18] Thus, at least in poikilotherms, the data clearly support fever as an important host defense mechanism. Experimental evidence for a beneficial effect of fever in mammals is less solid. However, in one study, rabbits that were able to develop fever in response to infection with *Pasteurella multocida* had increased survival.[19]

In order to better understand why fever may be blunted in the elderly, the pathogenesis of fever is briefly reviewed. Fever in man is mediated by a soluble leukocytic product first described by Beeson[20] which caused fever when injected into rabbits. Atkins and Wood later demonstrated that this pyrogenic mediator was released after injection with endotoxin, and termed the pyrogen *endogenous pyrogen*.[21]

Circulating mononuclear phagocytes, fixed tissue macrophages, and some tumor cells produce endogenous pyrogen.[22-24] However, lymphocytes do not make this pyrogenic substance, though lymphocytes may modify macrophage release of endogenous pyrogen. The release of endogenous pyrogen follows stimulation of macrophages by a wide variety of substances such as endotoxin, microorganisms, and antigen-antibody complexes. Endogenous pyrogen does not exist in a preformed state within the cell, and its production and release requires synthesis of new messenger RNA and protein[25] in an energy-requiring process. Hence, release of endogenous pyrogen occurs several hours post-stimulation. Following its release into the circulation, endogenous pyrogen acts on the preoptic area of the anterior hypothalamus to effect a "reset" of the thermoregulatory center "thermostat" to a higher temperature. The effect of endogenous pyrogen on the hypothalamus may be mediated by a wide variety of neurochemicals including prostaglandins (thus explaining the antipyrogenic effect of aspirin).[26-29] The hypothalamus then elicits a series of behavioral and physiologic responses which conserve body heat (ie, one feels cold and puts on some clothes; the metabolic rate is increased; and peripheral vasoconstriction occurs as well as shivering).[30,31]

Evidence has accumulated that endogenous pyrogen is closely related to or in part identical with interleukin-1 (IL-1).[32] Interleukin-1 has important immune functions, one of which includes stimulating lymphocytes to produce interleukin-2 (IL-2) (which is necessary for T lymphocyte proliferation). Interleukin-1 also mediates several acute phase reactions, which may be important host defense mechanisms.[32] Thus it can be inferred from the role(s) of IL-1 that there may be an interrelationship between fever response, immune reaction, and other host defense mechanisms, which supports the contention that fever has prognostic (and possibly therapeutic) value. Recently, evidence has been accumulated that indicate other cytokines, ie, tumor necrosis factor and interferon, act as endogenous pyrogens.[33]

Using the current model for the pathogenesis of fever, one mechanism for a blunted fever response to infection by some elderly persons could be from diminished release of endogenous pyrogen by old macrophages. There is some evidence for this possibility, as Inamizu et al[34] have shown decreased IL-1 production by macrophages with age in a murine model. Another potential mechanism for diminished febrile response may be a decreased response to endogenous pyrogen with age. For instance, this may occur at the anterior hypothalamus, perhaps at the receptor level, resulting in a lower reset temperature. Alternatively, older persons may be unable to mount adequate behavioral and physiologic thermoregulatory responses even with normal endogenous pyrogen–hypothalamic interaction. We have found, using a murine model, a reduced febrile response to endogenous pyrogen by old mice compared with young.[35] Which of these areas (anterior hypothalamus or heat conservation responses) is responsible for our observation has not yet been determined.

REFERENCES

1. Yoshikawa TT: Geriatric infectious diseases: an emerging problem. *J Am Geriatr Soc* 1983;31:34–39.
2. Yoshikawa TT: Aging and infectious diseases: state of the art. *Gerontology* 1984;30:275–278.
3. Williams ME: Clinical implications of aging physiology. *Am J Med* 1984;76:1049–1054.
4. Norman DC, Yoshikawa TT: Intraabdominal infections in the elderly. *J Am Geriatr Soc* 1983;31:677–684.
5. Reeves MM, Meredith D, Lewis FJ: Appendicitis in the older patient. *Surg Gynecol Obstet* 1958;106:610–612.
6. Verghese A, Berk SL: Bacterial pneumonia in the elderly. *Medicine* 1983;62:271–285.
7. Norman DC, Yoshikawa TT: Responding to septic arthritis. *Geriatrics* 1983;38:83–86.
8. Norman DC, Yoshikawa TT: Recognizing bacterial meningitis in the elderly. *Geriatr Med Today* 1984;3:85–88.
9. Gorse GJ, Thrupp LD, Nudleman KL, et al: Bacterial meningitis in the elderly. *Arch Intern Med* 1984;144:1603–1607.

10. Cunha BA, Gobbo PN, Beltran MD: The significance of fever. *J Crit Care* 1984;13:460–465.
11. Cantrell M, Yoshikawa TT: Aging and infective endocarditis. *J Am Geriatr Soc* 1983;31:216–222.
12. Finklestein MS, Petkin WH, Freedman ML, et al: Pneumococcal bacteremia in adults: age dependent difference in presentation and outcome. *J Am Geriatr Soc* 1983;31:19–27.
13. Bryant RE, Hood AF, Hood CE, et al: Factors affecting mortality of gram-negative rod bacteremia. *Arch Intern Med* 1971; 127:120–128.
14. Weinstein MP, Iannini PB, Stratton CW, et al: Spontaneous bacterial peritonitis. A review of 28 cases with emphasis on improved survival and factors influencing prognosis. *Am J Med* 1978;64:592–598.
15. Weinstein MP, Reller LB, Murphy JR, et al: The clinical significance of positive blood cultures: a comprehensive analysis of 500 episodes of bacteremia and fungemia in adults. II. Clinical observations with special reference to factors influencing prognosis. *Rev Infect Dis* 1983;5:54–70.
16. Roberts NJ: Temperature and host defense. *Microbiol Rev* 1979;43:241–259.
17. Kluger MJ, Ringler DM, Anver MR: Fever and survival. *Science* 1975;188:166–168.
18. Covert JB, Reynolds WW: Survival value of fever in fish. *Nature* 1977;267:43–45.
19. Kluger MJ, Vaughn LK: Fever and survival in rabbits infected with *Pasteurella multocida*. *J Physiol* 1978;282:243–251.
20. Beeson PB: Temperature-elevating effect of a substance obtained from polymorphonuclear leukocytes. *J Clin Invest* 1948;27:524.
21. Atkins E, Wood WB: Studies in the pathogenesis of fever. 1. The presence of transferable pyrogen in the bloodstream following the injection of typhoid vaccine. *J Exp Med* 1955;101:519–528.
22. Bodel P: Studies on the mechanism of endogenous pyrogen production. III. Human blood monocytes. *J Exp Med* 1974;140:954–965.
23. Bodel P: Spontaneous pyrogen production by mouse histiocytic and myelomonocytic tumor cell lines in vitro. *J Exp Med* 1978;147:1503–1516.
24. Bodel P, Ralph P, Wenc R, et al: Endogenous pyrogen production by Hodgkin's disease and human lymphoma cell lines in vitro. *J Clin Invest* 1980;65:514–518.
25. Nordlund JJ, Root RK, Wolff SM: Studies on the origin of human leukocytic pyrogen. *J Exp Med* 1970;131:722–742.
26. Feldberg W, Gupta KP, Milton AS, et al: Effect of pyrogen and antipyretics on prostaglandin activity in cisternal CSF of unanesthetized cats. *J Physiol* 1973; 234:279–303.
27. Stitt ST: Prostaglandin E_1 fever induced in rabbits. *J Physiol* 1973;232:163–179.
28. Harvey CA, Milton AS, Straughan DW: Prostaglandin E levels in cerebrospinal fluid of rabbits and the effects of bacterial pyrogen and antipyretic drugs. *J Physiol* 1975;248:26p–27p.
29. Dinarello CA, Bernheim HA: Ability of leukocytic pyrogen to stimulate brain prostaglandin synthesis in vitro. *J Neurochem* 1981;37:702–708.
30. Atkins E, Bodel P: Fever. *N Engl J Med* 1972;286:27–34.
31. Dinarello CA, Wolff SM: Pathogenesis of fever in man. *N Engl J Med* 1978;298:607–612.
32. Dinarello CA: Interleukin-1. *Rev Infect Dis* 1984;6:51–94.

33. Dinarello CA, Cannon JG, Wolff SM: New concept on the pathogenesis of fever. *Rev Infect Dis* 1988;10:168-189.
34. Inamizu T, Chang MP, Makinodan T: Influence of age on the production and regulation of interleukin-1 in mice. *Immunology* 1985;55:447-455.
35. Norman DC, Cantrell M, Ngo D, et al: The effect of age on the febrile response to endogenous pyrogen in a mouse model. *Fed Proc* 1984;43:1828.

SECTION II
CLINICAL SYNDROMES

4

Central Nervous System Infections

*Purnendu Sen
Donald B. Louria*

Infections of the central nervous system (CNS) are still associated with significant mortality and morbidity, particularly in neonates and the elderly (despite the availability of effective antimicrobial agents). The age-specific incidence of bacterial meningitis among adults is highest in the age group over 60 years of age — 1.2 per 100,000 population compared with 0.6 per 100,000 persons between the ages of 30 and 59.[1] Case fatality rates are also higher in older persons, at least for certain forms of meningitis; this may be in part due to delayed recognition of the presence of meningeal infection.

Many infections of the aging are related to anatomical abnormalities (eg, prostatic hypertrophy leading to urinary tract infections). There are no such predisposing anatomical defects in the CNS that develop as a consequence of aging. Ischemic changes due to atherosclerotic cerebral vessels is common in the elderly. Arterial or venous thrombosis also occurs in bacterial meningitis. This overlapping of vascular phenomena and neurologic findings may obscure the diagnosis of CNS infection in patients who have little fever.

Likewise, there are no abnormalities in the inflammatory response that would predispose to increased incidence or severity of CNS infection in the aged. Complement (C5) deficiency has been associated with *Neisseria* infection, particularly with recurrent episodes of meninogococcal meningitis; that is not a problem, however, in the elderly population. Similarly, immunoglobulin deficiency, such as low IgM, which has been reported in the elderly, does not seem to be an important predisposing factor in CNS infections in this age group.[2] Interestingly, Nerenberg and

Prasad reported that IgA and IgG in cerebrospinal fluid (CSF) increase with age but there is no evidence that those changes offer any protection against microbial infections involving the CNS.[3] Diminished antibody response to foreign antigen has been described in the elderly. This phenomenon may help to explain high mortality in aged individuals with Japanese B encephalitis.[4] Cell-mediated immune dysfunction is the only abnormality seen in the elderly that is linked with some specific CNS infection in this age group. Many studies have now demonstrated impairment of T lymphocyte functions in older animals and humans.[5-7] Resistance to infection with the intracellular pathogens, *Listeria monocytogenes, Salmonella typhimurium,* and *Toxoplasma gondii* have been shown to diminish in aging mice.[8] In vitro studies also have demonstrated that lymphocytes from elderly individuals sensitized to varicella zoster or *Mycobacterium tuberculosis* show less proliferation than lymphocytes from young persons.[9] These well-established T cell abnormalities could explain a proclivity to tuberculous, cryptococcal, and *Listeria* infections since in each of these infections delayed immune mechanisms constitute the major defense mechanism of the host.

In addition to intrinsic host defects accompanying the aging process that may predispose to infection, there is a gallimaufry of chronic diseases that are more prevalent in older persons and lead to increased susceptibility to infection. The long list includes diabetes, various forms of cancer, hematologic malignancies, and chronic liver disease. Each of these imposes host defects that promote certain infections. Additionally, some of these conditions require therapy with corticosteroids and other immunosuppressive agents that increase the hazard of superinfection. Some of the opportunistic infections that arise as a result of underlying disease or its treatment (eg, *Nocardia asteroides, Cryptococcus neoformans*) preferentially affect the CNS. Therefore, in elderly patients with chronic diseases, one must consider the possibility of infections with unusual pathogens if the CNS is involved. CNS infections in the abnormal host have been reviewed in detail elsewhere.[10]

Table 4-1 lists some underlying diseases that may supervene and the anticipated pathogens that may cause CNS infections, particularly in the geriatric population.

Fifty percent of the patients in many hospitals are over the age of 65 years. Hospitalized patients are, of course, often the victims of nosocomial bacteremia originating from the urinary tract, skin infections, decubitus ulcers, etc. Therefore, CNS infections with nosocomial pathogens such as *Escherichia coli,* other gram-negative bacteria, and staphylococci may also be seen in elderly patients. Neurosurgical procedures were responsible for 28% of bacterial meningitis in the elderly in one series.[11]

Infrequently, infection is acquired at a younger age but the manifestations involving the CNS do not appear until later years. Neurosyphilis,

Table 4-1
Superinfecting Pathogens in Patients with Specific Underlying Diseases

Underlying Diseases or Associated Conditions	Superinfecting Pathogens
Multiple myeloma	*Streptococcus pneumoniae, Haemophilus influenzae*
Chronic lymphatic leukemia	*St pneumoniae, H influenzae*
Hodgkin's disease and lymphoma	*Listeria monocytogenes, Nocardia* spp, *Mycobacterium tuberculosis, Legionella pneumophila, Cryptococcus neoformans,* herpes zoster, papovavirus (progressive multifocal leukoencephalopathy)
Organ transplantation and immunosuppressive therapy	
Diabetes mellitus	Zygomycetes, *Aspergillus, C. neoformans*

although now uncommonly observed, may not become apparent until the patient is over 60 years of age.

Similarly, there are slow viral infections such as Creutzfeldt-Jakob disease, that appear to arise in older people but have long latent periods and are likely to have been acquired many years earlier.[12]

CLINICAL MANIFESTATIONS

The clinical presentation of CNS infection in the aging population deserves special attention. The symptomatology is often atypical in this age group and there are other noninfectious diseases which may mimic an infectious process. Conversely, infection of the CNS may be misdiagnosed as cerebrovascular accident, brain tumor, or even psychosomatic illness.

The classic manifestations of acute meningitis, ie, high fever, headache, stiffness of the neck, may not be seen in the elderly. Confusion with low-grade fever may be the only manifestation of a serious CNS infection. Symptoms are often masked because of the patient's inability to communicate due to pre-existing cerebrovascular disease. Nuchal rigidity may be absent or might be misinterpreted as evidence of osteoarthritis of the cervical spine. However, complete neck rigidity is uncommon with cervical spondylosis[13] and when it is present, it should raise the possibility of meningitis. In community-acquired infection, a close family member might be the most helpful historian who would detect subtle mental changes, suspect something "unusual," and report to the physician. In a hospital setting, an elderly patient with multisystem disease, confusion, and mental changes may be felt to have a metabolic disturbance rather than infection. Dementia, a common feature in elderly patients with cerebrovascular diseases, and vitamin and endocrine disorders, may also be seen in chronic infections such as syphilis. The importance of any unexplained decrement in mentation as an early manifestation of meningitis cannot be overemphasized. Gorse et al[11] retrospectively studied bacterial meningitis in older and younger age groups. They found no significant difference in the initial neurologic examination except for severity of mental status abnormalities in the older age groups. Unexplained mentation changes should suggest CNS infection and, in the absence of contraindications, a lumbar puncture should usually be performed.

Many noninfectious disorders of the CNS in the aged, particularly acute cerebrovascular accidents and brain tumor, may present with fever, coma, seizures, and focal neurologic signs. In these patients, the initial evaluation of CSF may show pleocytosis, high protein, and even occasionally low sugar. These findings may be interpreted as indicating infection; this may result in unnecessary treatment with antimicrobial agents, but at times, such overtreatment is virtually unavoidable. Infectious agents in the elderly, as in all other age groups, may affect primarily the CNS but there are other infectious diseases occurring in the aged that affect multiple systems and in the process frequently involve the CNS. As a result, those individuals may present initially with either predominately extra-CNS or predominantly neurologic manifestations. Legionnaire's disease and infective endocarditis are two major examples in this category. In contrast, neurologic complications of some viral diseases occur far less often in aging persons. For example, Reye's syndrome, which is related to influenza B and less frequently to influenza A infection, is seen in children almost exclusively.

Recently, several comprehensive articles[11,13] on infections of the CNS in the elderly have been published. In this review, emphasis is placed on specific infectious agents and clinical presentations affecting older patients.

BACTERIAL INFECTIONS OF THE CNS

Parameningeal Focus of Infection

Brain abscess The incidence and etiologic agents are not different in the elderly compared with younger persons. Difficulty arises in the diagnosis of brain abscess in the aging because of nonspecific presentations. Fever may be absent in 50% of the patients,[14] and the other common symptoms and signs including headache, change in mental status, focal neurologic defects, and seizures may be misdiagnosed as cerebral tumors or cerebrovascular accident. The peripheral blood examination is usually unhelpful; the WBC count is ordinarily normal. Lumbar puncture, which may be dangerous, particularly in patients with focal signs, reveals nonspecific findings. Computed tomography (CT) is invaluable in the diagnosis of brain abscess but there are some reservations that deserve emphasis. The radiologic appearance of the "doughnut" ring lesion, detectable in 25% to 35% of brain abscesses,[15] may also be seen in cerebral infarction or necrotic tumors. Therefore, in patients in whom the index of suspicion is high, direct aspiration from the abnormal area remains the only method of diagnosis. In this situation, a clinician faces a difficult task, particularly in elderly patients in whom an invasive procedure may be associated with high mortality and morbidity.

In the very early stages of brain abscess with cerebritis, a technetium 99 brain scan may be more sensitive than the CT scan.[16] This may be the preferred investigative technique in a patient in whom CT scan shows no abnormality and the clinical features are highly suggestive of an infectious process. The most frequent pathogens in brain abscess in young and old alike include *Streptococcus* spp (often *S milleri*), *Bacteroides* sp, and Enterobacteriaceae.[14] *Streptococcus milleri* is an α-streptococcus that behaves like *Staphylococcus aureus* in its proclivity to abscess formation. Subdural empyema and epidural abscess, which arise mostly from infections in the paranasal sinuses, middle ear, or mastoids, are relatively infrequent in geriatric age groups. When suspected, CT scan and angiographic studies may be needed to establish the diagnosis.

There are two entities in which the CNS in the elderly can become involved from adjacent bone infection by contiguous spread. Malignant otitis externa seems to occur almost exclusively in elderly diabetics. In these patients, infection begins in the external auditory canal and then spreads to the soft tissues beneath the temporal bone and may lead to facial palsy, mastoiditis, osteomyelitis of the base of the skull, sigmoid sinus thrombosis, and multiple cranial palsies.[17,18] The clinical presentation is usually virtually diagnostic; an elderly diabetic presents with pain and tenderness around the ear and mastoid with drainage of purulent material from the external ear. There may be granulation tissue at the junction of the bony and cartilaginous portions of the external ear. In 50% of cases, facial nerve palsy develops.[18] Infrequently, the other cranial nerves, including the 10th, 11th, and 12th, may be involved. Rarely, meningitis has been described as a late complication. *Pseudomonas aeruginosa* is the predominant offending pathogen. It is important to recognize this entity early so that proper treatment can be initiated to avoid a high mortality rate.

Spinal epidural abscess, which may be a neurologic emergency situation, often results from vertebral osteomyelitis with extension into the spinal epidural space. This disease can occur in any age group, and may also arise secondary to hematogenous spread, or from trauma. Patients with vertebral osteomyelitis are predominately elderly male diabetics.[19] Patients may present acutely with backache and radicular pain or chronically as fever of unknown origin and then may rapidly develop neurologic manifestations with motor and sensory disturbances and even paraplegia.

Initial symptoms of vague back pain may be misinterpreted as osteoarthritis in elderly patients. Urinary tract infection is often the source in patients with vertebral osteomyelitis and gram-negative bacteria are usually the offending pathogens. *Staphylococcus* organisms are the other pathogens frequently involved in this infection. If treated aggressively and early with antibiotics and drainage, the prognosis for neurologic recovery is good.

Bacterial Meningitis in the Elderly

The spectrum of bacterial meningitis in the elderly is different from that seen in younger adult populations. The age-specific incidence is high and there is an inordinate frequency of unusual pathogens, perhaps due to the presence of associated chronic diseases. In various series, the percentage of unusual pathogens causing meningitis in older persons has been striking.[20,21] These include staphylococci, *L monocytogenes*, and enteric gram-negative pathogens. In one series,[1,3] 75% of the patients with meningitis over the age of 65 were found to have chronic diseases. In patients with these less usual pathogens, surgery, trauma, diabetes mellitus, and malignant diseases were the predominant underlying conditions. Nevertheless, *Streptococcus pneumoniae* and *Neisseria meningitidis* are still the two most frequent pathogens causing meningitis in the elderly.[22] In patients with pneumococcal meningitis, pneumonia is the most frequent source of infection. Other important sources include acute and chronic otitis media, mastoiditis, or fracture of skull and bones. In patients with pneumococcal pneumonia, 20% have positive blood cultures. Of these, 1% to 2% develop acute endocarditis[23] and subsequently meningitis. In these patients, it is obligatory on a daily basis to auscultate carefully for an aortic diastolic murmur. In elderly subjects with pneumococcal meningitis, multiple myeloma should be considered as a possible underlying disease, particularly in the patient who has been chronically ill with unexplained anemia and a high sedimentation rate. Like all other age groups, alcoholism and splenectomy are also important predisposing factors for pneumococcal meningitis in elderly patients.

Gorse et al[11] noted more frequent and more severe mental status changes in elderly patients with pneumococcal meningitis when compared with younger age groups.

In patients who have received antibiotics prior to lumbar puncture, counterimmunoelectrophoresis (CIE) for detection of *S pneumoniae* antigen is useful.[24] Blood cultures are positive in about 50% of cases.[25] Advancing age is associated with poor prognosis in patients with pneumococcal meningitis.[25,26] Other poor prognostic factors include coexisting illness, coma, and delay in therapy. Presence of demonstrable bacteremia[25] has also been associated with higher mortality. We have also found that bilateral persistent myoclonic twitches predict a bad outcome, as does the presence of large numbers of pneumococci in the spinal fluid on gram stain unaccompanied by a significant CSF polymorphonuclear pleocytosis.

Neisseria meningitidis, although more commonly seen in younger adults, still accounts for 16% of bacterial meningitis in the elderly.[22] There are no specific underlying diseases in the elderly that would predispose aged individuals to meningococcal infection. In institutionalized elderly persons, an epidemic of group B meninogococcal disease was reported in association with influenza virus[27]; 11 (20%) of 55 elderly individuals in the mental institution developed group B meninogococcal infection. A concurrent outbreak of A2 influenza was also documented in this population, suggesting that the virus had enhanced either the transmissability or pathogenicity of the meningococcus. In the absence of any epidemic, elderly individuals may contract the disease from asymptomatic carriers.

The diminished frequency of meningococcal disease in the elderly indicates a protective role of circulating antibodies in these persons. As in younger persons, the clinical course is often rapid and fatal. Serious complications such as adrenal insufficiency and myocarditis may develop more often in elderly patients.[22] As in pneumococcal infection, CIE can be extremely helpful for rapid detection of this pathogen when gram stain of CSF is unrewarding.[28,29]

Haemophilus influenzae (HI) infections in adults were once considered a rarity; but in the past decade, several reports of this infection in adults have been published.[30-33] In one series[34] of *H influenzae* infections in adults, almost half of the patients were 60 years of age or older. Various reports indicate that 55% of adult patients with HI meningitis may have active HI infection elsewhere or evidence certain predisposing factors. Extra-CNS HI infections include paranasal sinusitis, mastoiditis, otitis, epiglottitis, and pneumonia. Predisposing factors include splenectomy, multiple myeloma, and hypogammaglobulinemia. Alcoholism and diabetes mellitus have been mentioned as underlying conditions but a causal relationship has not been established. Some elderly patients with HI meningitis have no identifiable predisposing factors. The exact mechanisms of pathogenesis are not known but Norden[35] reported that bactericidal antibody is seen only in 21% of patients aged 20 years or older. However, apparent lack of such antibody may represent an artifact since more sensitive techniques suggest most adults possess circulating antibody against HI.

In addition, bactericidal antibody measured in vitro may not be protective. *Haemophilus influenzae* infections now have also been reported as nosocomial events among hospitalized adult patients.[33] Whatever may be the explanation, HI infections must be considered in the differential diagnosis of bacterial meningitis among elderly patients. The clinical presentation is similar to that observed in other causes of bacterial meningitis. Gram stain of CSF will identify the pathogen in 60% of cases, but here again, CIE is very helpful in rapid detection of the antigen; CIE studies are positive in 85% of the cases.[24] The most prevalent serotype causing serious infections in adults is type B.

Of the unusual pathogens causing meningitis in the elderly, *L monocytogenes* is the most interesting one. During a period of 8 years, 53 cases of listeria meningitis were reported to the New York City Health Department[36]; 77% of these patients were over 50 years of age. Frequently, the patients had chronic underlying diseases including chronic renal diseases, renal transplantation, cancer, connective tissue diseases, and alcoholism. In about 50% of patients, advanced age was the only risk factor for acquisition of the disease. As mentioned earlier, *L monocytogenes* is handled primarily by delayed immune mechanisms and diminished resistance to the pathogen has been demonstrated in aging mice.[8]

Clinically, patients may present acutely with fever, headache, neck stiffness, or with manifestations of cerebritis with focal neurologic defects. Infrequently, they may have evidence of chronic basal meningitis and in some patients there are few manifestations other than subtle mental decrement. Cerebrospinal fluid may show preponderance of neutrophils or lymphocytes. Microscopic presence of red blood cells in the CSF without trauma should suggest the diagnosis. Morphologically, this pathogen resembles diphtheroid bacilli and may be discarded as "contaminant" in the CSF. A very high mortality rate (83%) has been noted among persons over the age of 70.[36]

Gram-negative meningitis, predominately a disease of the newborn and infant, is now being reported increasingly among elderly patients.[36,37] There are no demonstrable immunologic deficits in the aging that would predispose them to gram-negative pathogens. Berk and McCabe[37] divided gram-negative meningitis in adults into two categories: one had underlying neurosurgical procedures and the other was designated as a "spontaneous" group; the urinary tract was a frequent source of infection in the latter group. It appears that even in the absence of trauma or neurosurgical procedures, elderly patients with gram-negative meningitis (with the exception of *Haemophilus* infection) often have focal or nosocomial systemic disease that predisposes to gram-negative bacteremia and/or meningitis. In patients with meningitis complicating neurosurgical procedures or occurring spontaneously, the mean ages were 59 and 57 years, respectively. In the spontaneous (or nontraumatic group), the course of the illness was often fulminant. *Escherichia coli* and *Klebsiella pneumoniae* are the predominant pathogens in adult gram-negative meningitis.[37,38] In one series,[38] neurologic complications developed in 64% of patients and were associated with a poor prognosis.

Staphylococcal infections involving the CNS in the elderly follow trauma or neurosurgical operations, including shunt procedures, or arise secondary to acute endocarditis. With staphylococcal endocarditis, there may be multiple brain abscesses or evidence of purulent meningitis.

Group B streptococcal infection of the CNS has been reported almost exclusively in neonates and infants. Serious infections, including endocarditis and meningitis, now have been described in adults and also among elderly patients.[39] This is now considered as an opportunistic pathogen in patients with diabetes mellitus, malignancies, cirrhosis of the liver, and chronic renal failure.[40] In patients with meningitis, rapid detection of the antigen may be possible with the use of a latex particle agglutination method.

Enterococcal meningitis, an uncommon entity, has been described in infants and the elderly.[41] Enterococcal bacteremia and endocarditis are usually seen in elderly patients and young drug addicts. In the former, the source of enterococcal infection is usually from either the genitourinary or the gastrointestinal tract. Although enterococcal endocarditis is more commonly seen in an aging population, CNS involvement is an uncommon event.

Tuberculosis of the CNS in the elderly is a serious disorder. Previously, it was a disease of the pediatric age group, but recent reports indicate[42-44] an increasing incidence of the disease in the elderly age group in the United States and other Western countries. In a review[42] of extrapulmonary tuberculosis, 8% of cases had tuberculous meningitis. In another series,[43] five (26%) of 19 patients with tuberculous meningitis were over the age of 55. CNS infection often occurs due to reactivation or rupture of a tubercle into the subarachnoid space, but may also occur as a consequence of seeding of the meninges through hematogenous dissemination. Miliary tuberculosis accompanies the meningitis in adults in the majority (50% to 80%) of cases.[42] In addition to meningitis, there may be arteritis involving the cerebral vessels.[10] Tuberculoma in the brain seems to be uncommon in elderly patients. In addition to defects in cell-mediated immunity in the aged, there are associated conditions in the elderly that may predispose to tuberculosis; these include corticosteroid therapy, uremia, malnutrition, and certain malignancies.

The clinical presentation is often puzzling. Patients may present with a picture of acute bacterial meningitis[45] or, more frequently, with low-grade fever, confusion, and lethargy with a duration of many weeks. Nuchal rigidity is absent in at least 40% of patients. Occasionally, the initial manifestations may be hemiplegia, cranial nerve palsies, seizures, intellectual disturbances, or hearing deficits[10]; these manifestations are probably secondary to tuberculous angiitis. We have seen a 72-year-old physician who presented with hemiparesis and low-grade fever. Despite CSF abnormalities and positive tuberculin tests, tuberculosis was not considered as a possible diagnosis. Autopsy findings showed extensive tuberculous meningitis. Hyponatremia secondary to inappropriate antidiuretic hormone secretion may further worsen the mental status in patients with tuberculous meningitis.

The chest x-ray film is normal in 50% of the patients. Of course, a negative tuberculin test, a frequent occurrence in elderly patients, by no means rules out the diagnosis of active tuberculosis in this age group. Cerebrospinal fluid findings are variable. The classic findings of lymphocytosis, low sugar, and high protein may not be present. Early in the course of the disease, predominance of polymorphonuclear leukocytes (PMNs) may be seen. Low sugar is not an invariable finding. Values less than 45 mg/100 mL have been reported only in 17% of patients.[46] The likelihood of finding a positive direct smear for acid-fast bacilli in CSF ranges from 15%[10] to 87%.[46] Most authors report that smears are positive in less than one third of cases. The yield seems to increase when serial spinal taps are done. Positive cultures from CSF vary from 45% to 90%; repeatedly negative cultures of CSF have been reported in patients who died and showed florid CNS tuberculosis at autopsy. In a patient with negative CSF cultures, one should look for other sources of positive cultures including sputum, urine, and bone marrow. Since there are not yet effective serologic tests for diagnosis of tuberculosis, in a suspected case, even if laboratory findings are negative, it is wise to start antituberculosis therapy without delay. Mortality of 60% has been reported in patients over the age of 50.[47]

Neurosyphilis The CNS is affected very early in the course of neurosyphilis when there is spirochetemia. Twenty to 30 percent of patients with secondary syphilis will have CSF abnormalities with a reactive VDRL test.[48] These patients may not have CNS symptoms. Acute meningitis may develop within the first 2 years of infection in untreated patients. Although syphilis can be contracted at any age, these early forms of neurosyphilis are rarely seen in elderly patients. Many patients with asymptomatic neurosyphilis probably have a spontaneous remission. Asymptomatic neurosyphilis is uncommon among elderly subjects.[49] The type of neurosyphilis that is more likely to be seen in aging persons is general paresis; among untreated patients with syphilis, 5% are likely to develop general paresis.[48] The average time duration for the onset of this neurologic complication is about 20 years.

Patients may present with personality changes which vary from very mild to severe, sometimes with complete disorientation. Some may manifest dementia or euphoria. Others may be seen by a psychiatrist for depression. Patients with tabes dorsalis are somewhat younger since this complication may develop 5 to 20 years after primary infection. The CSF in patients with neurosyphilis usually shows a positive VDRL but the VDRL may be negative in 10% to 20% of tabes dorsalis cases. Rarely, there may be a false-positive VDRL in the CSF. In some patients with neurosyphilis, the CSF VDRL may be negative but fluorescent treponemal antibody-absorption tests (FTA-ABS) are positive.[50] In these patients with a negative CSF VDRL, nontreponemal tests including VDRL, the rapid plasma reagin (RPR) test are usually negative in the serum. Physicians often ask about the need for CSF examination on the elderly whose serum VDRL and FTA-ABS tests are positive. The CSF examination is obligatory for syphilitic patients who have neurologic manifestations compatible with neurosyphilis.[49] For patients with positive serology for more than 1 year's duration but no abnormal neurologic manifestations, there are no clear indications for CSF examination.

FUNGAL AND YEAST INFECTIONS OF THE CNS

In the elderly, the yeast *Cryptococcus neoformans* causes the greatest concern. This organism is handled by the lymphocyte-macrophage system. Consequently an increased incidence and/or severity of this infection would be anticipated in an older population but in point of fact, there is no evidence that the disease is either more frequent or severe in the elderly. Two thirds of the patients with this disease are between the ages of 30 and 50 years.[51] Many patients with cryptococcal infections have no predisposing factors but 30% to 50% of the cases are associated with serious underlying diseases including Hodgkin's disease, sarcoidosis, and acquired immunodeficiency syndrome (AIDS). Corticosteroid and other immunosuppressive therapy also predisposes to cryptococcal superinfection. Although diabetes has been mentioned as a possible predisposing factor, the relationship is not firmly established. Many of the underlying diseases mentioned occur in the elderly and physicians involved with the care of geriatric patients must be aware of this infection.

Clinically, patients may present with occipital headache and confusion. In 5% of patients, mentation abnormality may be the only manifestation.[52] In 10%, there may be focal signs due to cryptococcal cerebral mass lesions. Fever is usually low grade or is absent. The CSF usually shows lymphocytic pleocytosis but a predominance of neutrophils may be seen. Elevated protein and low sugar are frequently found. India ink preparation is positive in about 30% of the cases. Cryptococcal antigen in CSF determined by a latex agglutination method is found in about 90% of the cases. A large volume of CSF may be required to obtain a positive culture, and it is important to emphasize that it may take four days to four weeks for the organism to grow in culture. Occasionally, the yeast is present in aberrant form and can be recovered in culture only by use of hypertonic media.[53]

Infrequently, *Candida albicans* or *Candida tropicalis* will cause meningitis in older persons, almost exclusively in those with diabetes or in those being treated for severe underlying diseases with corticosteroid and/or antibiotics.

OTHER INFECTIONS

There are other diseases in which the CNS is secondarily involved, but the predominant manifestations of the illness are due to the nervous system involvement. Infective endocarditis (IE) is an appropriate example in this group. Approximately 35% of the patients with IE are over 65 years of age.[54] In a series of 218 patients seen at Massachusetts General Hospital, 58 (69%) of 84 patients over the age of 50 years had neurologic complications.[55] Lerner and Weinstein[56] reported that 20% of patients with endocarditis had neurologic manifestations including major cerebral emboli, seizures, meningitis, subarachnoid hemorrhage, personality changes, obtundation, cortical blindness, and brain abscess. The pathogens most often involved are streptococci and staphylococci. This may be due to a higher frequency of endocarditis with these pathogens rather than an additional risk of CNS involvement. Purulent brain abscess and meningitis are uncommonly due to *Streptococcus viridans* and more often are caused by staphylococci and gram-negative bacteria. The value of blood cultures and echocardiograms cannot be overemphasized in an elderly patient who has CNS manifestations with fever and a heart murmur.

Legionnaire's disease is predominately seen in patients over the age of 50. This infection often presents with CNS involvement. In one group of nine patients with Legionnaire's disease with neurologic manifestations, five were over the age of 55.[57] There is a wide variety of neurologic manifestations. Abnormal mentation and headache are the most common presenting features. Infrequently, patients may present with seizures, cerebellar signs, or features of Guillain-Barré syndrome as the major manifestation of Legionnaire's disease. The CSF may show pleocytosis and elevated protein though usually the CSF shows no abnormal findings.

Infrequently, neurologic signs may precede the development of pulmonary infiltrates. Although *Legionella* has been cultured from brain tissue, it is not found in the CSF. Diagnosis is made from the serologic tests or either cultures or fluorescent antibody studies of sputum, tracheal aspirate, or pleural fluid.

Lyme disease, a tick-borne spirochetal disease, is now being described with increasing frequency among younger adults. The usual manifestations include a characteristic rash, joint pains and occasionally neurologic and cardiac abnormalities. This disease has been described among older persons who show various neurologic abnormalities.[58] Neurologic manifestations include meningitis, cranial nerve palsies, radiculoneuropathy, and encephalitis. It is possible that, as more data become available, Lyme disease will become an important consideration in the differential diagnosis of unexplained neurologic diseases, including aseptic meningitis, in any age group. The CSF usually shows increased lymphocytes and elevated protein but the diagnosis is ordinarily established by the serologic testing.

MANAGEMENT OF CNS INFECTIONS

Elderly patients with CNS infections often must be treated in the intensive care unit. In addition to their CNS problems, elderly patients often develop cardiorespiratory and renal problems that require close monitoring and observation.

The choice of antimicrobial agents is really no different from younger persons. However, several points need to be emphasized. Some of the manifestations of CNS infections are nonspecific and may be present in patients with bacterial meningitis as well as parameningeal infections (eg, brain abscess). It is important to make that distinction from clinical examination early since the choice of antimicrobial agents is dissimilar in pyogenic meningitis and brain abscess. This is due to the fact that common pathogens causing meningitis are rarely the etiologic agents in brain abscess where anaerobes are often the offending pathogens. Some of the antimicrobial agents used in meningeal infections, because of good penetration into the CSF, may not achieve adequate concentration in brain abscesses. Although studies on analysis of antibiotic concentrations in brain abscess pus are still somewhat controversial, several reports indicate[59,60] good penetration of penicillin (with a dose of 24 million units daily), chloramphenicol, and metronidazole, whereas levels of various cephalosporins and cloxacillin were poor. The role of third generation cephalosporins, of Trimethoprim-Sulfamethoxazole (TMP-SMX), and anti-pseudomonal penicillins, in the treatment of brain absess is not settled. Antimicrobial agents in CNS infection should be started promptly, often empirically, without culture results even if gram stain or CIE of CSF are negative. Choice must be made on the basis of epidemiologic history, physical examination, and preliminary CSF examination.

Ampicillin is the drug of choice in an elderly patient presenting with acute bacterial meningitis if no pathogen is found in the CSF by gram stain or CIE. This would be appropriate coverage for *Streptococcus pneumoniae, H influenzae,* and *Listeria* infections. This should be modified once the culture results are available.

The underlying diseases or associated conditions with CNS infections in the elderly, the possible pathogens and the empiric choice of antimicrobial agents are listed in Table 4-2.

In pneumococcal meningitis, penicillin still is the drug of choice but infrequently (about 2% of cases), pneumococci are resistant to penicillin. Therefore it is necessary to have all pneumococcal isolates from CSF tested for penicillin susceptibility. In adults with *H influenzae* infection, ampicillin resistance is not a major problem although this should be considered if *H influenzae* is acquired in the hospital setting.

One of the reasons for higher mortality in gram-negative bacillary meningitis has been the lack of effective antimicrobial agents with good penetration into the CSF. Aminoglycosides are the usual antibiotics of choice in serious systemic gram-negative infections but they do not penetrate well even if the meninges are inflamed. Such agents are therefore suboptimal unless given by the intralumbar or intraventricular route.

Recently, several third-generation cephalosporins have become available that have been effective for treatment of gram-negative bacillary meningitis; these include moxalactam and cefotaxime.[61,62] Moxalactam can be recommended only with considerable reservation because of the

Table 4-2
Initial Therapy of Meningitis in Adults in Various Circumstances

Underlying Diseases or Circumstances	Possible Pathogens	Initial Therapy
Mastoiditis, otitis media, and CT scan evidence of brain abscess	Streptococci (anaerobic and *S milleri*) *Bacteroides* spp	Penicillin + metronidazole or chloramphenicol
None	Pneumococcis, *Haemophilus influenzae*, meningococcis, *Listeria monocytogenes*	Ampicillin
Acute endocarditis	Staphylococci or streptococci	Pencillin + nafcillin
Hospital-acquired infections	Enterobacteriaceae, staphylococci	Nafcillin or vancomycin hydrochloride + gentamicin sulfate (both IV and intrathecal)*
Head trauma or neurosurgery	Enterobacteriaceae, *Pseudomonas* spp, staphylococci	Nafcillin or vancomycin + gentamicin (IV and intrathecal)*

* Anti-pseudomonal penicillins such as piperacillin or ceftazidime could be alternative choices.

potential toxic effects of the larger dosages needed to treat meningitis. Neither antibiotic is recommended for *Pseudomonas* infections nor effective in *Listeria* infections, and moxalactam is not predictably effective in pneumococcal infections. There are many new antibiotics being introduced but their efficacy in meningitis is unestablished except for ceftriaxone which is at least as effective as moxalactam and cefatoxime, and has the virtue of requiring administration only once or twice a day. Trimethoprim-sulfame-thoxazole has also been remarkably effective in some of these gram-negative CNS infections and is adequate for *Listeria* infections.[63]

There have been major controversies concerning treatment of neurosyphilis. Several authors have questioned the efficacy of standard benzathine penicillin. Many physicians now prefer to treat those patients with high doses of intravenous (IV) penicillin.

Several articles offer additional details of the treatment of CNS infection and have been recently published.[13,61,62,64] The antimicrobial agents of choice in the elderly for the treatment of CNS infections is summarized in Table 4-3.

Table 4-3
Antimicrobial Agents of Choice in Treatment of CNS Infections in the Elderly

Pathogens	Antimicrobial Agents Preferred	Alternate Choice
Pneumococcus	Penicillin G IV 20 – 24 million units daily in divided doses every 3 – 4 h	Chloramphenicol IV 4-6 g daily in 4 divided doses
Meningococcus	Penicillin G IV 20 – 24 million units daily in divided doses every 3 – 4 h	Chloramphenicol IV 4 – 6 g daily in 4 – 6 divided doses
Haemophilus influenzae	Ampicillin IV 12 g daily in divided doses (in betalactam-negative *H influenzae*) Chloramphenicol 4 – 6 g IV daily in divided doses (betalactam-positive *H influenzae*)	Moxalactam disodium 4 g daily in divided doses or cefotaxime sodium 12 g daily in 6 divided doses
Listeria monocytogenes	Ampicillin 12 g daily in 6 divided doses	Trimethoprim-sulfamethoxazole
Staphylococcus aureus	Nafcillin sodium IV 12 g daily in 6 divided doses	Vancomycin hydrochloride IV 2 g daily in 4 divided doses
Enterobacteriaceae (*Escherichia coli, Klebsiella, Pneumoniae*)	Cefotaxime sodium 12 g daily in divided doses in 6 divided doses	Trimethoprim (10 mg/kg/day)-sulfamethoxazole 50 mg/kg/day

Pathogens	Antimicrobial Agents Preferred	Alternate Choice
Pseudomonas aeruginosa	Gentamicin sulfate IV 5 mg/kg/day + gentamicin sulfate (intrathecal) 2−4 mg/day	Piperacillin sodium or azlocillin 18−24 g daily in 6 divided doses or ceftazidime IV in 3 divided doses
Mycobacterium tuberculosis	Isoniazid 300 mg PO daily + rifampin 600 mg PO daily + pyrazinamide 20−35 mg/kg/day in 4 divided doses	
Treponema pallidum (neurosyphilis)	Penicillin G IV 12−24 million units daily in 6 divided doses for 2 weeks	Tetracycline hydrochloride 500 mg 4 times daily for 30 days
Lyme disease with CNS manifestations	Penicillin G IV 20 million units daily in 6 divided doses	Tetracycline 500 mg PO 4 times daily

SUMMARY

Central nervous infections in the elderly are often caused by unusual pathogens including gram-negative bacteria, *Mycobacterium tuberculosis,* and *Cryptococcus neoformans.* This is probably ordinarily related to associated chronic illness in this age group rather than any defect in host defense mechanisms. Many noninfectious disorders that affect the CNS in the aging population can produce manifestations that also may be seen with infectious diseases of the CNS. Infectious etiologics are often not considered for lack of specific presentations and therefore appropriate tests are not pursued with consequent increase in mortality and morbidity. With a high index of suspicion, sophisticated laboratory tests, and proper radiologic procedures, early diagnosis of CNS infections can be achieved. A variety of effective antimicrobial agents including third-generation cephalosporins, IV trimethoprim-sulfamethoxazole, antituberculosis agents, and antiviral agents with reasonable CSF penetration are now available. These agents obviously will be helpful in reducing the high mortality of many CNS infections.

REFERENCES

1. Mortality morbidity weekly report, United States, 1978. *MMWR* 1979;28:277−279.
2. Murasko DM, Nelson BJ, Silver R , et al: Immunologic response in an elderly population with a mean age of 85. *Am J Med* 1986;81:612−618.
3. Nerenberg ST, Prasad R: Radioimmunoassays for Ig classes G, A, M, D,

and E in spinal fluids: Normal values of different age groups. *J Lab Clin Med* 1975;86:887—898.
4. Sabin AB, Ginder DR, Matumoto M, et al: Serological response of Japanese children and old people to Japanese B encephalitis mouse brain vaccine. *Proc Soc Exp Biol Med* 1947;65:135—140.
5. Waldorf DS, Wilkins RF, Decker JL: Impaired delayed hypersensitivity in aging population. Association with antinuclear reactivity and rheumatoid factor. *JAMA* 1968:203;831—834.
6. Inkeles B, Innes JB, Kuntz MM, et al: Immunologic studies of aging. Cytokinetic basis for the impaired response of lymphocytes from aged humans to plant lectins. *J Exp Med* 1977;145:1176—1187.
7. Menon M, Jaroslow BN, Koesterer R: The decline of cell mediated immunity in aging mice. *J Genontol* 1974;29:499-505.
8. Gardner ID, Remington JS: Age-related decline in the resistance of mice to infection with intracellular pathogens. *Infect Immun* 1977;16:593—598.
9. Miller AE: Selected decline in cellular immune response to varicella-zoster in the elderly. *Neurology* 1980;30:582—587.
10. Smith L: Host deficiency states and central nervous system infections, in Grieco MH (ed): *Infections in the Abnormal Host*. New York, Yorke Medical Books, 1980, pp 623—652.
11. Gorse GJ, Lauri DT, Nudleman KL, et al: Bacterial meningitis in the elderly. *Arch Intern Med* 1984;144:1603—1607.
12. Harter DH, Petersdorf RG: Pyogenic infections of the central nervous system, in Braunwald E, Isselbacher D, Petersdorf RG, et al (eds): *Harrison's Principles of Internal Medicine,* ed 11. New York, McGraw-Hill Book Co, 1987, pp. 1980-1987.
13. Roeltgen DP: Infections and the nervous system in the elderly. *Geriatrics* 1983;38:105—113.
14. Sheld WM, Winn HR: Brain abscess, in Mandell GL, Douglas RG Jr, Bennett JE (eds): *Principles and Practice of Infectious Diseases*, ed. 2. New York, Wiley Medical Publications, 1985, pp. 585-592.
15. Crocker ER, McLaughlin AF, Morris JG, et al: Technetium brain scanning in the diagnosis and management of cerebral abscess. *Am J Med* 1974;56: 192—201.
16. Mascucci EF, Sauerbrunn BJL: The evolution of a brain abscess. The complementary roles of radionuclide and computed tomography scans. *Clin Nucl Med* 1982;7:166—170.
17. Chandler JR: Malignant external otitis: Further considerations. *Ann Otol Rhinol Laryngol* 1977;86:417—428.
18. Zaky DA, Bentley DW, Lowy K, et al: Malignant external otitis: A severe form of otitis in diabetic patients. *Am J Med* 1976;61:298—302.
19. Sapico FL, Montgomerie JZ: Pyogenic vertebral osteomyelitis: Report of nine cases and review of the literature. *Rev Infect Dis* 1979;1:754—776.
20. Harter DH, Petersdorf RG: Pyogenic infections of the central nervous system, in Braunwald E, Isselbacher K, Petersdorf RG, et al (eds): *Harrison's Principles of Internal Medicine*, ed 11. New York, McGraw-Hill Book Co, 1987, pp 1980—1987.
21. Eigler JOL, Wellman WE, Rooke ED, et al. Bacterial meningitis: A general review: *Mayo Clin Proc* 1961;36:357—365.
22. Berk SL, Smith JK: Infectious diseases in the elderly. *Med Clin North Am* 1983;67:273—293.
23. Austrian R: Pneumococcal endocarditis, meningitis and rupture of the aortic valve. *Arch Intern Med* 1957;99:539—544.

24. Kaplan SL: Antigen detection in cerebrospinal fluid — Pros and cons. *Am J Med* 1983;75:109–118.
25. Swartz MN, Dodge PR: Bacterial meningitis — A review of selected aspects. *N Engl J Med* 1965;272:779–787.
26. Weiss W, Figueroa W, Shapiro WH, et al: Prognostic factors in pneumococcal meningitis. *Arch Intern Med* 1967;120:517–524.
27. Young LS, LaForce FM, Head JJ, et al: A simultaneous outbreak of meningococcal and influenza infection. *N Engl J Med* 1972;287:5–9.
28. Feldman HA: The meningococcus: A twenty-year perspective. *Rev Infect Dis* 1986;8:288–294.
29. Whittle HC, Greenwood BM, Davidson NM, et al: Menin-gococcal antigen in diagnosis and treatment of group A meningococcal infections. *Am J Med* 1975;58:823–828.
30. Eykyn SJ, Thomas RD, Phillips I: *Haemophilus influenzae* meningitis in adults. *Br Med J* 1974;2:463–465.
31. Hirschmann JV, Everett ED: *Haemophilus influenzae* infections in adults: Report of nine cases and a review of the literature. *Medicine* 1979;58:80–94.
32. Van Dijk JM, Burger A: *Haemophilus influenzae* meningitis in the elderly. *J Am Geriatr Soc* 1986;34:530–532.
33. Simon HB, Southwick FS, Moellering RC, et al: *Haemophilus influenzae* in hospitalized adults: Current perspectives. *Am J Med* 1980;69:219–226.
34. Spagnuolo PJ, Ellny JJ, Lerner PI: *Haemophilus influenzae* meningitis: The spectrum of disease in adults. *Medicine* 1982;62:74–85.
35. Norden CW: Prevalence of bactericidal antibodies to *Haemophilus influenzae*, type B. *J Infect Dis* 1974;130:489–494.
36. Cherubin CE, Marr JS, Sierra MF, et al: Listeria and gram negative bacillary meningitis in New York City, 1972–1979. *Am J Med* 1981;71:199–209.
37. Berk SL, McCabe WR: Meningitis caused by Gram negative bacilli. *Ann Intern Med* 1980;93:253–260.
38. Mangi RJ, Quintiliani R, Andriole VT: Gram-negative bacillary meningitis. *Am J Med* 1975;59:829–836.
39. Lerner PI, Gopalakrishna KV, Wolinsky E, et al: Group B streptococcus (*S. agalactiae*) bacteremia in adults: Analysis of 32 cases and review of the literature. *Medicine* 1977;56:457–473.
40. Duma RJ, Weinberg AN, Medrik TF, et al: Streptococcal infection. A bacteriologic and clinical study of streptococcal bacteremia. *Medicine* 1969;48:87–127.
41. Bayer AS, Seidel JS, Yoshikawa TT, et al: Group D enterococcal meningitis. *Arch Intern Med* 1976;136:883–886.
42. Weir MR, Thornton GF: Extrapulmonary tuberculosis: Experience of a community hospital and review of the literature. *Am J Med* 1985;79:467–478.
43. Haas EJ, Madhavan T, Quinn EL, et al: Tuberculosis meningitis in an urban general hospital. *Arch Intern Med* 1977;137:1518–1521.
44. Iseman MD: Tuberculosis in the elderly: Treating the "white plague." *Geriatrics* 1980;35:90–107.
45. Sen P, Kapila J, Salaki J, et al: The diagnostic enigma of extra-pulmonary tuberculosis. *J Chronic Dis* 1977;30:331–350.
46. Kennedy DH, Fallon RJ: Tuberculosis meningitis. *JAMA* 1979;241:264–268.
47. Munt PW: Miliary tuberculosis in the chemotherapy era: With a clinical

review in 69 American adults. *Medicine* 1972;51: 139 – 155.
48. Fiumara NJ: Diagnosis and treatment of latent and late syphilis: Evaluation of the reactive serologic test for syphilis, in McCormack WM (ed): *Diagnosis and Treatment of Sexually Transmitted Diseases*. Littleton, Mass, John Wright PSG Inc, 1983 pp 127 – 142.
49. Jaffe HW, Kabins SA: Examination of cerebrospinal fluid in patients with syphilis. *Rev Infect Dis* 1982;4:5842 – 5847.
50. Kolar OJ, Burkhart JE: Neurosyphilis. *Br J Vener Dis* 1977;53:221 – 225.
51. Salaki JS, Louria DB, Chmel H: Fungal and yeast infections of the central nervous system. A clinical review. *Medicine* 1984;63:108 – 132.
52. Sen P, Louria DB: Higher bacterial and funal infections, in Grieco MH (ed): *Infections in the Abnormal Host*. New York, Yorke Medical Books, 1980, pp 325 – 359.
53. Louria DB, Kaminski T, Kapila R, et al: Study on the usefulness of hypertonic culture media. *J Clin Microbiol* 1976;4:208 – 213.
54. Berk SL, Alvarez S: Bacterial infections in the elderly. Special consideration for a special patient population. *Postgrad Med* 1985;77:168 – 173.
55. Pruitt AA, Rubin RH, Karchmer AW, et al: Neurologic complications of bacterial endocarditis. *Medicine* 1978;57:329 – 343.
56. Lerner PI, Weinstein L: Infective endocarditis in the antibiotic era. *N Engl J Med* 1966;274:259 – 266.
57. Johnson JD, Raff MJ, VanArsdall JA: Neurologic manifestations of Legionnaire's disease. *Medicine* 1984;63:303 – 310.
58. Reik L Jr, Burgdorfer W, Donaldson JO: Neurologic abnormalities in Lyme disease without erythema chronicum migrans. *Am J Med* 1986;81:73 – 78.
59. Delouvois J, Gortvai P, Hurley R: Antibiotic treatment of abscess of the central nervous system. *Br Med J* 1977;2:985 – 987.
60. Ingham HR, Selkon JB, Roxby CM: Bacteriologic study of otogenic cerebral abscess: Chemotherapeutic role of metronidazole. *Br Med J* 1977;2:991 – 993.
61. Cherubin CE, Eng RH: Experience with the use of cefotaxime in the treatment of bacterial meningitis. *Am J Med* 1986;80:398 – 404.
62. Corrado ML, Gombert ME, Cherubin CE: Designing appropriate therapy in the treatment of Gram-negative bacillary meningitis. *JAMA* 1982;248: 71 – 74.
63. Levitz RE, Quintiliani R: Trimethoprim-sulfamethoxazole for bacterial meningitis. *Ann Intern Med* 1984;100:881 – 890.
64. Henry K, Crossley K: Meningitis, principles of diagnosis, advances in treatment. *Postgrad Med* 1986;80:59 – 66, 69 – 71.

5

Encephalitis

Reisa F. Ullman
Burke A. Cunha

Encephalitis is essentially an inflammation of the brain, frequently accompanied by inflammation of the meninges, and is not as uncommon as is usually perceived. Its importance lies in the significant overall mortality, the frequency of residual neurologic deficits, and the possibility of specific treatment in certain instances. While there are many diverse causes of encephalitis, including various viral, bacterial, and fungal etiologies, only the four major clinical entities will be discussed in this section. They have been found to be important causes of encephalitis in the older age groups and physicians must become increasingly aware of their existence in order to help differentiate their signs and symptoms from those frequently attributed simply to other illnesses and the concomitant complications of advancing age itself.

Although arboviruses are considered by some to be the most common cause of encephalitis in the United States (and among these, St Louis encephalitis appears to affect the elderly more frequently), they are commonly overlooked in the differential diagnosis. Herpes simplex viral encephalitis is important to recognize early because of the improved survival with antiviral therapy, and *Mycoplasma pneumoniae* and Legionnaires' disease, although not as frequently seen, can cause confusion for the physician because of their multisystem involvement. The majority of patients present with fever, headache, and mental status changes, and it is usually difficult to differentiate the various encephalidites solely on the basis of clinical features. Examination of the CSF is essential, and EEG, computed tomography (CT) scans, and brain scans have frequently been helpful in localizing sites of pathologic changes. However, the diagnosis usually depends on specific serology or culture of the organism, and in certain cases, on brain biopsy. The physician must therefore maintain a high level of suspicion for these entities in the evaluation of an older patient with fever, headache, and mental status changes.

ST LOUIS ENCEPHALITIS

St Louis encephalitis was first recognized when epidemics occurred in St Louis, Missouri, and southern Illinois during 1932 and 1933. Subsequent outbreaks have occurred in Texas, Florida, California, Washington, New Jersey, and the Ohio-Mississippi Valley, with the emergence of two epidemiologic patterns being noted. The first is found in the West where outbreaks of St Louis encephalitis were found mostly in irrigated rural areas, and the second pattern has been noted to occur primarily in urban-suburban locations, the latter of which has been characterized by a significantly higher incidence of encephalitis in persons over 50 years of age.[1-4] Both sexes are usually equally affected. The virus is transmitted through a cycle of wild bird—mosquito—wild bird, with humans acting as an accidental host. The mosquito vector has been shown to be *Culex tarsalis* in the western United States, *Culex pipiens* in the eastern United States, and *Culex nigripalpus* in Florida. St Louis encephalitis virus has also been found in tropical America, but only sporadic clinical infection has been reported.

Infection with St Louis encephalitis virus usually occurs from midsummer to early fall, and most commonly produces inapparent infection. However, among the patients with confirmed disease, about three quarters have clinical encephalitis, and almost all patients older than 40 years of age develop encephalitis, with increased severity of the disease found with advancing age.[1,2,5] The initial symptoms of fever, malaise, headache (most often frontal), and myalgias usually occur abruptly after an incubation period of 4 to 21 days. Within the following 24 hours, evidence of confusion and disorientation usually appears.[1,2,5] Subsequent changes in mentation may range from mild lethargy and subtle abnormalities noted on mental status examination, to stupor and coma. Other symptoms may include nausea with vomiting and photophobia. Tremors of the extremities, face, and tongue are common, especially in patients more than 40 years old, and may be continuous or intention in type.[2,3,6] Pathologic reflexes including suck and snout reflexes, and exaggerated palmomental reflexes are present in about 50% of the patients. Less commonly, cranial nerve abnormalities causing nystagmus, oculomotor muscle paresis, and facial weakness may occur. Stiff neck, positive Kernig's sign, motor weakness, changes in deep tendon reflexes, and varying plantar responses may also be found, but sensory deficits are rare. Seizures occur in about 10% of patients and have been shown to be a poor prognostic sign.[1,3] The severity of the illness corresponds closely to the duration and severity of fever, and temperatures of 102° to 105°F for more than five or six days are associated with a poor prognosis. Urinary tract involvement including sterile pyuria, dysuria, and hematuria may also occur.[3,5] The syndrome of inappropriate secretion of antidiuretic hormone with resultant hyponatremia and serum hypo-osmolarity has occurred in about one third of patients, and usually responds well to water restriction.[7]

Cerebrospinal fluid is usually under moderate pressure, is clear, and shows a predominant lymphocytosis, normal glucose, and elevated protein. The cell count usually ranges from about 50−250 cells/µL, and an early polymorphonuclear cell predominance may be noted.[3,6] CSF protein ranges from 25−500 mg/mL. Other laboratory findings have variably included peripheral leukocytosis, elevated BUN, elevated serum transaminases, and elevated serum aldolase, along with abnormal electromyographic (EMG) studies.[3,6] In most patients, the EEG shows diffuse generalized slowing occasionally associated with focal lesions, but no correlation has been found between the severity of the disease and the extent of the EEG changes. The brain scan and CT scan are usually normal. The major pathologic changes found in the CNS of fatal cases of St Louis encephalitis are perivascular mononuclear infiltration, perineural or perivascular proliferation of the microglia, and degeneration of the neurons.[8] These lesions predominate in the substantia nigra, but are also found in the anterior horn cells, thalamus, cerebral cortex, corpus striatum, and cerebellum.

The case fatality rate averages about 8% in this illness,[9] with deaths occurring most frequently in the elderly.[1] The majority of patients who survive have a complete recovery from the immediate illness which lasts from 1 to 3 weeks. However, some patients experience a prolonged convalescent period and may complain of fatigue, irritability, and loss of memory, all of which improve with the passage of time.[10]

The diagnosis of St Louis encephalitis should be suspected when a patient, especially one more than 50 years old, develops clinical encephalitis in the summer or fall, and has a CSF lymphocytosis with increased protein and normal glucose.[4] St Louis encephalitis must be differentiated from enteroviral infections which are usually milder, have a flulike prodrome for several days, and may be accompanied by one or more of their nonneurologic manifestations such as gastroenteritis, rashes, and upper respiratory infections. The other arboviral encephalitides must also be differentiated from St Louis encephalitis, especially western equine encephalitis (WEE), eastern equine encephalitis (EEE), and California encephalitis. However, each of these occur more commonly, or are more devastating, in children, and WEE and EEE may be preceded by infection in horses.[4,9] Since it is difficult to differentiate these on a clinical basis, the ultimate diagnosis must be established serologically by hemagglutination inhibition and complement fixation with acute and convalescent titers. Virus isolation is usually unsuccessful; however, a few cases have been documented of premortem isolation of the virus from the CSF, blood, and the throat of affected individuals.[6] Treatment is usually supportive since no specific antiviral therapy is available at this time, and no vaccine has yet been developed. Specific attention should be paid to the treatment of possible complications which may occur, such as superimposed bacterial infection and pulmonary embolus, which may contribute to the morbidity and mortality of this illness. Early diagnosis and immediate reporting of cases may help detect outbreaks and promote the institution of prompt control measures, such as limiting exposures to mosquitoes in the high-risk groups and eradication of the mosquito vector.[5,11]

HERPES SIMPLEX ENCEPHALITIS

Herpes simplex encephalitis is a serious infection of the CNS most frequently caused by herpes simplex virus type 1 (HSV-1), and is generally considered the most common cause of sporadic cases of acute viral encephalitis.[12,13] This illness occurs in all age groups, both sexes, and shows no seasonal predilection, but the identification of patients on clinical grounds who are more likely to have proven disease has been found to be higher in persons more than 50 years old.[13,14] The mortality rate varies from about 30% to 70% in most studies, with a significant decrease in these rates being found among those treated with antiviral therapy.[15-19]

The clinical course of herpes simplex encephalitis usually begins with a prodrome of symptoms including fever (often to 104°–106°F), headache, malaise, nausea, vomiting, sore throat, memory loss, and speech difficulty.[13,20] This is usually followed by disorientation, lethargy, auditory and olfactory hallucinations, photophobia, facial or major motor seizures, and personality changes. As the patient becomes progressively more impaired, changes in the level of consciousness from lethargy to stupor and coma may occur. Various neurologic signs including dysphasia, motor paralysis, ataxia, bowel and bladder incontinence, pathologic reflexes, nuchal rigidity, cranial nerve palsies, visual field loss, and signs of increased intracranial pressure (ie, papilledema) may also become evident.[14-17,20] A history of recurrent HSV infection (mostly herpes labialis) was found in about 22% of patients with proven HSV encephalitis in one study.[14]

Laboratory analysis usually shows a mild leukocytosis with a shift to the left, and examination of the CSF may reveal elevated pressure and normal or slightly increased protein. CSF glucose is usually normal, but hypoglycorrhachia may occur.[14] An elevated WBC count is usually present and consists of a mixture of polymorphonuclear leukocytes

(PMNs) and lymphocytes, with the latter predominating later in the course of the disease.[21] Red blood cells have frequently, but not always, been found in the CSF of patients with HSV encephalitis, and in a recent study, about 42% of patients had more than 50 RBCs in the CSF. Infectious HSV has been isolated from the CSF of patients with encephalitis only on rare occasions, and therefore absence of the virus does not rule out the diagnosis, and thus the need to define new noninvasive means of identification of this illness still persists. Interferon has been found in the CSF and brain biopsy specimens of patients with HSV encephalitis[22]; however, the usefulness of this finding in making the diagnosis is not yet known. Antibody studies have shown that levels in the CSF increase significantly within the first month of onset of symptoms in most patients, and lowered ratios of serum to CSF antibody have also been found.[21,23] However, since these rises in titer, and changes in serum:CSF ratios do not occur early enough in the course of illness, they are only of use for the retrospective diagnosis of HSV encephalitis, and therefore do not help in the decision concerning therapy.[21,24]

Other diagnostic tests which may be useful in suggesting the diagnosis of HSV encephalitis in a patient with the above signs and symptoms include the EEG, brain scan, and CT scan. The EEG has been found to be the most helpful of these techniques, showing localization of disease in 81% of biopsy-proven HSV encephalitis versus 50% with brain scan, and 59% with CT scan.[14] The most common EEG findings consist of spiked and slow waves localized in the area of brain involved, usually one of the temporal-frontal regions.[25] Abnormal brain scan findings may include enhanced uptake of radionuclide in the affected area of the brain, and CT scans most commonly show a low density lesion within one or both temporal lobes, frequently accompanied by mottled and irregular contrast enhancement at the edge of the lesion, localized edema, mass effect, and possibly hemorrhage.[14] Before CT scanning became available, cerebral arteriography was used as a diagnostic study, and typically revealed a space-occupying lesion in the temporal lobe.[20] This technique may still be useful in the delineation of a brain biopsy site along with determination of the affected region by CT scan and EEG.

At this time, detection of HSV in brain biopsy specimens still remains the most definitive method for diagnosis of HSV encephalitis.[14,16-18,21] Demonstration of the virus may be done by the fluorescent antibody test, electron microscopy, or tissue culture. The fluorescent antibody test is the most rapid and specific, and is relatively sensitive, but the identification of virus in tissue culture within two to three days by its typical cytopathic effect is the hallmark for establishing the diagnosis. Despite the controversy surrounding brain biopsy, studies have shown that false-negative biopsies are rare, the morbidity and mortality, either short-term or long-term, are relatively low, and in patients with negative brain biopsy findings for HSV, the brain biopsy was useful in establishing alternative diagnoses, some of which were treatable.[16,18] The most common among these other diseases are vascular disease, cryptococcal infection, coxsackievirus encephalitis, other viral encephalitides, abscess, tuberculosis, tumor, Reye's syndrome, subacute sclerosing panencephalitis, and toxoplasmosis.[14,16,24]

The pathologic features of HSV encephalitis are similar to other viral encephalitides; however, the inflammatory and necrotic changes are characteristically most marked in the orbitofrontal and temporal lobes.[20,22,26] The infection produces a necrotizing process involving both gray and white matter, with either unilateral or bilateral involvement. Microscopically, perivascular lymphocytic cell infiltration and microglial reaction may be seen in less severely involved areas, while increased numbers of macrophages may be present in more severely affected areas. The typical eosinophilic Cowdry type A intranuclear inclusion bodies are usually seen in neurons, oligodendrocytes, and astrocytes during the acute phase of illness. The finding of these inclusions may be helpful in establishing the diagnosis, and in one study these were found in 56% of patients with brain biopsy-proven HSV encephalitis.[24] However, these inclusion bodies are not unique to HSV encephalitis, and may also be seen in infection caused by coxsackievirus, Epstein-Barr virus, cytomegalovirus, varicella zoster virus, measles virus, lymphocytic choriomeningitis, subacute sclerosing panencephalitis, and Reye's syndrome.[20,24] The manner in which HSV spreads to the CNS of humans is still a subject for speculation. Some investigators hypothesize that HSV-1 results from intranasal spread to the olfactory tract and subsequently to the temporal and/or frontal lobes, unilaterally or bilaterally.[22] In older individuals, HSV encephalitis appears to result more often from recurrent infection than primary infection according to serologic findings,[13,18,24] and the possible relationship between HSV encephalitis and reactivation of latent infection has also been proposed.[27]

The treatment of HSV encephalitis includes the basic supportive measures as well as control of seizures with anticonvulsants, and management of increased intracranial pressure with mannitol, steroids, or surgical decompression. However, the most important part of therapy has only recently come about due to studies with antiviral agents. Until recently, vidarabine (ara-A) was considered the treatment of choice for HSV encephalitis. In patients with biopsy-proven HSV encephalitis, treatment with ara-A at a dose of 15 mg/kg/day for ten days via a continuous intravenous (IV) infusion over 12 hours resulted in a mortality of 28% compared with a 70% mortality in placebo-treated patients.[17] Investigators have shown that mental status at the time of treatment, and age, are important in predicting outcome. Patients who were lethargic at the time of presentation did much better than those in coma, and increasing age adversely affected the prognosis.[16,17] Residual neurologic sequelae, including speech and cognitive deficits, seizures, paralysis, ataxia, and postinfectious encephalopathy may occur, although neurologic status has been found to improve during the first few months after therapy, and may continue for at least a year. However, older patients who are comatose at the initiation of treatment may die during the first few months secondary to complications such as bacterial infection and pulmonary embolism.[16]

Vidarabine is thought to specifically inhibit HSV DNA polymerase and possibly ribonucleotide reductase, both of which are necessary for DNA synthesis. This drug is deaminated to the active metabolite Arahypoxanthine and is cleared by the kidney, with maximal urinary excretion of an IV dose of ara-A at four hours and half the dose being cleared by 24 hours.[28] Since ara-A has a low water solubility, it must be administered with a relatively large amount of fluid and at a recommended concentration of not greater than 700 mg/L.[29,30] Fluid overload is therefore a concern, and patients must be monitored closely for signs of increased intracranial pressure, seizures, electrolyte imbalance, congestive heart failure, and other related problems. The frequency and severity of side effects have been shown to be dose-related and include nausea and vomiting, weight loss, weakness, megaloblastic anemia, skin rash, diarrhea, tremors, thrombocytopenia, and transient elevation of liver function tests and serum creatinine.[16,30-32] These side effects can be minimized though by following the above recommended 12-hour infusion and adjusting the dosage at the first signs of toxicity.

Acyclovir, a newer and more water-soluble antiviral compound, is a guanosine analog and has been shown to selectively inhibit HSV replication and have a high in vitro therapeutic index. Clinical trials done both in Sweden and the United States comparing the efficacy of acyclovir versus vidarabine have concluded that acyclovir is superior to vidarabine for the treatment of herpes simplex encephalitis. Using doses of acyclovir of 10 mg/kg infused IV over one hour every eighth hour for ten days, and vidarabine 15 mg/kg/day infused over a 12-hour period for ten days, there was variably a 19% and 28% mortality in the acyclovir-treated group in contrast to a 50% and 54% mortality in the vidarabine-treated patients, respectively.[18,19,33] As noted in previous studies, patients with advanced age and decreased level of consciousness had a poor outcome. Although renal, gastrointestinal (GI), bone marrow, and CNS toxicities have been reported with the use of acyclovir, especially in patients with abnormal renal function, the drug was well tolerated in both studies, and the acyclovir-treated group developed fewer abnormal laboratory values than the vidarabine-treated group.[18,19,33] Thus, at this time, acyclovir is the preferred drug for treatment of HSV encephalitis and that early diagnosis and institution of antiviral therapy are key in therapy.

MYCOPLASMA ASSOCIATED ENCEPHALITIS

Mycoplasma pneumoniae infection is a well-recognized cause of pneumonia and upper respiratory tract illness in the general population, occurring commonly in fall and winter, and characterized by intrafamily spread. Although it is usually a benign and self-limited disease not requiring hospitalization, severe pulmonary disease may occur as well as disease involving other organ systems including the GI tract, the hematologic, cardiovascular, musculoskeletal, neurologic, and dermatologic systems, as well as reports of associated acute glomerulonephritis, hepatitis, and pancreatitis.[34-36] The disease occurs commonly in children and young adults,[35,37] but has been reported in older patients as well, with about 25% of patients older than 40 years of age in one study.[34,36-38] The reported cases of complications of *M pneumoniae* infection appear to occur more commonly in patients older than those with classic pneumonia, and seem to predominate with multiorgan system involvement.[39]

Central nervous system complications of atypical pneumonia were initially described in 1938, when the causative organism was not yet known to be *M pneumoniae*. Over the years, many reports of neurologic involvement have appeared in the literature and seem to be the most frequently reported extrapulmonary manifestations of this disease[37]; they include encephalitis, meningitis, myelitis, polyradiculitis, and acute psychosis.[40,41] The incidence of CNS involvement occurring with *M pneumoniae* infections is estimated to be 0.1%, but is increased to about 7% among hospitalized patients,[42,43] and of these, encephalitis appears to be the most frequent manifestation of CNS disease.[37,44]

Concurrent or antecedent respiratory infection is common, and the majority of patients present with fever, chills, nonproductive cough, headache, and malaise.[34,36,38,45-47] Chest roentgenogram frequently reveals a lower lobe infiltrate, although no specific pattern in pathognostic.[37,48] The onset of neurologic signs and symptoms is variable, ranging from one to fourteen days, with an average of ten days after the above systemic symptoms appear. These CNS manifestations then progress over a period of a few hours to a few days, and may include headache, lethargy, confusion, altered mental status, nuchal rigidity, brisk reflexes, and a variety of other signs ranging from cerebellar and focal cranial nerve signs to diffuse motor and sensory abnormalities and possibly coma with decerebrate posturing.[37,43,44]

Laboratory studies usually reveal a normal WBC count, but mild leukocytosis may occur, and occasionally a shift to the left appears in the differential.[34,36,41,42,45-49] The ESR is usually elevated and cold agglutinins (IgM autoantibody that agglutinates human type O erythrocytes at

4°C) are positive at greater than 1:64 in 33% to 76% of patients.[34-36] They usually become positive at about day 7, will show a rise in titer and reach a peak at about 4 weeks, and thereafter decrease, becoming negative at about 4 months. This appears to correspond to the severity and duration of infection. It should be noted, however, that cold agglutinins are not specific for *M pneumoniae* infection, and they may be found in low titres, eg., 1:64 in a variety of other conditions including influenza, infectious mononucleosis, rubella and adenovirus, psittacosis, liver disease, peripheral vascular disease, and dysproteinemias.[34] Specific serum anti-*M pneumoniae* complement fixation titers of greater than 1:64 or a fourfold rise in titer should also be found and will confirm the diagnosis.[36,41,42,46,47,49] This titer will usually begin to rise about seven to nine days after infection begins and will peak about 3 to 4 weeks later, and may remain near this peak for about 4 to 6 months and then decline over about 2 to 3 years. A subclinical anemia also appears to be common, with approximately 83% of patients having positive direct Coombs' tests and 64% showing a reticulocytosis.[34]

Sputum culture may be positive for *M pneumoniae*, although frequently it is not. Examination of the CSF usually reveals normal or slightly elevated pressure, pleocytosis with a variable percentage of lymphocytes and polymorphonuclear leukocytosis, normal or moderately increased protein level, and a normal glucose level, although one case of hypoglycorrhachia has been reported.[34,44-47,49,50] Diffuse bilateral cerebral dysfunction is frequently present on EEG in the form of slow waves, although this test is not always done.[34,41,44] While brain and CT scans are usually normal, those with positive findings are consistent with cerebral edema and cerebritis appearing as an expanding central lesion.[41,44,47,48]

Isolation of *M pneumoniae* from neural tissue and CSF is difficult, and only a few cases have been reported in which *Mycoplasma* was cultured from the CSF,[46,50] although it has been cultured more frequently from the nasopharynx of some patients with CNS disease.[34,50] Thus the diagnosis of *M pneumoniae*-associated encephalitis is frequently a presumptive one and must be distinguished from other viral and bacterial encephalidites by a number of studies including negative viral serology and virus isolation, negative spinal fluid cultures, the clinical picture of an atypical pneumonia with encephalitis, and positive serology for *M pneumoniae*. Complement fixation antibody titers to *M pneumoniae* may be found in the CNS, although uncommon,[46,49] and the organism has been demonstrated in the CSF utilizing sophisticated radioisotropic and immunofluorescent techniques which are not generally available.[51]

Because of the difficulty in identifying this organism in the CNS, several mechanisms have been proposed for the pathogenesis of neurologic involvement as well as the other extrapulmonary manifestations in *M pneumoniae* infection. Among these are possible generation of a neurotoxin by the organism, production of autoantibodies, altered or suppressed immune responsiveness induced by *Mycoplasma*, and direct invasion by the organism into the CNS.[46,50,52] Since the majority of *Mycoplasma* infections are benign, the number of autopsy and biopsy specimens are limited, but of those brain tissue sections that have been studied, the pathologic findings have included edema, vascular microthrombi, demyelination, free hemosiderin-filled macrophages, inflammation, and nonspecific changes of astrocytes and microglial cells.[46,47] Many of these pathologic features are those of a postinfectious encephalitis and thus are not specific for *M pneumoniae* infection. Therefore the mechanism of neurologic involvement remains to be elucidated, although studies with animal models suggest the possibility that *M pneumoniae* may cause blood-borne infection of the brain, and occur more readily in compromised patients.[40]

Recovery from this illness may be slow, varying from weeks to months, but it is usually complete. However, residual deficits including depression, intellectual impairment, memory loss, and evidence of specific neurologic dysfunction may occur, and seem to appear more commonly in the older age groups.[34,41,42,47] Death has also been reported and again is more common in the older patients. Therapy consists of general supportive measures as well as specific antibiotic treatment. Although IV tetracycline or erythromycin remain the drugs of choice for this infection, their effectiveness in altering the course of neurologic disease is still unknown.[41,42,47]

LEGIONNAIRES' DISEASE

Legionnaires' disease is a serious respiratory illness which was recognized as a distinct entity only after an outbreak of pneumonia at an American Legion convention in Philadelphia in 1976.[53] The causative organism has been found to be *Legionella pneumophila,* a fastidious, obligately aerobic, gram-negative bacillus which has been shown to be responsible for both epidemic and sporadic cases of pneumonia throughout the world.[54-56] Over the years, one of the most important features of this infection has emerged as its propensity for multisystem involvement including the GI tract, renal impairment, hematologic changes, as well as neurologic manifestations. It has been estimated to account for about 10% of cases of "atypical" community-acquired pneumonia, and although the disease may develop during any time of the year, it occurs most commonly between the months of July and October.[54-56] *Legionella pneumophila* appears to cause disease most frequently in patients more than 50 years old, with males slightly more commonly affected than females (about 2.5:1.0 in some studies).[56] Several other predisposing factors have come to be recognized since the original case descriptions, and include increased frequency in states of immunosuppression, either from drugs which affect cellular immunity or from the primary disease itself, smoking, alcohol consumption, and increased incidence among patients with some significant underlying condition such as diabetes, cancer, chronic pulmonary disease, chronic cardiac disease, chronic renal failure with dialysis, renal and bone marrow transplants, as well as the acquired immunodeficiency syndrome (AIDS).[54-56] In one study, 70% of patients had some underlying disease at the time they developed Legionnaires' disease.[56]

Legionella pneumophila are ubiquitous organisms that appear to grow best in areas of stagnant warm water, and infections due to this organism seem to be transmitted through the air from contaminated sites such as air conditioning systems, plumbing systems, and cooling towers.[54,55,57] This probably accounts for the more common occurrence of illness in large buildings, that is, hotels and hospitals. After an incubation period of from two to ten days, patients usually experience the gradual onset of prodromal symptoms characterized by weakness, malaise, lethargy, anorexia, and headache.[53-56,58] Within 48 hours, about 90% to 95% of patients will develop high unremitting fevers, with temperatures of 104° F and higher occurring in at least 50% of them.[54,56] Despite these high temperatures, a relative bradycardia (inappropriate pulse response to an increase in temperature) has been noted to occur in about two thirds of patients.[58] This is usually accompanied by recurrent shaking chills and onset of a dry nonproductive cough, although upper respiratory symptoms such as rhinitis, coryza, and sore throat are uncommon.[54-56,58] After the first 48 hours of illness, the cough may become productive and purulent sputum may be noted in one half of patients, while hemoptysis may be seen in about one third of patients.[54] Pleuritic chest pain and dyspnea may also occur in one third of patients. Gastrointestinal symptoms are a frequent accompaniment of this infection and include painless, watery diarrhea which may occur in the first week of illness in about one half of patients, nausea and vomiting, and occasionally associated abdominal pain or tenderness.[55,56,58] After the first four days, most patients appear acutely ill with evidence of tachypnea, rhonchi, and rales found on physical examination in about 75% of cases.[56] Small pleural effusions, with signs of consolidation and pleural friction rubs, have been reported less frequently.[56,59]

CNS manifestations are among the most important and diverse of the extrapulmonary findings of Legionnaires' disease, and have been reported in about one third of patients, and in an even higher percentage of fatal cases of the disease.[55,56] Changes in mental status ranging from confusion, personality changes, disorientation, depression, and stupor to coma, are the most common findings reported and are generally believed to be out of proportion to the metabolic derangements which these patients experience.[60-62] Memory loss, visual and auditory hallucinations, and slurred speech have also been reported, but headache, usually severe and frontal in type, is probably the second most common neurologic finding.[60] Neck stiffness and seizures have been described occasionally, but focal neurologic involvement is thought to be uncommon. However, cases of hemiparesis, dysphasia, proximal muscle weakness, motor and sensory peripheral neuropathies, cranial nerve palsies, hypo- and hyperreflexia, Babinski's sign, and urinary incontinence have been noted in the literature several times.[60-64] Cerebellar ataxia and dysarthria, as well as nystagmus, photophobia, dizziness, vertigo, tremors, and papilledema have also been reported to occur in Legionnaires' disease.[60,65]

Although the laboratory findings in Legionnaires' disease are not specific for this illness, they may be helpful clues in pointing to the diagnosis. The WBC count is usually increased and often reveals a shift to the left of granulocytic precursors.[54,56] The ESR is usually increased and elevated levels of liver function tests as well as a slight increase in bilirubin seem to occur commonly. Both hyponatremia, possibly secondary to the syndrome of inappropriate antidiuretic hormone (SIADH), and hypophosphatemia have been noted to occur in about one half of patients. Elevations of serum creatinine phosphokinase and aldolase have also been noted infrequently. The sputum gram stain usually reveals few cells and no predominant organism, although Giménez staining of transtracheal or bronchoscopic washings may reveal gram-negative bacilli. Culture of *L pneumophila* can now be done on selective media with special technique, with growth occurring in about two to seven days, and the yield appears to be higher from transtracheal aspirates than from bronchoscopic lavage samples.[54] Several extrapulmonary sites have also grown *Legionella* in culture, including blood, kidney, liver, dialysis graft sites, and bowel abscess. Urinalysis frequently reveals hematuria and/or proteinuria, and hemoglobinuria and myoglobinuria have been reported with renal failure.[55] Evidence of an acute pulmonary infiltrate is found in almost all patients (91% in one study), and unilateral, unilobar, and lower lobe involvement are usually the more common findings. The most common radiographic pattern is that of rapid, asymmetrical progression from an interstitial infiltrate to alveolar infiltrate. Pleural effusions have also been found in from 18% to 50% of patients and may develop before the infiltrates.[54,55]

Despite the diversity and severity of neurologic findings associated with this illness, specific diagnostic procedures have not been particularly helpful. Examination of the CSF is frequently normal, but among those that have been abnormal (about 25% in one series), only a mild pleocytosis of neutrophils or monocytes have been found.[60,64] Brain scans and CT scans have infrequently revealed some nonspecific abnormalities, but the EEG has been found to be abnormal in about 40% of cases in which it was performed, and most commonly has shown diffuse slowing and dysrhythmias compatible with encephalopathy. Electromyography and nerve conduction velocities have been done in a group of patients and were abnormal in all of them, some of whom had asymptomatic neuropathies which disappeared with resolution of the illness.[60,61] Autopsies have generally revealed normal or nonspecific findings, but interestingly, two cases have been reported in which the typical *L pneumophila* bacillus was seen within the brain and cultured from the brain tissue itself.[60] However, *Legionella* has not yet been found on special staining or grown in culture from the CSF.

The ultimate diagnosis of Legionnaires' disease depends on the finding of a fourfold or greater rise in antibody titer (to at least 1:128), usually done by the indirect immunofluorescent method using paired serum samples obtained during the acute and convalescent phases.[54-56] However, this method of diagnosis may take several weeks to months, since the titer may take from 1 to 8 or 9 weeks to develop a fourfold rise. Sputum samples, lung tissue, or other tissues or fluids may be tested for the bacteria by use of the direct fluorescent antibody examination and may yield results within a few hours. This test for sputum has been found to be very sensitive, but only moderately specific for *L pneumophila*.[54,55] Two newer tests appear promising for clinical use in the detection of Legionnaires' disease. Both of these utilize urine to check for soluble antigens, one by radioimmunoassay and the second by enzyme-linked immunosorbent assay (ELISA), giving similar results to those done by radioimmunoassay.

Therapy for Legionnaires' disease includes various types of supportive measures for some of the severe complications which tend to occur. These may include artificial ventilation for respiratory failure and development of the adult respiratory distress syndrome (ARDS), dialysis for renal failure, and appropriate treatment for any superimposed bacterial or viral infection that may occur. Specific treatment includes erythromycin 4 g/day given IV in four divided doses for 2−4 weeks; as this is considered the drug of choice at the present time. In the severely ill patient, rifampin given orally in a dose of 1200 mg/day in two divided doses may be added to the regimen. Alternately, doxycycline may be given IV in an initial dose of 200 mg followed in 12 hours by 100 mg and then 100 mg every 12 hours thereafter. Again, in the severely ill patient, rifampin may be used in combination with doxycycline. With the appropriate therapy, most patients will feel better within a few days, along with resolution of fever, but clearing of infiltrates on chest roentgenograms may be slow, and may take from a few weeks to a few months to return to normal. Patients with severe neurologic symptoms may suffer some residual impairment, such as peripheral neuropathy, memory deficits, weakness, and signs of cerebellar dysfunction.[60,63–65] Since only two patients have had documented invasion of the CNS by *Legionella*, the cause of these neurologic manifestations remains unclear, and it has been suggested that toxins or some immunologic reactions may be responsible.[60,64]

Further studies must be done before the full explanation of these extrapulmonary manifestations becomes known, and thus no other specific therapy is recommended at this time. The overall case fatality rate is about 20%, and increases dramatically to about 80% in immunosuppressed patients who have not been treated. Thus the prognosis appears to be affected primarily by the use of appropriate antibiotic therapy as well as the presence of an underlying illness and increased age.[54–56]

REFERENCES

1. Altman R, Goldfield M: The 1964 outbreak of St Louis encephalitis in the Delaware Valley: I Description of outbreak. *Am J Epidemiol* 1968;87:457–469.
2. Powell KE, Blakey DL: St Louis encephalitis: The 1975 epidemic in Mississippi. *JAMA* 1977;237:2294–2298.
3. Southern PM Jr, Smith JW, Luby JP, et al: Clinical and laboratory features of epidemic St Louis encephalitis. *Ann Intern Med* 1969;71:681–689.
4. Hughes E, Lauerman L, Birch WE, et al: Arboviral infections of the central nervous system — United States, 1985. *MMWR* 1986;35:341–350.
5. Nelson DB, Kappus KD, Janowski HT, et al: St. Louis encephalitis — Florida 1977, patterns of a widespread out-break. *Am J Trop Med Hyg* 1983;32:412–416.
6. Brady MT, May R: Premortem isolation of Saint Louis encephalitis virus: case report and implications for hospital and laboratory personnel. *Pediatr Infect Dis* 1985;4:548–550.
7. White MG, Carter NW, Rector FC, et al: Pathophysiology of epidemic St Louis encephalitis. I. Inappropriate secretion of antidiuretic hormone. *Ann Intern Med* 1969;71:691–702.
8. Suzuki M, Phillips CA: St Louis encephalitis. *Arch Pathol* 1966;81:47–54.
9. McGowan JE Jr, Bryon JA, Gregg MB: Surveillance of arboviral encephalitis in the United States, 1955–1971. *Am J Epidemiol* 1973;97: 199–207.
10. Finley KH, Riggs N: Convalescence and sequelae, in Monath TP (ed): *St Louis Encephalitis*. Washington, American Public Health Association, 1980.
11. Miller JR, Horter DH: Acute viral encephalitis. *Med Clin North Am* 1972;56:1393–1398.
12. Harter DH, Petersdorf RG: Viral diseases of the central nervous system: Aseptic meningitis and encephalitis, in Braunwald E, Isselbacher K, Petersdorf RG (eds): *Harrison's Principles of Internal Medicine* ed 11. New York, McGraw-Hill Book Co, 1987, 1987–1995.
13. Corey L, Spear PG: Infections with herpes-simplex viruses (pt 2). *N Engl J Med* 1986;314:749–757.
14. Whitley RJ, Soong SJ, Linnemann C Jr, et al: Herpes simplex encephalitis. Clinical assessment. *JAMA* 1982;247:317–320.

15. Williams BB, Lerner AM: Some previously unrecognized features of herpes simplex virus encephalitis. *Neurology* 1978;28:1193–1196.
16. Whitley RJ, Soong SJ, Hirsch MS, et al: Herpes simplex encephalitis. Vidarabine therapy and diagnostic problems. *N Engl J Med* 1981;304:313–318.
17. Whitley RJ, Soong SJ, Dolin R, et al: Adenine arabinoside therapy of biopsy-proved herpes simplex encephalitis. *N Engl J Med* 1977;297:289–294.
18. Whitley RJ, Alford CA, Hirsch MS, et al: Vidarabine versus acyclovir therapy in herpes simplex encephalitis. *N Engl J Med* 1986;314:144–149.
19. Sköldenberg B, Forsgren M, Alestig K, et al: Acyclovir versus vidarabine in herpes simplex encephalitis. *Scand J Infect Dis* 1985;547:89–96.
20. Miller JK, Hesser F, Tompkins VN: Herpes simplex encephalitis. Report of 20 cases. *Ann Intern Med* 1966;64:92–103.
21. Koskiniemi M, Vaheri A, Taskinen E: Cerebrospinal fluid alterations in herpes simplex virus encephalitis. *Rev Infect Dis* 1984;6:608–618.
22. Legaspi RC, Gatmaitan B, Bailey EJ, et al: Interferon in biopsy and autopsy specimens of brain. *Arch Neurol* 1980;37:76–79.
23. Hayashi K, Yanagi K, Takagi S: Detection of herpes simplex virus type I — IgM immune complexes in the brain of a patient with prolonged herpes encephalitis. *J Infect Dis* 1986;153:56–63.
24. Nahmias AJ, Whitley RJ, Visintine AN, et al: Herpes simplex virus encephalitis: Laboratory evaluations and their diagnostic significance. *J Infect Dis* 1982;145:829–836.
25. Upton A, Gumpert S: Electroencephalography in the diagnosis of herpes simplex encephalitis. *Lancet* 1970;1:650–652.
26. Davis LE, Johnson RT: An explanation for the localization of herpes simplex encephalitis? *Ann Neurol* 1979;5:2–5.
27. Leider W, Magoffin RL, Lennette EH, et al: Herpes simplex encephalitis and its possible association with reactivated latent infection. *N Engl J Med* 1965;273:341–349.
28. McKendall RR: Pharmacology of antiviral chemotherapeutic agents useful in human viral infections of the nervous system. *Clin Neurol Pharmacol* 1982;5:115–129.
29. Shope TC, Kauffman RE, Bowman D, et al: Pharmaco-kinetics of vidarabine in the treatment of infants and children with infections due to herpesviruses. *J Infect Dis* 1983;148:721–725.
30. Sköldenberg B, Alustig K, Burman L, et al: Acyclovir versus vidarabine in herpes simplex encephalitis. Randomized multicenter study in consecutive Swedish patients. *Lancet* 1984;2:707–711.
31. Ross AH, Julia A, Balakrishnan C: Toxicity of adenine arabinoside in humans. *J Infect Dis* 1976;133:192–198.
32. Sachs SL, Smith JL, Pollard RB, et al: Toxicity of vidarabine *JAMA* 1979;241:28–29.
33. Whitley RJ, NIAID Collaborative Antiviral Study Group: Interim summary of mortality in herpes simplex encephalitis and neonatal herpes simplex virus infections: vidarabine versus acyclovir. *J Antimicrob Chemother* 1983;12:105–112.
34. Murray HW, Masur H, Senterfit LB, et al: The protean manifestations of mycoplasma pneumonia infection in adults. *Am J Med* 1975;58:229–242.
35. Cassell GH, Cole BC: Mycoplasmas as agents of human disease. *N Engl J Med* 1981;304:80–89.

36. Ali NJ, Sillis M, Andrews BE, et al: The clinical spectrum and diagnosis of *Mycoplasma pneumoniae* infection. *Q J Med* 1986;58:241–251.
37. Ponko A: The occurrence and clinical picture of serologically verified *Mycoplasma pneumoniae* infections with emphasis on central nervous system cardiac and joint manifestations. *Ann Clin Res* 1979;11:1–60.
38. Izumikawa K, Hara K: Clinical features of *Mycoplasma pneumoniae* in adults. *Yale J Biol Med* 1983;56:505–510.
39. Lind K: Manifestations and complications of *Mycoplasma pneumoniae* disease: a review. *Yale J Biol Med* 1983;56:461–468.
40. Ogata S, Kitamoto O: Clinical complications of *Mycoplasma pneumoniae* disease — central nervous system. *Yale J Biol Med* 1983;56:481–486.
41. Linz DH, Tolle SW, Elliot DL: *Mycoplasma pneumoniae* pneumonia—experience at a referral center. *West J Med* 1984;140:895–900.
42. Cotton EM, Strampfer MJ, Cunha BA: Legionella and mycoplasma pneumonia — a community hospital experience. *Clin Chest Med* 1987;8: 441–453.
43. Sterner G, Biberfeld G: Central nervous system complications of *Mycoplasma pneumoniae* infection. *Scand J Infect Dis* 1969;1:203–208.
44. Hodges GR, Fass RS, Saslow S: Central nervous system disease associated with *Mycoplasma pneumoniae* infection. *Arch Intern Med* 1972;130:277–282.
45. McCarthy BE: Encephalitis associated with pneumonia due to *Mycoplasma pneumoniae*. *Ir Med J* 1983;76:459–460.
46. Fisher RS, Clark AW, Wolinsky JS, et al: Postinfectious leukoencephalitis complicating *Mycoplasma pneumoniae* infection. *Arch Neurol* 1983;40:109–113.
47. Plotkin GR, Slovak JP Jr, Lenz PE: Case report: *Mycoplasma* pneumonia presenting as meningoencephalitis and hemolytic anemia. *Am J Med Sci* 1979;278:235–242.
48. Wright RA, Hill MR: Pneumonia and meningoencephalitis in a female adolescent. Case report. *Mo Med* 1984;81:660–661,666.
49. Klimek JJ, Russman BS, Quintiliani R: *Mycoplasma pneumoniae* meningoencephalitis and transverse myelitis in association with low cerebrospinal fluid glucose. *Pediatrics* 1976;58:133–135.
50. Kashara I, Otsubo Y, Yanase T, et al: Isolation and characterization of *Mycoplasma pneumoniae* from cerebrospinal fluid of a patient with pneumonia and meningoencephalitis. *J Infect Dis* 1986;58:241–251.
51. Bayer AS, Galpin JE, Theofilopoulos AN, et al: Neurologic disease associated with *Mycoplasma pneumoniae* pneumonitis. *Ann Intern Med* 1981;94:15–20.
52. Fernald GW: Immunologic mechanisms suggested in the association of *M pneumoniae* infection and extrapulmonary disease: a review. *Yale J Biol Med* 1983;56:475–479.
53. Fraser DW, Tsai TR, Orenstein W, et al: Legionnaires' disease. Description of an epidemic of pneumonia. *N Engl J Med* 1977;297:1189–1197.
54. Edelstein PH, Meyer RD: Legionnaires' disease. A review. *Chest* 1984;85:114–120.
55. Meyer RD: *Legionella* infections. A review of five years of research. *Rev Infect Dis* 1983;5:258–278.
56. Helms CM, Viner JP, Weisenburger DD, et al: Sporadic Legionnaires' disease: clinical observations of 87 nosocomial and community-acquired cases. *Am J Med Sci* 1984;288: 2–12.

57. Woo AH, Yu VL, Goetz A: Potential in-hospital modes of transmission of *Legionella pneumophila*. *Am J Med* 1986;80:567–573.
58. Cunha BA (ed): Legionnaires' Disease. *Semin Respir Infect* 1987;2:189–279.
59. Davis GS, Winn WC Jr, Beaty HN: Legionnaires' disease: infections caused by *Legionella pneumophila* and *Legionella*-like organisms. *Clin Chest Med* 1981;2:145–166.
60. Johnson JD, Raff MJ, Van Arsdell JA: Neurologic manifestations of Legionnaires' disease. *Medicine* 1984;63:303–310.
61. Weir AI, Bone I, Kennedy DH: Neurologic involvement in legionellosis. *J Neurol Neurosurg Psychiatry* 1982;45:603–608.
62. Kennedy DH, Bone I, Weir AI: Early diagnosis of Legionnaires' disease: Distinctive neurological findings. *Lancet* 1981;1:940–941.
63. Lees AW, Tyrell WF: Severe cerebral disturbance in Legionnaires' disease. *Lancet* 1978;2:1336–1337.
64. Harris LF: Legionnaires' disease associated with acute encephalomyelitis. *Arch Neurol* 1981;38:462–463.
65. Maskill MR, Jordan EC: Pronounced cerebellar features in Legionnaires' disease. *Br Med J* 1981;283:276.

6
Upper Respiratory Tract Infections in the Elderly

Constance A. Benson
Stuart Levin

Infections of the respiratory tract are among the most common infections in all age groups, including the elderly. Alterations in host defenses, both mechanical and immunologic, and age-dependent modifications of respiratory tract flora are included as proposed mechanisms for a noted increase in the susceptibility to respiratory tract pathogens.[1] Mechanical alterations in host defense of the upper respiratory tract with advancing age include a decrease in the efficiency of elimination of foreign particles by the nasopharyngeal and tracheobronchial tree. This may result from poor respiratory muscle tone, decreased cough reflexes, and impaired mucociliary transport.[1,2] Mucosal barrier defenses may be overcome by such senile changes as decreased cell surface fibronectin,[2] decreased salivary gland flow and volume, increased salivary protease concentration,[3] decreased tear volume and enzyme secretion,[4] and a decrease in local IgA production.[2] Local IgA assists in agglutination of bacteria, improving their mechanical removal and inhibiting their adherence to respiratory epithelial cells, thereby reducing local colonization.[2] A decrease in local IgA levels may interfere with this mechanism of defense.[2]

Such changes in mechanical and mucosal physiologic function may be responsible for subtle differences in oral and nasopharyngeal microbial flora in the aged. Valenti et al report an increase in oropharyngeal colonization with gram-negative bacilli in patients over age 65 years and correlate this rise with the patient's decreasing level of independent functioning.[5] Healthy elderly patients were colonized at a prevalence rate of 6% to 9%, rising to 22% in patients in a skilled care facility, and to 40% to 60% in an acute care hospital setting.[5] Decreases in local IgA, cell surface fibronectin, and protease content of saliva coupled with altered mucosal characteristics may facilitate acquisition of environmental organisms by modifying adherence properties of gram-negative bacilli.

Although significant changes in mechanical and mucosal barriers are apparently age-dependent, most investigations have focused attention on abnormalities of the senescent immune system. Most authors agree that cell-mediated immunity is most profoundly affected by aging. Documented changes include increased anergy to common skin test antigens,[6,7] decreased mitogen-responsive T cell populations with decreased clonal proliferation in vitro,[8,9] increased T suppressor cell activity, and decreased production of interleukin-2 (IL-2) or T cell growth factor.[10] Alterations in humoral immunity have been less well documented and might seemingly result from decreased T helper cell function.[11] Possible abnormalities may also relate to intrinsic B cell dysfunction and include a depressed primary response to new antigens,[12] decreased lymphocyte production of immunoglobulins on exposure to pokeweed mitogen in vitro, and increased IgG and IgA levels and decreased IgM levels with age.[13,14] A small subset of the elderly in one study had increased IgG levels, which were associated with an increased mortality compared with controls.[14] There is general agreement that polymorphonuclear leukocyte and monocyte function are not significantly affected by aging, although depressed phagocytosis in vitro due to alterations in oxidative metabolism and abnormal phagocytosis in hospitalized elderly patients have been reported.[15,16]

Although a specific causal relationship between senescent changes in mechanical and immunologic host defenses and increased susceptibility to respiratory pathogens is difficult to demonstrate, these alterations are likely to be significant factors in the development of upper respiratory tract infection.

COMMON CERVICOFACIAL INFECTIONS

Acute Bacterial Parotitis

Acute bacterial parotitis primarily affects the elderly, debilitated, or postoperative patient. The most common infecting organism is reported to be *Staphylococcus aureus*.[17,18] A number of case reports include oral anaerobes such as *Bacteroides, Fusobacterium, Peptostreptococcus*, and *Eikenella* as possible etiologic agents.[17,19] In addition, colonization of the aged, particularly hospitalized elderly patients, with aerobic gram-negative bacilli requires their consideration as etiologic agents.[5] Clinically, patients report the sudden onset of brawny, painful, erythematous swelling of the parotid gland and pre- and postauricular areas with loss of the angle of the mandible, followed by fever, chills, and systemic toxicity. If untreated, swelling may progress involving other structures of the neck.

Treatment will require combined surgical decompression, drainage, and appropriate antibiotic coverage. An antistaphylococcal agent combined with agents active against oral anaerobes and gram-negative bacilli should be used. Choices may include clindamycin combined with a third generation cephalosporin or aminoglycoside or combination agents such as ticarcillin-clavulanic acid or ampicillin-sulbactam.

Sialoadenitis

Infection of the salivary gland tissue may be more common in the elderly due to age-dependent decreases in salivary flow, increases in salivary viscosity, and the prevalence of sialolithiasis, all of which may lead to ductal obstruction and subsequent suppuration.[3,20] Infection occurs more commonly in the submandibular gland due to the smaller caliber of Wharton's duct and its greater propensity for obstructive sialolithiasis.[20] (Etiologic microorganisms will reflect the oral microbial flora, as outlined in Table 6-1.) Symptoms are those of the initial obstruction with pain on salivation during meals, followed by the onset of swelling, localized erythema, tenderness, and fever. Therapy requires alleviation of the obstruction and drainage of necrotic material combined with appropriate antibiotic coverage, discussed in detail in a later section of this chapter.

**Table 6-1
Predominant Oral Microbial Flora in Adults**

Anaerobic	
Gram-positive cocci	*Peptostreptococcus*
Gram-negative cocci	*Veillonella*
Gram-positive bacilli	*Actinomyces*
	Eubacterium
	Lactobacillus
	Leptotrichia
Gram-negative bacilli	*Fusobacterium*
	Bacteroides
	Campylobacter
Spirochetes	*Treponema*
Facultative and aerobic	
Gram-positive cocci	*Streptococcus (S mutans, S sanguis, S mitior, S salivarius)*
Gram-negative cocci	*Branhamella*
Gram-positive bacilli	*Lactobacillus*
	Corynebacterium
Gram-negative bacilli	*Enterobacteriaciae*

Reproduced with permission from Chow et al.[21]

HERPES ZOSTER

Herpes zoster arising from reactivation of varicella zoster virus latent in dorsal root ganglia occurs most commonly in the elderly with a peak occurrence in the fifth to seventh decades.[22] The disease is found at a rate of ten cases per 1000 patients after age 70.[22] The trigeminal and cervical dermatomes are affected in 16% and 8%, respectively.[23] The ophthalmic branch of the fifth cranial nerve may be the most often affected of the facial and cervical dermatomes. Eye involvement occurs in 50% of those with ophthalmic branch disease, heralded by dermatomal involvement of the tip of the nose.[23] Although 90% of elderly subjects in one study had humoral antibodies to varicella zoster, only 64% had a measurable varicella zoster-specific immune response, which may provide a partial explanation for the increase in the incidence of this disease in the aged.[24] Clinically, the disease is characterized by a four- to five-day prodrome of malaise, fever, headache and lancinating pain, burning, or dysesthesia in a dermatomal distribution. The prodrome is followed by a papular eruption on an erythematous base which rapidly becomes, in order, vesicular, pustular, crusted, and then scabbed, over a five- to seven-day period. The rash occurs in a distinct dermatomal distribution that respects the mid-line. Dissemination of infection, while usually associated with immunosuppression of the host, may occur in up to 15% of otherwise healthy elderly patients.[25] Complications include ophthalmologic infection such as keratouveitis, iridocyclitis or scleritis, encephalitis, cerebral angiitis with contralateral hemiparesis, and postherpetic neuralgia.[22,26-28] Postherpetic neuralgia is the most common sequela, affecting 25% to 30% of infected elderly patients.[23,26]

Treatment is dependent on the dermatome involved and on underlying host factors. Because of the relatively high rate of dissemination and the significant morbidity associated with ophthalmologic infections or CNS involvement, systemic treatment may be considered in this population. In one study, intravenous (IV) acyclovir infused in a dose of 500 mg/m^2 3 times daily for seven days resulted in more rapid healing, fewer days of pain, shorter duration of viral shedding, and reduction of progression or development of cutaneous and visceral dissemination than placebo control.[29] There did not appear to be a significant difference between acyclovir and vidarabine in this study.[29] Intravenous acyclovir alone was not sufficient to treat coexistent ocular involvement and, in one study, had no effect on two patients with delayed contralateral hemiparesis due to herpes zoster associated with cerebral angiitis.[28,30,31] Topical acyclovir in the treatment of herpes zoster keratouveitis decreased the required duration of therapy, accelerated resolution of corneal disease, and decreased recurrence rates after discontinuation of therapy as compared to standard topical steroid therapy.[30]

Systemic short-course steroid therapy has been advocated by some for use in the immunocompetent patient for prevention of postherpetic neuralgia.[22,23] The utility of acyclovir or vidarabine in prevention of this complication has not yet been fully established. Acyclovir is associated with fewer side effects than vidarabine and should be the preferred antiviral agent when treatment is necessary. Vidarabine requires IV administration while acyclovir is available in an oral and an IV form. Oral acyclovir should be administered in doses of 600-800 mg five times daily for therapeutic effect in treating varicella-zoster virus infections. Given the available data, however, elderly patients may benefit significantly from antiviral therapy. Treatment is advocated for those who are immunosuppressed or at greater risk of dissemination or significant postherpetic morbidity.

ERYSIPELAS

Erysipelas is a bacterial facial lymphangitis usually caused by ß-hemolytic streptococcal infection, although staphylococcal organisms may cause the syndrome in approximately 10% of cases.[32,33] It occurs most frequently in the elderly. The microorganisms may invade through an infected wound, local trauma, or by contiguous extension from another site. Often the original site of infection is obscure. Clinically, the patient presents with warm, tender, indurated, erythematous swelling of facial skin. The border of the rash is sharply demarcated with scalloped edges which are pink to deep red in color. Systemic symptoms include fever as high as 104° to 105°F, headache, nausea, and vomiting. Approximately 25% of patients may be bacteremic. Treatment with parenteral penicillin usually results in rapid improvement. Antistaphylococcal agents may be added initially until culture data are available. In a small percentage of patients, erysipelas will recur, usually at the same site.

UNCOMMON CERVICOFACIAL INFECTIONS

Suppurative Thyroiditis

Thyroid gland infection is rare, possibly owing to the substantial blood supply of the gland and the presence of high concentrations of iodine-containing compounds within the gland which may have an antibacterial effect.[34] Infection rarely occurs by hematogenous spread but may occur slightly more often by direct extension from contiguous structures. The single most important determinant appears to be pre-existent thyroid disease, which is present in 61% of those with suppurative thyroiditis.[34] The age at onset ranges from 4 months to 80 years with a mean age of 32.8 years. Twenty percent of cases occur in patients over age

65.[34] Clinically, patients present with fever, chills, anterior neck pain, hoarseness, dysphagia, and a warm, erythematous, tender, fluctuance over the involved lobe of the thyroid. Sixty-nine percent of cases will have concurrent pharyngitis or pharyngeal pain.[34] Leukocytosis and a "cold" area on a thyroid scan may be noted. Of the 224 cases reviewed in a recent study, 159 were bacterial with streptococci and staphylococci causing 42% and 35% of cases respectively.[33] Gram-negative bacilli, anaerobes, and syphilitic infections accounted for the remainder.[34] There were 33 fungal, 21 mycobacterial, 11 parasitic, and two actinomycotic infections reported. Treatment with the appropriate antimicrobial agent and surgical drainage of abscesses were successful in the majority; however, the mortality rates ranged from 8.6% to 25% depending on which study was reviewed.[34] Death was generally the result of tracheal obstruction or perforation, abscess rupture, metastatic infection, or sepsis.

Cervicofacial Actinomycosis

Cervicofacial actinomycosis most commonly arises from an odontogenic source. It may also arise from soft tissue trauma and may present insidiously, becoming clinically overt at a time distant from the original insult. Infections are generally reported in younger age groups, the majority occurring between ages 30 and 60 years, but because of the increased incidence of dental caries and periodontal disease in the aged,[35] it must be considered as a possible cause of cervicofacial infections in this population as well. Infection is caused most often by *Actinomyces israelii*, a common oral organism.[36] It is an anaerobic, branching, filamentous gram-positive organism, not usually pathogenic, which may invade and cause disease under conditions of pre-existent infection, lowered host resistance, or reduced tissue oxygen tension.

Clinically, the disease may present with one of two distinct patterns: (1) a painless, enlarging, fluctuant mass at the border of the mandible, and (2) a more acute, pyogenic submandibular or cervical cellulitis with abscess formation. Cutaneous fistulas or sinus tracts may occur although intraoral drainage is more common. Cases have been reported involving the palate, tongue, larynx, trachea, salivary glands, maxilla, and paranasal sinuses.[36,37] There may be actinomycotic involvement of bone as well. The diagnosis is based on culture of the organism or demonstration of sulfur granules or masses of gram-positive filamentous organisms in tissue specimens. Treatment requires a combination of surgical drainage, excision of sinus tracts, and prolonged, high-dose penicillin. Initial therapy IV with penicillin G in a dose of 10 to 20 million units per day for 4 to 6 weeks may be followed by oral penicillin 2 – 4 g/day for 6 to 12 months.[36] Alternative drugs which have proved useful include tetracycline, erythromycin, and clindamycin.

Haemophilus Influenzae Cellulitis

This disease is primarily one of children aged 6 months to 3 years; however, the recognition of *Haemophilus* organisms as significant pathogens in adults in recent years has led to increasing case reports of this disease in older patients, including those over age 65.[38,39] The infection presents typically as a diffuse unilateral facial cellulitis which is indurated, tender, and has a distinctive purplish hue. It may occur concomitant with or following a febrile upper respiratory tract infection and in adults has been reported in association with epiglottitis.[37] A similar syndrome has also been reported due to *Streptococcus pneumoniae*.[40-42] Treatment recommendations usually include ampicillin and chloramphenicol or a third-generation cephalosporin until antibiotic sensitivities are known.

THE COMMON COLD AND INFLUENZA SYNDROME

Investigations of the common cold specific to the geriatric age group are lacking. Information available from general reviews suggests that the annual rate of upper respiratory illness decreases with advancing age.[43] However, while the annual rate may decrease, the potential morbidity associated with upper respiratory illnesses, particularly in the form of pneumonia and its sequelae, rises in elderly populations either due to age-related disease of the cardiorespiratory system or immunologic changes as discussed. Control of the common cold may be of greater significance, therefore, to this population.

Etiology

Etiologic microorganisms remain the same in the elderly as in other adults; however, the host response may differ from that of the younger adult. Rhinoviruses are responsible for the largest percentage of colds in adults — approximately 30% in most studies.[44] Coronavirus, parainfluenza viruses, adenoviruses, respiratory syncytial virus, and influenza viruses may account for from 5% to 15% of colds in adults.[43-45] A number of other viruses have been implicated as causative agents in isolated cases and include the enteroviruses, rubella, rubeola, varicella, and Epstein-Barr viruses.[43-45]

Epidemiology

Adults in general suffer from 2.0 to 2.5 upper respiratory illnesses per patient per year in temperate climates.[43] Rates may rise during peak seasons to four to six illnesses per year. Institutionalized or debilitated elderly patients appear to be at increased risk for infection with influenza viruses and respiratory syncytial viruses. Institutional outbreaks with increased morbidity and mortality due to secondary pneumonia have been reported for both.[46,47]

Although precise mechanisms of transmission have not been delineated for all implicated viruses, rhinoviruses have been reported to spread most efficiently by direct contact and self-inoculation.[44,48,49] Other investigators have suggested that adenovirus and influenza virus may be better transmitted via aerosolized droplets.[50]

Clinical Syndromes

Symptoms due to the common cold and influenza have been well described elsewhere.[45] The particular danger of such infections in the elderly is the resultant modification of host defense mechanisms that may allow involvement of the lower respiratory tract or allow secondary bacterial invasion. Lower respiratory tract complications occur in approximately 10% of patients, primarily in those over age 65.[45] Influenza viruses have been demonstrated to impair neutrophil chemotaxis, chemiluminescence, and bacterial killing after intranasal inoculation of volunteers with influenza virus and pneumococci.[51] Other studies have shown depression of systemic macrophage function, depression of numbers of circulating T cells, impairment of delayed cutaneous hypersensitivity, and impairment of mucociliary clearance mechanisms.[51] Similar impairment of mucociliary clearance has been noted with respiratory syncytial virus infection.[44,52] Such alterations may compound preexisting age-dependent abnormalities of these systems. Such changes may contribute to secondary bacterial colonization and invasion of lower respiratory tract structures.

Prevention and Treatment

Inactivated influenza virus vaccine parenterally administered is available to the general public for prophylaxis against influenza A and B. Reported efficacy rates for the vaccine range from 67% to 92%.[53] The frequent antigenic shift of hemagglutinin and neuraminidase components of influenza A viruses occurs more commonly than with influenza B and generally requires modification in composition and readministration of the vaccine yearly. Recommendations for administration of the vaccine include the elderly in chronic care facilities in the highest priority followed by those over age 65 who have underlying chronic illnesses such as diabetes or cardiopulmonary disease.[54] Immunization of all healthy individuals over age 65 is recommended but on a lower priority basis.

Adenovirus vaccines containing serotype 4, 7, and 21 for prophylactic use are currently available only for military recruits and are not suggested for the geriatric population.[45]

Environmental control measures with frequent handwashing, environmental decontamination, and avoidance of contact combined with supportive measures in the form of salicylates for fever, nasal phenylephrine or oxymetazoline hydrochloride for decongestion, dextromethorphan containing cough syrup, bed rest, and fluids may be of most practical benefit in prevention of spread and in treatment of viral upper respiratory illness.

The use of interferon-α_2 for control of rhinovirus infection is currently under investigation. Its most practical use may be for administration in a family or institutional setting during peak seasons or once an index case has been identified within a given population.[55]

The only available therapeutic agent for treatment of viral upper respiratory infection at present is amantadine hydrochloride, which has been shown to reduce the duration of influenza virus illness by approximately 50%.[56] Recommended dosing begins with 200 mg initially followed by 100 mg bid for three to five days in patients at high risk with symptoms suggestive of an influenzalike illness. A new congener with fewer side effects, rimantidine, may be of equal efficacy but is not yet available.[57] Unfortunately, the elderly have a higher drug-induced neurologic complication rate, primarily ataxia,[56] which may limit the usefulness of these drugs.

PHARYNGITIS

Inflammation of the pharynx is a common illness for which more than 40 million patients seek medical attention in the United States each year.[58] Viruses remain the most common etiologic agents causing pharyngitis in the elderly.[59] Influenza and rhinovirus are most often implicated. Group A ß-hemolytic streptococci may account for only 5% to 10% of pharyngeal infections in patients over age 40.[58,60] Rare causes of pharyngitis in the general population such as diphtheria may be seen with slightly greater frequency in the elderly due to altered immune mechanisms or waning specific immunity with advancing age.[61-63] The importance of diagnosis of pharyngitis and its etiology lies in the recognition of treatable diseases and the prevention of significant sequelae. Discussion will range from those infections likely to be seen with greater frequency to those of lesser frequency occurring in the geriatric population.

Etiology, Clinical Presentation, and Diagnosis

Viral pharyngitis The majority of viral-induced pharyngeal infections in the elderly occur in association with the common cold or influenza syndromes. Viruses associated with pharyngeal inflammation as part of their symptom complex include rhinoviruses, coronaviruses, adenoviruses, parainfluenza viruses, enteroviruses, Epstein-Barr virus, cytomegaloviruses, and influenza A and B viruses.[43-45] Pharyngitis associated with the common cold is generally mild. Rhinorrhea and nasal congestion with cough, malaise, or other mild systemic symptoms generally accompany the sore throat. Physical findings are usually limited to nasal and pharyngeal mucosal edema and hyperemia, without exudation or lymphadenopathy. Pharyngitis associated with influenza is accompanied by headache, malaise, fever, severe myalgias, and cough, which may last five to seven days or longer. The pharynx may appear hyperemic and injected but exudates and adenopathy again are rare. In the elderly, the systemic complaints may overshadow the pharyngeal discomfort.

Infectious mononucleosis The mononucleosis syndrome due to Epstein-Barr virus (EBV) infection may occur in the elderly as a primary event in an incidence of from 0.76% to 2.2%.[64] The disease appears to differ in older patients with prominent symptoms being more protracted fever, more marked hepatobiliary disease, and less peripheral adenopathy than that associated with disease in young adults.[64] Pharyngitis may be a prominent feature in only 55% of patients.[64] Examination of the pharynx may be unremarkable or may reveal exudation and erythema. Diagnosis is based on clinical presentation; however, the disease may be more difficult to recognize in the aged because of its atypical presentation.[65,66] Serologic evaluation with measurement of EB viral capsid antigen, IgG and IgM, and EBV early antigen will confirm the diagnosis. The appearance of heterophil antibody may be delayed in the elderly.[64] Cytomegalovirus (CMV) may cause a similar syndrome, although the incidence of primary or reactivation infection in the elderly is unknown.

Streptococcal pharyngitis Acute streptococcal pharyngitis is less common in the elderly than in younger age groups. Group A ß-hemolytic streptococci may be isolated in as few as 5% to 9% of patients over age 40 who present with pharyngitis.[60,61] The classic presentation has been well described previously.[67] As is true in younger populations, symptoms and signs in the elderly may be indistinguishable from those of the viral pharyngitides. The diagnosis is established by throat culture.

Diphtheria Surveys of elderly populations have reported that from 44% to 48% of those over age 60 may have unprotective levels of diphtheria antitoxin[62,63] and, in at least one study, 17.3% of reported diphtheria cases over a 10-year period occurred in patients over age 50.[62] The incidence of the disease has decreased significantly over past decades although the case fatality ratio remains as high as 10%.[68] Disease associated with *Corynebacterium diphtheriae* may begin insidiously, with the average duration of symptoms prior to hospitalization being 7.2 days.[69] Sore throat is the chief complaint in approximately 70% of patients with fever and dysphagia each noted in 50% of patients.[69] Cough, hoarseness, chills, and rhinorrhea may occur in approximately 25% of patients. In a study of 44 reported cases from the University of Washington, only 54.8% had an obvious diphtheritic membrane,[69] characteristically grayish and firmly adherent to the tonsil and pharyngeal mucosa. Neuropathic sequelae developed in 9.5% of this population. Five deaths occurred, three of which were in patients older than age 65. Older age at onset, the presence of a diphtheritic membrane, especially involving the larynx, and the presence of dyspnea at onset were associated with a poorer prognosis.[69] The presence of a rapidly evolving pharyngeal or tonsilar exudate (hour by hour) or laryngeal stridor with pharyngeal exudate are as important and specific signs of diphtheria as the classic extensive pharyngeal membrane. Other corynebacteria associated with a membranous pharyngitis that mimic diphtheria include *C hemolyticum* and *C ulcerans*.[70-72] Diagnosis rests on clinical presentation and culture or demonstration of the organism in tissue.

Complications of Pharyngitis

Probably the most common suppurative complication of acute pharyngitis in the elderly is peritonsillar abscess characterized by severe odynophagia, dysphagia, and low-grade fever, with medial displacement of the tonsil on the involved side. Bilateral disease may cause respiratory embarrassment. Unchecked infection may extend to the deep pharyngeal and fascial spaces with their attendant complications, discussed in detail elsewhere in this chapter. Other less common suppurative complications include otitis media, mastoiditis, and jugular vein septic thrombophlebitis with metastatic infection, a syndrome associated with *Fusobacterium necrophorum*.[73] Acute rheumatic fever and poststreptococcal glomerulonephritis are thought to be immunologic complications of group A ß-hemolytic streptococcal infection, and are rare in geriatric patients.

Treatment

Viral pharyngitis requires only symptomatic treatment with rest, fluids, and aspirin or other analgesics. Influenza A may be alleviated to a considerable degree with early amantadine therapy, as previously discussed. Active immunization is available for influenza A and B and is recommended for those over age 65, especially those who are institutionalized or have chronic underlying illnesses.

Streptococcal pharyngitis should be treated with either a single 1.2-million unit injection of benzathine penicillin or a ten-day course of penicillin V 250 mg every six hours. Erythromycin may replace penicillin in those who are allergic to it. Treatment within 1 week of onset of illness will prevent acute rheumatic fever.

The treatment of diphtheria requires administration of antitoxin, available only in horse serum, and appropriate antibiotic therapy to eradicate nasopharyngeal carriage. Useful antibiotics include penicillin, erythromycin, clindamycin, tetracycline, and rifampin. A ten-day to 2-week course may be necessary for eradication from the nasopharynx.[69]

LARYNGITIS AND EPIGLOTTITIS

Laryngitis is an acute inflammation of the larynx associated with hoarseness and dysphonia. Epiglottitis is a rapidly progressive infection of the larynx localized to the epiglottis and adjacent structures. While previously thought to be an uncommon, benign disease in adults, increasing reports indicate that epiglottitis is neither as rare nor as benign as thought. The actual incidence of these infections in patients over age 65 is unknown; however, several patients in this age group are included in most reviews.[38,39,42,74-77]

Etiology

Acute laryngitis generally occurs in association with a viral upper respiratory illness. Causative viruses may include rhinoviruses, adenoviruses, parainfluenza viruses, influenza A and B, coronavirus and respiratory syncytial virus.[43,45] Bacterial laryngitis appears to be less common as a primary illness but may result from secondary bacterial invasion following a viral laryngitis. Implicated bacterial agents include *Branhamella catarrhalis*, *Streptococcus pneumoniae*, and group A ß-hemolytic streptococci.[78] Granulomatous laryngitis may result from tuberculosis, histoplasmosis, actinomycosis, syphilis, *Klebsiella rhinoscleromatis*, and *Mycobacterium leprae* infections.[79] Of these, the mycobacteria and *Klebsiella rhinoscleromatis* may be seen more commonly in an aging population. *Candida* laryngitis has been reported in elderly immunocompromised hosts.[80]

Acute epiglottitis is most often a bacterial infection. *Haemophilus influenzae* type B remains the most common etiologic organism in adults; however, infections have been reported due to a number of other bacteria as well, including *Streptococcus pneumoniae*, *Staphylococcus aureus*, *Streptococcus pyogenes*, *B catarrhalis*, *F necrophorum*, *Pasteurella multocida*, and *Kelbsiella pneumoniae*.[38-42,81-83] Epiglottitis due to *S pneumoniae* has been particularly associated with underlying malignancy in adults.[40,41] A single case of epiglottitis due to *Candida albicans* has been reported in an otherwise healthy 75-year-old woman.[83]

Clinical Presentations

Acute laryngitis presents with hoarseness and varying degrees of dysphonia, often with other symptoms of viral upper respiratory illness. Respiratory obstruction with viral laryngitis is rare. There are no clinical features which distinguish one etiology from another.

Granulomatous and other chronic laryngitides generally present as insidious diseases characterized by intermittent hoarseness, odynophagia, odynophonia, and variable symptoms of respiratory obstruction with or without fever.[78] Tuberculous laryngitis most often occurs in the setting of concomitant pulmonary tuberculosis.[84] Hyperemic mucosa with multinodular lesions progressing to epithelial ulceration resembling carcinoma may occur. Laryngeal tuberculosis has a predilection for the posterior surfaces of the vocal cords, arytenoid cartilages, and laryngeal surface of the epiglottis.[79,84] Disseminated histoplasmosis and blastomycosis may affect the larynx in from 15% to 30% of cases.[79] Clinically, they appear similar to tuberculous laryngitis with the exception that they more commonly affect the anterior surfaces of the larynx. Blastomycosis may also be associated with a thin grayish membrane covering the mucosa. Rhinoscleromatous laryngitis occurs in the course of progressive upper respiratory rhinoscleroma. The glottic and subglottic regions may be affected by large granulomatous masses or infiltration. Persistent hoarseness and insidious respiratory obstruction are primary laryngeal symptoms.[85,86] Lepromatous and syphilitic laryngeal diseases are rare and the systemic symptoms of the diseases generally overshadow laryngeal involvement.

Acute epiglottitis in the adult presents with symptoms similar to those which occur in children. It is characterized by the rapid progression of fever, dysphagia, odynophagia, and respiratory distress. Pharyngeal pain may occur out of proportion to the degree of abnormality noted on examination of the pharynx.[75] The duration of symptoms prior to seeking medical attention may range from eight to 72 hours, longer than is generally seen in children.[75] Symptoms are thought to be generally milder than in children; however, there are numerous reports of sudden respiratory obstruction and death in adults with acute epiglottitis.[74,76,77,81,87] One study reports a 50% mortality rate associated with adult epiglottitis.[81] The symptoms and signs do not differ significantly from one bacterial etiology to another.

Physical examination may reveal a toxic patient in mild to moderate respiratory distress. Inspiratory stridor may be heard. Fever may range from 100° to 103°F. Several cases of concomitant cervical cellulitis have been reported in elderly patients.[38,39,42] The throat may appear benign. The epiglottis, when visualized, is hyperemic, described as "fiery red," and swollen, often with pooled secretions in the valecula. *Candida* epiglottitis may have white patches extending across the epiglottis and aryepiglottic folds. Progressive edema of the epiglottic structures combined with reflex-induced laryngeal spasm and retained secretions are thought to be responsible for acute airway obstruction.[74] If adequately treated early, most patients recover without sequelae.

Diagnosis

The diagnosis of laryngitis rests on recognition of the clinical symptoms. Granulomatous laryngitis will require laryngeal biopsy for differentiation from laryngeal carcinoma. Demonstration of organisms in laryngeal tissue will confirm the diagnosis.

Acute therapy of the patient with epiglottitis may be necessary prior to establishing an etiology. The disease must be recognized by the clinical syndrome and treated empirically until culture data are available. Bacteremia occurs at a rate of 20% to 30% in adults, similar to that associated with pneumococcal pneumonia.[40-42] Combined culture of the epiglottis and bloodstream may yield an organism in only 40% to 60% of cases in adults, the remainder being culture-negative.[42]

Radiographic evaluation is useful in confirming the diagnosis of acute epiglottitis. Soft tissue neck radiographs should be taken in an upright position to avoid compromise of an endangered airway. Swelling of the epiglottis, aryepiglottic folds, arytenoids, and prevertebral soft tissue may be seen. As the epiglottis swells it forms a posteriorly facing C-shape with a central groove made by a pencil-thin column of air.[81,88]

The epiglottis may be visualized directly with the use of a tongue depressor applied as far posteriorly as the tonsillar pillar. Even in adults, however, this manipulation may accentuate laryngeal spasm and result in airway obstruction. It is recommended that radiographs and physical examination of the epiglottis be undertaken in the operating room or in the presence of facilities for and personnel capable of rapid intubation or tracheostomy.

Treatment

Supportive measures suffice in the therapy of routine laryngitis. Granulomatous laryngitis responds to appropriate antimicrobial therapy of the underlying organism. In addition to supportive care and airway management, epiglottitis requires specific antimicrobial therapy aimed at the commonly implicated organisms. Initial coverage should include agents active against *H influenzae* type B, *Streptococcus pneumoniae*, *Staphylococcus aureus*, and group A ß-hemolytic streptococci. Ampicillin and chloramphenicol, with or without a semisynthetic penicillin, are the traditional agents used; however, the third-generation cephalosporins should be the drugs of choice to cover all the possible pathogens once further clinical experience is obtained. When *H influenzae* type B is isolated, rifampin should be given prophylactically to household contacts and probably to the patient at discharge for eradication of carriage.[77]

SINUSITIS

Acute sinusitis is an infection of one or more of the paranasal sinuses, most often of bacterial origin, and often complicating a viral upper respiratory illness or odontogenic infection. Little has been written about sinusitis in an elderly population.

Etiology

A number of organisms have been implicated as causative agents in acute sinusitis. *Streptococcus pneumoniae* and untypeable *H influenzae* remain the most common isolates in acute community-acquired infection in the elderly.[89,90] The incidence of infection due to aerobic gram-negative bacilli and *Staphylococcus aureus* may rise with age as does the naso- and oropharyngeal colonization with these organisms, particularly in those aged patients who are debilitated or institutionalized.[5] *Branhamella catarrhalis* and oral anaerobes, alone or in mixed culture, may be implicated in a small number of acute sinus infections.[90,91] The etiology of nosocomial sinusitis is generally representative of environmental flora including *Pseudomonas, Klebsiella, Enterobacter, S aureus*, and *Escherichia coli*.[92,93] Though unproved, a number of unusual pathogens of the nasopharynx and paranasal sinuses may have a slightly greater predilection for the elderly, particularly in the presence of chronic underlying illnesses such as diabetes or of the waning cell-mediated immunity recognized with aging. These include *Klebsiella ozaenae, Klebsiella rhinoscleromatis*, and the Phycomycetes.[85,86,94–98]

Clinical Presentation and Diagnosis

The symptoms, signs, and radiologic abnormalities of acute community-acquired bacterial sinusitis have been well described elsewhere[99] and do not differ in the aged patient. *Klebsiella ozaenae* in the elderly or chronically debilitated patient usually causes an atrophic rhinitis syndrome with a chronic mucoid nasal discharge. Acute maxillary and frontal sinusitis due to this organism has been described and has been associated with septicemia in an elderly patient.[94,95] Rhinoscleroma due to *K rhinoscleromatis* is endemic to eastern Europe, the Middle East, and Central and South America, although with immigration, it has been reported with increasing frequency in the United States. The insidious onset and long course of the disease may delay its diagnosis and increase the likelihood of its recognition in older populations. The disease presents with varying degrees of nasal obstruction, nasal deformity, epistaxis, hoarseness, and dysphagia. Physical examination may demonstrate granular, erythematous, edematous mucosa with crusting of the mucous membranes, initially of the nose, progressing to involve the palate, pharynx, paranasal sinuses, larynx, and trachea. Granulomatous involvement may be followed by extensive fibrosis and gradual airway narrowing and obstruction.[85,86]

Rhinocerebral phycomycosis occurs predominantly in the debilitated, immunosuppressed patient and in poorly controlled diabetics, categories which encompass many of the elderly. Symptoms referable to intraoral, nasopharyngeal, or paranasal sinus disease are most often presenting complaints. The disease spreads via arterial invasion with a necrotizing vasculitis of contiguous structures. Facial swelling, intranasal necrosis, and eschar formation, fever, and headache are common signs and symptoms. These symptoms may be accompanied by cranial nerve palsies, decreased vision, proptosis and obtundation as lesions rapidly involve intracranial structures. Nonseptate branching hyphae of *Rhizopus* or *Mucor* may be demonstrated in tissue.[96-98]

The diagnosis of acute sinusitis rests on the clinical presentation, radiographic abnormalities, and culture of appropriate clinical material. Sinus puncture is unnecessary in the management of routine sinusitis and therapy may be based on the knowledge of microbial etiologies previously described. However, sinus puncture may be of use in nosocomial sinusitis, in patients who do not respond to empiric therapy, or in immunosuppressed patients who may have unusual pathogens.

Complications of acute sinusitis will depend on the location of the sinus involved. Frontal, ethmoid, and maxillary sinusitis may be complicated by orbital cellulitis or abscess, cavernous sinus thrombosis, mucocele formation, osteomyelitis of the skull, purulent meningitis, and intracranial suppuration primarily of the frontal lobe.[99-102] Brain abscess would appear from the literature to be a less common complication in the elderly than in those aged 10 to 30 years.[100] Sphenoid sinusitis may be complicated by cavernous sinus thrombosis, retro-orbital abscess, involvement of the optic tract or pituitary gland, and basilar meningitis.[103,104]

Treatment

Ampicillin, amoxicillin, trimethoprim-sulfamethoxazole, and the cephalosporins have been used successfully in the routine treatment of acute sinusitis.[89] Nosocomial sinusitis will generally require a second- or third-generation cephalosporin or an antipseudomonal penicillin and an aminoglycoside until culture data are available.[92,93] A ten-day course is recommended based on sinus aspiration data.[92,93] *Klebsiella ozaenae* is susceptible to cephalothin, gentamicin, and chloramphenicol.[94,95] *Klebsiella rhinoscleromatis* is susceptible to streptomycin, kanamycin, tetracycline, chloramphenicol, and possibly cephalosporins.[85,86] Prolonged therapy for 9 to 12 months may be necessary.[86] A combination of amphotericin B, surgical resection, and control of underlying illnesses will generally be required for the successful treatment of the phycomycoses.[96-98] Persistent complaints following adequate treatment for sinusitis may dictate the need for sinus drainage or lavage for diagnostic and therapeutic purposes. Chronic sinus symptomatology may not be infectious in origin and surgical decompression or mucosal resection may be necessary for relief of symptoms.[99]

OTITIS EXTERNA, OTITIS MEDIA, AND MASTOIDITIS

Otitis Externa

Acute otitis externa is an infection of the external ear canal caused by organisms indigenous to the canal, that is, *Staphylococcus epidermidis*, *S aureus*, diphtheroids, and anaerobic gram-positive cocci.[105] Gram-negative bacilli, particularly *Pseudomonas aeruginosa*, are also frequently grown in culture.[105] The decreased water content of aging skin, increased epithelial sloughing, and increased production of thicker, drier cerumen with age may increase local debris and the potential for obstruction with subsequent development of external ear infection. The involved ear canal may be pruritic, reddened, edematous, and increasingly painful, often in association with purulent drainage on examination. Treatment with local antibiotic instillation of ear drops containing polymixin or gentamicin, combined with a steroid preparation, has been successful.[106]

A virulent form of external otitis, *malignant otitis externa*, has a particular predilection for elderly diabetic patients.[105,107,108] This is a necrotizing vasculitic infection most often caused by *P aeruginosa*. The mean age at onset is approximately 69 years.[105] Ninety percent of patients have diabetes mellitus, usually of long standing, with evidence, locally or systemically, of diabetic or atherosclerotic microvascular disease.[105,107] Impaired cellular immunity has been demonstrated concomitant with the infection.[108] The combination of poor local perfusion and impaired immunity is felt to create an optimal environment for proliferation of *Pseudomonas*.[108,109]

Clinically, the patient presents with otalgia, external ear drainage, swelling, and erythema of the external canal and/or surrounding structures. Granulation tissue may be visible in the canal. The tympanic membrane is usually normal. Neurologic deficits were present at the onset in approximately 39% of patients in one study.[105] These ranged from an isolated facial nerve palsy to multiple cranial nerve deficits, basilar meningitis, or CNS suppuration. Culture revealed *P aeruginosa* in nearly 100% of patients in most studies.[105,107,110,111] However, *Aspergillus fumigatus* was implicated in an isolated case report.[112] Useful diagnostic studies include CT scanning, which may best delineate the extent of soft tissue, cartilage, and bone damage, and bone or gallium scanning which may help define the presence of bony involvement and inflammation early in the course of the disease.[113-115] CT scanning is the most useful study for following the progression of disease and gallium scanning for following the efficacy of therapy.[113-115]

Therapy generally requires the combination of an aminoglycoside, an antipseudomonal penicillin and extensive surgical debridement.[105,107,116] Some success has been reported with the third-generation cephalosporins when used alone,[117] but this requires further study. Long-term treatment of 6 to 8 weeks is generally required. Mortality rates appear to depend on the extent of disease at the time of recognition and the institution of appropriate therapy. Overall mortality rates range from 15% to 35%.[105] Those with no cranial nerve involvement may have an overall survival of 85% while those with one or more cranial neuropathies may have a survival of only about 50%.[105]

Otitis Media and Mastoiditis

The middle ear is a structure in continuity with the nasopharynx, eustachian tubes, and mastoid air cells. These contiguous structures are lined with respiratory epithelium subject to the age-related alterations in the respiratory tract previously noted: decreased production and increased **viscosity of mucus, decreased local IgA production, and decreased** mucociliary clearance.[1-4] Such changes may theoretically predispose to accumulation of fluid and an increased propensity for microbial contamination. Subsequent obstruction of drainage through the eustachian tube from mucosal edema or thickened secretions may allow invasion and suppuration.

Etiology Infection of the middle ear and mastoid is uncommon in the elderly. No investigations have defined differences in the microbiology of otitis media in the aged as a distinct patient population. Investigational data suggest that increased colonization of the upper respiratory tract with aerobic gram-negative bacilli in the elderly may increase the contribution of these organisms to middle ear infection. In one study of gram-negative bacillary middle ear infection, groups at extremes of age were those most commonly affected.[118] The organisms isolated most often, however, are *Streptococcus pneumoniae*, found in 31% of cases; nontypeable *H influenzae* in 27%; and group A ß-hemolytic streptococci, *Staphylococcus aureus*, and *B catarrhalis* in 2% to 5% each.[119] Approximately one third of aspirated middle ear cultures are negative and viruses and anaerobes have been implicated as contributing agents in some of these cases.[119-121] Tuberculous otitis media has been well described and with the increased prevalence of reactivation tuberculosis in the aged, tuberculosis should be considered in the differential diagnosis.[122-125] The occurrence of acute otitis media in the adult without a history of previous episodes at a younger age suggests underlying nasopharyngeal carcinoma or lymphoma. Acute serous otitis media in older adults, ranging from 46 to 74 years old, has been associated with later development of a necrotizing vasculitis.[126]

Clinical manifestations and treatment The clinical presentation of acute suppurative otitis media and mastoiditis has been discussed in detail in several reviews.[127,128] Tuberculous otitis media has an insidious onset with chronic otorrhea followed by profound hearing loss.[122,123,125] Otalgia is present in 50% of cases.[122] Physical examination demonstrates multiple perforations which become coalescent. Abundant granulation tissue and purulent discharge may be seen.

Antimicrobial agents useful in the therapy of acute otitis media include ampicillin or amoxicillin, above or in combination with ß-lactamase inhibitors such as sulbactam and clavulanic acid, trimethoprim-sulfamethoxazole, cefaclor, and an erythromycin-sulfonamide combination.[127] Tuberculous otitis responds well to two-drug antituberculous chemotherapy.[122,123]

OROFACIAL, ODONTOGENIC, AND DEEP CERVICAL INFECTIONS

Microbiologic Considerations

Orofacial and deep cervical infections are most often of odontogenic origin. The etiologic organisms involved generally reflect the existing oral flora. Subtle differences may be noted when these infections occur in an elderly population based on the changes in oral microbial flora and physiologic function that occur with aging. Table 6-1 outlines the prevalent microbial environment in adults. Studies delineating changes in the aged focus on the observed increase in oropharyngeal colonization with gram-negative bacilli. Valenti et al report a 6% to 9% prevalence rate of colonization with gram-negative bacilli in healthy patients over age 65 who function independently,[5] compared with a 3% rate in healthy controls under age 65. This rate increased as the level of care required by the elderly patient increased rising to 40% to 60% in those hospitalized on an acute care ward.[5] Underlying illnesses were associated with increased colonization with gram-negative bacilli only if they limited the patient's ability to function independently.[5] The most common gram-negative bacilli isolated from elderly patients in this study included *Klebsiella* organisms, *E coli, Enterobacter* organisms, *Pseudomonas*, and *Proteus* organisms.[5] Certain sites in the oral cavity may favor colonization by specific organisms.[21] The tooth surface is often colonized with *Streptococcus sanguis, S mitis*, and *Actinomyces viscosus*, the tongue and buccal mucosa with *Veillonella* organisms and *S salivarius*, and the gingival crevices with *Bacteroides* and *Fusobacterium* organisms.

Alterations in the microbial flora in the aged may relate to a number of host factors including nutritional changes, decreases in mucociliary transport, and clearance of microorganisms,[1,2] decreases in salivary gland flow and volume, increases in salivary viscosity,[3] and alterations in local secretory IgA levels with advancing age.[2] The presence of periodontal disease, which increases progressively with advancing years,[35] may also shift the predominant flora.

The etiology of odontogenic infections reflects the existing oral flora. Chow et al, in a prospective study of 31 patients with orofacial odontogenic infections,[21] isolated obligate anaerobes from 94% of patients and aerobes from 55%. Fifty-two percent of patients had mixed aerobic and anaerobic infections. While *Bacteroides, Peptostreptococcus,* and *Streptococcus* were the most common isolates from such infections in the study,[21] facultative aerobic gram-negative bacilli may assume an increasingly important role as oropharyngeal colonization with them rises with age.

Anatomical and Physiologic Considerations

Although localized dentoalveolar and periodontal infections are significant in the elderly, contiguous spread to deeper fascial spaces and the potential suppurative complications of such spread may be more devastating. Mucosal, bony, and soft tissue changes in the elderly may make the local containment of infection and the early recognition of suppurative complications more difficult. Soft tissue odontogenic infection generally extends along pathways of least resistance from involved teeth to contiguous potential spaces.[21,129] Age-dependent thinning of mucosal epithelium, decreases in capillary number and flow, and decreases in soft tissue content of water, hyaluronic acid, collagen, and ground substance may combine to reduce local barriers to spreading infection and to reduce the elderly host's ability to repair injured tissue.[35] Perforation of alveolar bone by pus may be more easily accomplished through aged osteoporotic bony tissue allowing access to deeper fascial compartments. Similar decreases in skin and soft tissue hydration, blood flow, collagen, and ground substance may reduce skin elasticity and tone, making local swelling more difficult to appreciate early in the course of infection.

Clinical Syndromes

Dentoalveolar, gingival, and periodontal infections Dental caries and pulpal infections increase with age owing to the previously discussed anatomical and physiologic alterations.[35] Apical migration of gingival tissue may lead to gradual exposure of the tooth root increasing the predilection to periapical infection.[35] The incidence of periodontal disease also rises with age, approaching 58% in those over 65 years of age.[35] A spectrum of clinical disease beginning with dental caries progresses in order to pulpal infection, periapical infection or abscess, gingivitis, and periodontitis.[129] Clinically, the patient may be asymptomatic until a generalized pulpitis develops. The tooth involved may then be sensitive to percussion and hot or cold stimuli. If the pulp is not drained, periapical infection may develop and extend to the gingiva or localize with abscess formation. Once infected, the gingiva may appear dusky with swelling and increasing friability of the free gingival margin. Pain is generally not prominent. As infection advances, the gingiva may separate from the teeth and pus may be expressed from periodontal pockets. As the periodontitis advances, infection becomes generalized with destruction of supporting tissue and eventual loss of teeth. Chronic progressive periodontal disease is the most common cause of tooth loss in the elderly.[35,129]

Acute necrotizing ulcerative gingivitis, although an uncommon disease, may occur more frequently in an elderly population than in other groups because of the abnormalities of salivary flow and content, altered blood flow, altered immune function, and progressive increase in periodontal disease in the aged, factors which have been related to the occurrence of this disease.[129,130] The patient may note the acute onset of pain in the gingiva, which interferes with mastication, followed by fever, malaise, and local lymphadenopathy. Necrosis of the gingiva produces a punched-out appearance with formation of a grayish pseudomembrane. Halitosis and taste alteration may accompany the infection.

Treatment of dentoalveolar, gingival, and periodontal infections includes local debridement or drainage, extraction of involved teeth, and antibiotic therapy for advanced infection. Penicillin remains the antibiotic of choice as most oral bacteria remain sensitive to it. However, increasing resistance of some oral *Bacteroides* spp[21,129] and the greater prevalence of facultative aerobic gram-negative bacilli in the elderly, may dictate a change in antibiotic coverage if a lack of adequate response to penicillin is noted. Cefoxitin may be a useful antibiotic alone. Clindamycin and metronidazole may be used in combination with most betalactams when resistant *Bacteroides* spp are implicated in infection. Ampicillin, amoxicillin and ticarcillin combined with ß-lactamase inhibitors are also reasonable choices in appropriate clinical situations.

Deep fascial compartment infections As discussed previously, the anatomical and physiologic changes which occur with advancing age may limit the ability of the elderly patient to contain the spread of odontogenic infection. Potential spaces around the face include the masticator, buccal, canine, and parotid spaces. The suprahyoid regions include the sublingual, submandibular, and lateral pharyngeal spaces. The infrahyoid and total neck spaces include the retropharyngeal, danger, pretracheal, and prevertebral spaces. These spaces all potentially communicate with one another and may become infected with contiguous spread of unchecked infection.[21,129] While infection of these spaces does not differ significantly in the elderly from those in other adult age groups, one must be cognizant of the alterations in microbiologic flora, the increased prevalence of dental caries and periodontal disease, and therefore the increased potential in the elderly for fascial space infections.

Clinical manifestations

Masticator space infection The masticator spaces may be further subdivided into the masseteric, pterygoid, and temporal spaces, all of which intercommunicate with one another. Infections of these spaces generally derive from the second and third molar teeth. Clinically, the patient experiences pain in the body or ramus of the mandible associated with marked trismus. When visible, swelling appears brawny and indurated. Extension into the temporal space may produce swelling over the zygomatic arch, preauricular area, and into the periorbital area, involving the whole side of the face. The temporal space communicates with the orbit via the inferior orbital fissure and unchecked infection may extend to orbital structures.

Canine, buccal, and parotid space infection Infections of these spaces commonly arise from the maxillary or mandibular canine and premolar teeth. Clinically, involvement of the canine space will produce swelling and induration of the upper lip that may extend along the nasolabial fold to the lower eyelid. Involvement of the buccal space will be determined by the location of the tooth root apices with respect to the origin of the buccinator muscle in the maxilla or mandible. If the root apices lay below the maxillary origin or above the mandibular origin of this muscle, pus will drain into the oral cavity. If the opposite exists, infection will extend laterally into the buccal space. This is associated clinically with marked swelling and induration over the cheek with minimal trismus. Parotid space infection generally results from extension of masseteric or buccal space infection. Clinically, the patient experiences intense pain and dramatic swelling of the angle of the jaw without trismus, accompanied by fever and chills. The proximity of the parotid space to the lateral pharyngeal space posteriorly increases the potential for contiguous spread into the other fascial spaces of the neck.

Sublingual, submandibular, and lateral pharyngeal space The myelohyoid muscle forming the floor of the mouth separates these spaces from one another. Infections from the sublingual space generally arise from the mandibular incisors. Clinically, the patient notes brawny, indurated swelling of the floor of the mouth from the mandible to the mid-line. Since there is only a loose connective tissue separation at the mid-line, infection easily moves across to involve bilaterally the sublingual space. Elevation of the tongue may occur resulting in respiratory embarrassment. Posteriorly, the sublingual space may communicate with the mandibular and lateral pharyngeal spaces. Infection of the submandibular space may arise from contiguous extension of sublingual space infection or, more commonly, from the mandibular second and third molars. Brawny edema and swelling occurs. Infection involving both the submandibular and sublingual spaces bilaterally is termed Ludwig's angina. A devastating infection first described in 1836, this complication produces extensive tissue swelling and edema pressing the tongue backward and upward, encroaching on the larynx, inducing dysphonia, hoarseness, and respiratory impairment. Fever, chills, and systemic symptoms may be marked. Prior to the advent of antibiotics, this disease was fatal. Dental infection has been reported as the causative factor in 90% of cases,[129] and as dental infection becomes more prevalent with advancing age, Ludwig's angina, when seen today, may occur more commonly in the elderly.

Lateral pharyngeal space infection may result from a number of other sources in addition to odontogenic infections including pharyngitis, tonsillitis, otitis, mastoiditis, and parotitis. Clinically, the patient may present with pain, swelling extending medially into the pharyngeal wall, dysphagia, and mild trismus when the anterior portion of the space is involved. With involvement of the posterior region, trismus may not be prominent and swelling may not be visible, but respiratory impairment and extension into the jugular and carotid sheath, which lie in proximity, may occur.

Retropharyngeal, danger and prevertebral spaces These spaces lie behind the esophagus and extend inferiorly communicating with one another and via the danger space with the upper mediastinum caudally and the base of the skull cephalad. Infection of these spaces arises from nasal, pharyngeal, and odontogenic sources. Symptoms may be variable depending on the location of the infection and proximate structures. Clinically, manifestations include dysphagia, regurgitation of fluids through the nose, neck pain, nuchal rigidity, dyspnea, hoarseness, heaache, and systemic symptoms of fever, chills, and malaise. Bulging of the posterior pharyngeal wall may be visible deep in the throat. Lateral radiographs of the neck will demonstrate widening of the involved spaces.

Treatment considerations The principles of treatment of fascial space infections may be generalized. Surgical drainage and debridement of necrotic tissue and extraction of involved teeth are of utmost importance. Antibiotic therapy should be governed by gram stain and culture of appropriate clinical material and knowledge of pre-existing oral flora. The principles are the same as those noted for odontogenic infections. Penicillin remains the drug of choice with the understanding that a small subset of oral *Bacteroides* spp may be resistant.[21] Clindamycin and cefoxitin have been used successfully.[21] The prevalence of oropharyngeal colonization with gram-negative bacilli in the debilitated elderly patient may dictate combination therapy with an aminoglycoside or a third-generation cephalosporin and penicillin or clindamycin. Ticarcillin-clavulanic acid, amoxicillin-clavulanic acid or ampicillin-sulbactam may also be useful alternatives. Adjunctive therapy with topical irrigation of open wounds with hydrogen peroxide or utilization of hyperbaric oxygen have been advocated by some,[21,129] but the paucity of well-controlled studies limit these as general recommendations.

Complications

Osteomyelitis of the jaws Conditions affecting host resistance and jaw vascularity are major determinants in the development of osteomyelitis of the jaws. Osteoporosis of bone, decreased bone vascularity, poor nutritional status, and the presence of other chronic underlying diseases in many elderly patients make this a more common complication in this age group than in younger individuals. Osteomyelitis of the jaw results primarily from contiguous extension of periodontal and odontogenic infections. The maxillary bone is less commonly affected as an isolated event because of its paucity of medullary tissue, its thin cortical plates, and its less extensive vascular supply,[21,129] allowing easier access of pus into soft tissue. The mandible more readily confines infection to the bone because of its well-developed medullary cavity vascularity and periosteum.

Earlier studies report staphylococci as the most common etiologic organisms.[21,130] More recent studies suggest that anaerobes and mixed aerobic-anaerobic infections of oral origin are more important etiologic agents.[21,130] In the elderly, facultative aerobic gram-negative bacilli must also be considered. The age-dependent increase in the incidence of reactivation tuberculosis suggests *Mycobacterium tuberculosis* as a possible causative agent as well. There are three major clinical presentations:

1. Acute suppurative osteomyelitis presents clinically with deep pain, high fever, and hypoesthesia of the mental nerve. Swelling is minimal. As the syndrome evolves, malaise and anorexia may develop, teeth in the involved area begin to loosen, and pus may track through the gingival sulcus, mucosa, or skin. An indurated cellulitis of the cheek or chin may develop. Regional lymphadenopathy is present. Laboratory studies may show a leukocytosis and elevated ESR, and radiographs will begin to show raising of the periosteum and early lytic lesions within ten to 21 days. Bone scan and gallium scan may be positive early in the course. A definable source of infection can often be identified.
2. Secondary chronic osteomyelitis is a continuation of the acute phase and may result from incomplete therapy of the acute infection. Clinical characteristics include continued bone pain and tenderness, cutaneous fistula formation, and gradual development of bone sequestra.
3. Primary, chronic osteomyelitis presents as a chronic low-grade infection, insidious in onset, with no acute phase. It may be caused by less virulent microorganisms and symptoms of progressive bone pain or fistula formation may be its hallmarks.

Clinical history, physical examination, radiographic studies, technetium or gallium bone scanning, and routine laboratory studies can usually establish the diagnosis of osteomyelitis of the jaw. Computed tomographic (CT) scanning may be helpful in difficult cases. A microbiologic diagnosis will be necessary to guide adequate therapy and most often will require a bone biopsy specimen. Cutaneous or other external draining sites may not reflect the true microbiologic flora involved. The antibiotic regimen of choice should depend on the organisms isolated from bone. Empiric choices, if necessary, should cover the organisms indigenous to local flora and any others to which a particular host may be especially susceptible. This may necessitate coverage for gram-negative bacilli or mycobacterial organisms in the elderly. Therapy requires prolonged antibiotic treatment, in most cases from 6 to 12 weeks. Surgical debridement and drainage may also be necessary.

Suppurative jugular thrombophlebitis and carotid artery erosion This complication generally results from infection of the lateral pharyngeal space containing these structures. Clinically, the patient presents with fever, chills, tenderness, pain, and swelling of the angle of the mandible and along the sternocleidomastoid muscle. There may be associated neck rigidity. Symptoms of involvement of the lateral pharyngeal space will be present as well. Septic embolization may be noted. The capability of some *Bacteroides* and *Fusobacterium* organisms to degrade heparin and accelerate coagulation has been postulated as an explanation for the prevalence of these organisms as causative agents in this complication.[73,131,132]

Septic cavernous sinus thrombosis Infection involving the maxillary teeth and the masticator spaces are the most common odontogenic source of this complication. In addition to the signs and symptoms of masticator space infection, clinically the patient presents with venous engorgement of the retina, conjunctiva, and periorbital tissue, paresis of cranial nerves III, IV, and VI, and evidence of meningeal irritation. Treatment requires early surgical decompression and antibiotic therapy.

Mediastinitis This suppurative complication usually arises via extension from the lateral pharyngeal or retropharyngeal spaces which communicate through the danger space with the mediastinum. Fatal mediastinitis has been reported following involvement of these spaces with odontogenic infection.[133]

Maxillary sinusitis Maxillary sinusitis is a potential suppurative complication of dental infection and has been discussed elsewhere.

SUMMARY

The paucity of investigational data with specific regard to upper airway infection in the elderly necessitates extrapolation of information from more generalized investigational literature. While acute bacterial parotitis, sialoadenitis, facial herpes zoster infection, erysipelas, and malignant otitis externa may have an age-dependent prevalence in the elderly, odontogenic infections and their complications secondary to periodontal disease may be the most serious and common infections of the aged in the upper respiratory tract. The other infections discussed in this chapter, while continuing to occur with regularity in elderly patients, may be less frequent than in other populations. The age-related changes in host defense, physiologic function, and microbial flora discussed in this chapter may lend a different perspective to one's view of these infections and dictate a less traditional approach to them.

The authors express their gratitude to Sandra Blanch for preparation of this manuscript.

REFERENCES

1. Gardner ID: The effect of aging on susceptibility to infection. *Rev Infect Dis* 1980;2:801–810.
2. Phair J: Host defense in the aged, in Gleckman RA, Gantz NM (eds): *Infections in the Elderly*. Boston, Little, Brown & Co, 1983; pp 1–12.
3. Drummond JR, Chisholm DM: A qualitative and quantitative study of the ageing human labial salivary glands. *Arch Oral Biol* 1984;29:151–155.

4. McGill JI, Linkos GM, Goulding N, et al: Normal tear protein profiles and age-related changes. *Br J Ophthalmol* 1984;68:316–320.
5. Valenti WM, Trudell RG, Bentley DW: Factors predisposing to oropharyngeal colonization with gram negative bacilli in the aged. *N Engl J Med* 1978;298:1108–1111.
6. Weksler ME: Senescence of the immune system *Med Clin North Am* 1983;67:263–272.
7. Czlonkowska A, Korlak J: The immune response during aging. *J Gerontol* 1979;34:9–14.
8. Phair JP: Aging and infection: A review. *J Chronic Dis* 1979;32:535–540.
9. Inkeles B, Innes JB, Kuntz MM, et al: Immunological studies of aging — III. Cytokinetic basis for the impaired response of lymphocytes from aged humans to plant lectins. *J Exp Med* 1977;145:1176–1187.
10. Gillis S, Kozak R, Durante M, et al: Immunological studies of aging. Decreased production of and response to T cell growth factor by lymphocytes from aged humans. *J Clin Invest* 1981;67:937–942.
11. Pahwa SG, Pahwa RN, Good RA: Decreased *in vitro* humoral immune responses in aged humans. *J Clin Invest* 1981;67:1094–1102.
12. Phair J, Kauffman CA, Bjornson A, et al: Failure to respond to influenza vaccine in the aged: correlation with B-cell number and function. *J Lab Med* 1978; 92:822–828.
13. Phair JP, Kauffman CA, Bjornson A, et al: Host defense in the aged: evaluation of components of the inflammatory and immune responses. *J Infect Dis* 1978;138:67–73.
14. Buckley CS III, Buckley EG, Dorsey FC: Longitudinal changes in serum immunoglobulin levels in older humans. *Fed Proc* 1974;33:2036–2039.
15. Antonaci S, Jirillo E, Ventura MT, et al: Nonspecific immunity in aging: Deficiency of mono cyte and polymorphonuclear cell-mediated functions. *Mech Ageing Dev* 1984;24:367–375.
16. Gardner ID, Lim ST, Lawton JWM: Monocyte function in ageing humans. *Mech Ageing Dev* 1981;16:233–239.
17. Richmond JB (ed): Symposium on child's mouth. *Pediatr Clin North Am* 1956;3:845–1072.
18. Brook I, Finegold SM: Acute suppurative parotitis caused by anaerobic bacteria: Report of two cases. *Pediatrics* 1978;62:1019–1020.
19. Bissell P, Glew RH, Liland JB: Parotitis associated with *Eikenella corrodens* in a healthy adult. *Arch Otolaryngol* 1983;109:772–773.
20. Goldberg MH: Infections of the salivary glands, in Topazian RG, Goldberg MH (eds): *Management of Infections of the Oral and Maxillofacial Regions*. Philadelphia, WB Saunders Co, 1981, pp 304–307.
21. Chow AW, Roser SM, Brady FA: Orofacial odontogenic infections. *Ann Intern Med* 1978;88:392–402.
22. Lass JL: Herpes zoster: Protecting older patient's vision. *Geriatrics* 1984;39:79–80,85–87,91–94.
23. Smith IM: Infectious disease problems in the elderly, in Reichel W (ed): *Clinical Aspects of Aging*. Baltimore, Williams & Wilkins Co, 1983 pp 218–234.
24. Berger R, Florent G, Just M: Decrease of the lymphoproliferative response to varicella-zoster virus antigen in the aged. *Infect Immun* 1981;32:24–27.
25. Bentley DW: Management of infection in the elderly, in Cape RDT, Coe RM, Rossman T (eds): *Fundamentals of Geriatric Medicine*. New York, Raven Press, 1983, pp 204–205.
26. Jemsek J, Greenberg SB, Taber L, et al: Herpes zoster-associated

encephalitis: Clinicopathologic report of 12 cases and review of the literature. *Medicine* 1983;62:81–97.
27. Doyle PW, Gibson G, Dolman CL: Herpes zoster ophthalmicus with contralateral hemiplegia: identification of cause. *Ann Neurol* 1983;14:84–85.
28. Hilt DC, Buchholz D, Krumholz A, et al: Herpes zoster ophthalmicus and delayed contralateral hemiparesis caused by cerebral angiitis: Diagnosis management approaches. *Ann Neurol* 1983;14:543–553.
29. Balfour HH, McMonigal KA, Bean B: Acyclovir therapy of varicella-zoster virus infections in immunocompromised patients. *J Antimicrob Chemother* 1983;12(suppl B):169–179.
30. McGill J, Chapman C, Copplestone A, et al: A review of acyclovir treatment of ocular herpes zoster and skin infections. *J Antimicrob Chemother* 1983;12(suppl B):45–49.
31. McGill J, Chapman C: A comparison of topical acyclovir with steroids in the treatment of herpes zoster keratouveitis. *Br J Ophthalmol* 1983;67:746–750.
32. Topazian RG: Uncommon infections of the oral and maxillofacial regions, in Topazian RG, Goldberg MH (eds): *Management of Infections of the Oral and Maxillofacial Regions*. Philadelphia, WB Saunders Co, 1981; p 286.
33. Swartz MN: Cellulitis and superficial infections, in Mandell GL, Douglas RG, Bennett JE (eds): *Principles and Practice of Infectious Diseases*, ed 2. New York, John Wiley & Sons, 1985; p 603.
34. Berger SA, Zonszein J, Villamena P, et al: Infectious diseases of the thyroid gland. *Rev Infect Dis* 1983;5:108–122.
35. Koopmann CF, Coulthard SW: The oral cavity and aging. *Otolaryngol Clin North Am* 1982;15:293–312.
36. Weese WC, Smith IM: A study of 57 cases of actinomycosis over a 36-year period. *Arch Intern Med* 1975;135:1562–1568.
37. Hartley JH, Schatten WE: Cervicofacial actinomycosis. *Plast Reconstr Surg* 1973;51:44–47.
38. Allen RKA, Faulks LW: Empyema due to beta-lactamase producing *Haemophilus influenzae* type b complicating severe laryngopharyngitis and cervical cellulitis. *Aust NZ J Med* 1983;13:377–379.
39. Drapkin MS, Wilson ME, Shrager SM, et al: Bacteremic *Haemophilus influenzae* type b cellulitis in the adult. *Am J Med* 1977;63:449–452.
40. Lederman MM, Lauder J, Lerner PI: Bacteremic pneumo-coccal epiglottitis in adults with malignancy. *Am Rev Respir Dis* 1982;125:117–118.
41. Kessler HA, Schade R, Trenholme GM, et al: Acute pneumococcal epiglottitis in immunocompromised adults. *Scand J Infect Dis* 1980;12:207–210.
42. Rose FB, Garman RF, Falkenberg KJ, et al: Acute epiglottitis, cellulitis, and *Streptococcus pneumoniae* bacteremia. *Scand J Infect Dis* 1982;14:301–303.
43. Mento AS, Ullman BM: Acute respiratory illness in an American community: The Tecumseh study. *JAMA* 1974;227:164–169.
44. Gwaltney JM: Epidemiology of the common cold. *Ann NY Acad Sci* 1980;353:54–60.
45. Anderson LJ, Patriarca PA, Hierholzer JC, et al: Viral respiratory illnesses. *Med Clin North Am* 1983;67:1009–1030.
46. Mathur U, Bentley DW, Hall CB: Concurrent respiratory syncytial virus and influenza A infections in the institutionalized elderly and chronically ill. *Ann Intern Med* 1980;93(pt 1):49–52.
47. *MMWR* 1977;26:351.

48. Hendley JO, Wenzel RP, Gwaltney JM: Transmission of rhinovirus colds by self-inoculation. *N Engl J Med* 1973;288:1361 – 1364.
49. Gwaltney JM, Moskalski PB, Hendley JO: Hand-to-hand transmission of rhinovirus colds. *Ann Intern Med* 1978;88:463 – 467.
50. Couch RB, Cate TR, Douglas RG, et al; Effect of route of inoculation on experimental respiratory viral disease in volunteers and evidence for airborne transmission. *Bacteriol Rev* 1966;30:517 – 529.
51. Couch RB: The effects of influenza on host defense. *J Infect Dis* 1981;144:284 – 291.
52. Hall WJ, Hall CB, Speers DM: Respiratory syncytial virus infection in adults: Clinical, virologic and serial pulmonary function studies. *Ann Intern Med* 1978;88:203 – 205.
53. Douglas RG, Betts RF: Influenza virus, in Mandell GL, Douglas RG, Bennett JE (eds): *Principles and Practice of Infectious Disease*, ed 2. New York, John Wiley & Sons, 1985; pp 846-868.
54. Immunization Practices Advisory Committee of the Centers for Disease Control: Prevention and control of influenza. *MMWR* 1984;33:253 – 260.
55. Hayden FG, Gwaltney JM: Intranasal interferon $\alpha 2$ for prevention of rhinovirus infection and illness. *J Infect Dis* 1983;148:543 – 550.
56. LaMontagne JR, Galasso GJ: Report of a workshop on clinical studies of the efficacy of amantadine and rimantidine against influenza virus. *J Infect Dis* 1978;138:928 – 931.
57. Dolin R, Reichman RC, Madore HP, et al: A controlled trial of amantidine and rimantidine in the prophylaxis of influenza A infection. *N Engl J Med* 1982;307:580 – 584.
58. Komaroff AL, Aronson MD, Pass TM, et al: Serologic evidence of chlamydial and mycoplasmal pharyngitis in adults. *Science* 1983;222:927 – 928.
59. Corcoran JG, Axline SG: Infectious diseases in the geriatric patient. *Otolaryngol Clin North Am* 1982;15:421 – 438.
60. Levy ML, Ericsson CD, Pickering LK: Infections of the upper respiratory tract. *Med Clin North Am* 1983;67:153 – 171.
61. Nelson LA, Peri BA, Rieger CHL, et al: Immunity to diphtheria in an urban population. *Pediatrics* 1978;61:703 – 710.
62. Weiss BP, Strassberg MA, Feeley JC: Tetanus and diphtheria immunity in an elderly population in Los Angeles County. *Am J Pub Health* 1983;73:802 – 804.
63. Kerttula Y, Nors T, Kuronen T, et al: Immunity to diphtheria in Helsinki in 1975. *Scand J Infect Dis* 1980;12:37 – 39.
64. Horwitz CA, Henle W, Henle G, et al: Infectious mononucleosis in patients aged 40 to 72 years: Report of 27 cases, including 3 without heterophil antibody responses. *Medicine* 1983;62: 256 – 262.
65. Ginsburg AD, Ginsburg JC: Infectious mononucleosis in older patients. *Can Med Assoc J* 1982;127:1103 – 1105.
66. McKendrick MW, Geddes AM, Edwards JMB: Atypical infectious mononucleosis in the elderly. *Br Med J* 1979;2:970.
67. Bisno AL: *Streptococcus pyogenes*, in Mandell GL, Douglas RG, Bennett JE (eds): *Principles and Practice of Infectious Diseases*, ed 2. New York, John Wiley & Sons, 1985, pp 1124 – 1132.
68. Munford RS, Ory HW, Brooks GF, et al: Diphtheria deaths in the United States, 1959 – 1970. *JAMA* 1974;229:1890 – 1893.
69. Dobie RA, Tobey DN: Clinical features of diphtheria in the respiratory tract. *JAMA* 1979;242:2197 – 2201.

70. Lipsky BA, Goldberger AC, Tompkins LS, et al: Infections caused by nondiphtheria cornynebacteria. *Rev Infect Dis* 1982;4:1220−1235.
71. Kovatch AL, Schuit KE, Michaels RH: *Corynebacterium hemolyticum* peritonsillar abscess mimicking diphtheria. *JAMA* 1983;249:1757−1758.
72. Green SL, LaPeter KS: Pseudodiphtheritic membranous pharyngitis caused by *Corynebacterium hemolyticum. JAMA* 1981;245:2330−2331.
73. Seidenfeld SM, Sutker WL, Luby JP: *Fusobacterium necrophorum* septicemia following oropharyngeal infection. *JAMA* 1982;248:1348−1350.
74. Andreassen UK, Husum B, Tos M, et al: Acute epiglottitis in adults. A management protocol based on a 17-year material. *Acta Anesthesiol Scand* 1984;28:155−157.
75. Russel GAL Acute epiglottitis in adults not due to *Haemophilus. J Laryngol Otol* 1985;99:1035-1038.
76. Johnstone JM, Lawy HS: Acute epiglottitis in adults due to infection with *Haemophilus influenzae* type b. *Lancet* 1967;2:134−135.
77. Glode MP, Halsey NA, Murray M, et al: Epiglottitis in adults: Association with *Haemophilus influenzae* type b colonization and disease in children. *Pediatr Infect Dis* 1984;3:548−551.
78. Schalen L, Christensen P, Kamme C, et al: High isolation rate of *Branhamella catarrhalis* from the nasopharynx in adults with acute laryngitis. *Scand J Infect Dis* 1980;12:277−280.
79. Caldarelli DD, Friedberg SA, Harris AA: Medical and surgical aspects of the granulomatous diseases of the larynx. *Otolaryngol Clin North Am* 1979;12:767−781.
80. Lawson R, Bodey G, Luna M: Case report. *Candida* infection presenting as laryngitis. *Am J Med Sci* 1980;280:173−174.
81. Schabel SI, Katzberg RW, Burgener FA: Acute inflammation of epiglottis and supraglottic structures in adults. *Radiology* 1977;122:601−604.
82. Branefors-Helander P, Jappsson PH: Acute epiglottitis. A clinical, bacteriological and serological study. *Scand J Infect Dis* 1975;7:103−111.
83. Haberman RS, Becker ME, Ford CN: *Candida* epiglottitis. *Arch Otolaryngol* 1983;109:770−771.
84. Bachman AL, Zizmor J, Noyek AM: Tuberculosis of the larynx. *Semin Roentgenol* 1979;14:325−327.
85. Miller RH, Shulman JB, Canalis RF, et al: *Klebsiella rhinoscleromatis*: A clinical and pathogenic enigma. *Otolaryngol Head Neck Surg* 1979;87:212−221.
86. Shum TK, Whitaker CW, Meyer PR: Clinical update on rhinoscleroma. *Laryngoscope* 1982;92:1149−1153.
87. Linaker BD: Acute epiglottitis requiring tracheostomy in an adult. *Br Med J* 1976;2:1045.
88. Harris RD, Berdon WE, Baker DH: Roentgen diagnosis of acute epiglottitis in the adult. *J Assoc Can Radiol* 1970;21:270−272.
89. Hamory BH, Sande MA, Sydnor A, et al: Etiology and antimicrobial therapy of acute maxillary sinusitis. *J Infect Dis* 1979;130:197−202.
90. Evans FO, Sydnor JB, Moore WEC, et al: Sphenoid sinusitis of the maxillary antrum. *N Engl J Med* 1975;293:735−739.
91. Frederick J, Brande AI: Anaerobic infection of the paranasal sinuses. *N Engl J Med* 1974;290:135−137.
92. Pope TL, Stelling CB, Leitner YB: Maxillary sinusitis after nasotracheal intubation. *South Med J* 1981;74:610−612.
93. Caplan ES, Hoyt NJ: Nosocomial sinusitis. *JAMA* 1982;247:639−641.
94. Murray KA, Clements BH, Keas, SE: *Klebsiella ozaenae* septicemia

associated with Hansen's disease. *J Clin Microbiol* 1981;14:703 – 705.
95. Goldstein EJC, Lewis RP Martin WJ, et al: Infections caused by *Klebsiella ozaenae*: A changing disease spectrum. *J Clin Microbiol* 1978;8:413 – 418.
96. Rosenberger RS, Wast BC, King JW: Case Report. Survival from sinoorbital mucormycosis due to *Rhizopus rhizopodiformis*. *Am J Med Sci* 1983;286:25 – 30.
97. Meyers BR, Wermser G, Hirschman SZ, et al: Rhinocerebral mucormycosis: remortem diagnosis and therapy. *Arch Intern Med* 1979;139:557 – 560.
98. Parfrey NA: Improved diagnosis and prognosis of mucormycosis. A clinicopathologic study of 33 cases. *Medicine* 1986;65:113 – 123.
99. Sable NS, Hengerer A, Powell KR: Acute frontal sinusitis with intracranial complications. *Pediatr Infect Dis* 1984;3:58 – 61.
100. Bradley PJ, Manning KP, Shaw MDM: Brain abscess secondary to paranasal sinusitis. *J Laryngol Otol* 1984;98: 719 – 725.
101. Kaufman DM, Litman N, Miller MH: Sinusitis: Induced subdural empyema. *Neurology* 1983;33:123 – 232.
102. Morgan PR, Morrison WV: Complications of frontal and ethmoid sinusitis. *Laryngoscope* 1980;90:661 – 666.
103. Lew D, Southwick FS, Montgomery WW, et al: Sphenoid sinusitis. A review of 30 cases. *N Engl J Med* 1983;309:1149 – 1154.
104. Tisdale BA, Mackenzie IJ: The complications of sphenoid sinusitis. *J Laryngol Otol* 1983;97:661 – 670.
105. Doroghazi RM, Nadol JB, Hyslop NE, et al: Invasive external otitis. Report of 21 cases and review of the literature. *Am J Med* 1981;71:603 – 614.
106. Weinstein L: Diseases of the upper respiratory tract, in Braunwald E, Isselbacher D, Petersdorf RE (eds): *Harrison's Principles of Internal Medicine*, ed 11.New York, McGraw-Hill Book Co, 1987, pp 1111 – 1115.
107. Cohn AM: Progressive necrotizing otitis. *Arch Otolaryngol* 1974;99:136 – 139.
108. Yust I, Radiano C, Tartakovsky B, et al: Impairment of cellular immunity in patients with malignant external otitis. *Acta Otolaryngol* 1980;90:398 – 403.
109. Ostfeld E, Segal M, Czernobilsky B: Malignant external otitis: Early histopathologic changes and pathogenic mechanism. *Laryngoscope* 1981;91:965 – 970.
110. Raines JM, Schindler RA: The surgical management of recalcitrant malignant external otitis. *Laryngoscope* 1980;90:369 – 378.
111. Sutherland GE: Malignant external otitis in a nondiabetic adult. *South Med J* 1981;74:516.
112. Petrak RM, Pottage JC, Levin S: Invasive external otitis caused by *Aspergillus furmigatus* in an immunocompromised patient. *J Infect Dis* 1985;151:196.
113. Gold S, Som PM, Lucente FE, et al: Radiographic findings in progressive necrotizing "malignant" external otitis. *Laryngoscope* 1984;94:363 – 366.
114. Mendelson DS, Som PM, Mendelson MH, et al: Malignant external otitis: The role of computed tomography and radionuclides in evaluation. *Radiology* 1983;149:745 – 749.
115. Strashum AM, Negatheim M, Goldsmith SJ: Malignant external otitis: Early scintigraphic detection. *Radiology* 1984;150:541 – 545.
116. Strauss M, Aber RC, Couner GH, et al: Malignant external otitis: Long term (months) antimicrobial therapy. *Laryngoscope* 1982;92:397 – 405.
117. Haverkos H, Caparosa R, Yu VL, et al: Moxalactam therapy. Its use in

chronic suppurative otitis media and malignant external otitis. *Arch Otolaryngol* 1982;108:329 – 333.
118. Ostfeld E, Rubinstein E: Acute gram-negative bacillary infections of middle ear and mastoid. *Ann Otol* 1980;89:33 – 36.
119. Schwartz RH: Bacteriology of otitis media: A review. *Oto-laryngol Head Neck Surg* 1981;89:444 – 450.
120. Brook I, Schwartz R: Anaerobic bacteria in acute otitis media. *Acta Otolaryngol* 1981;91:111 – 114.
121. Henderson FW, Collier AM, Sanyal MA, et al; A longitudinal study of respiratory viruses and bacteria in the etiology of acute otitis media with effusion. *N Engl J Med* 1982;306:1377 – 1383.
122. Windle-Taylor PC, Bailey CM: Tuberculous otitis media: A series of 22 patients. *Laryngoscope* 1980;90:1039 – 1044.
123. Plester D, Pusalkar A, Steinbach E: Clinical records. Middle ear tuberculosis. *J Laryngol Otol* 94:1415 – 1421.
124. Jeang MK, Fletcher EC: Tuberculous otitis media. *JAMA* 1983;249:2231 – 2232.
125. Brutuco RL, Spencer MJ: Tuberculous otomastoiditis: An old disease renewed. *West J Med* 1980;133:69 – 71.
126. Sergent JS, Christian CL: Necrotizing vasculitis after acute serous otitis media. *Ann Intern Med* 1974;81:195 – 199.
127. Klein JO: Management of acute and chronic otitis media, in Remington JS, Swartz MN (eds): *Current Clinical Topics in Infectious Diseases*. New York, McGraw-Hill Book Co, 1981, pp 278 – 294.
128. Klein JO: Otitis externa, otitis media, mastoiditis, in Mandell GL, Douglas RG, Bennett JE (eds): *Principles and Practice of Infectious Diseases*, ed 2. New York, John Wiley & Sons, 1985; pp. 364-369.
129. Goldberg MH, Topazian RG: Odontogenic infections and deep fascial space infections of dental origin, in Goldberg MH, Topazian RG (eds): *Management of Infections of the Oral and Maxillofacial Regions*. Philadelphia, WB Saunders Co, 1981, pp 173 – 231.
130. Topazian RG: Osteomyelitis of the Jaws, in Goldberg MH, Topazian RG (eds): *Management of Infections of the Oral* and *Maxillofacial Regions*. Philadelphia, WB Saunders Co, 1981, pp 232 – 266.
131. Cogen RB, Stevens AW, Cohen-Cole S, et al: Leukocyte function in the etiology of acute necrotizing ulcerative gingivitis. *J Periodontol* 1983;54:402 – 407.
132. Newman MG: Anaerobic oral and dental infections. *Rev Infect Dis* 1984;6 (suppl 1):S107 – S114.
133. McCurdy JA, MacInnis EL, Hays LL: Fatal mediastinitis after a dental infection. *J Oral Surg* 1977;35:726 – 729.

7

Atypical Pneumonias

Paul N. Gobbo
Burke A. Cunha

Although the majority of infectious pneumonias in the elderly, both community-acquired and nosocomial, are caused by the more common bacterial pathogens, not infrequently one of the atypical pneumonia agents may be responsible. The recognition of atypical pneumonias in the aged population is especially important, since many of the responsible organisms will not respond to those antibiotics used empirically for the more common bacterial pneumonias. The atypical agents may cause severe pulmonary disease in the elderly, many of whom already have a diminished respiratory reserve.[1] Thus early appropriate antibiotic therapy is especially crucial in the elderly, since they usually tolerate the added insult poorly.[2]

The atypical pneumonias originally included those nonbacterial agents which failed to respond to routine antibiotic therapy (ie, penicillin or sulfonamides), and included *Mycoplasma pneumoniae*, *Chlamydia psittaci* (psittacosis), and *Coxiella burnetii* (Q fever). Since then, additional atypical agents have been added, including *Francisella tularensis* (tularemia), viruses (mainly influenza virus A and B, respiratory syncytial virus, parainfluenza virus, and adenovirus), and most recently, *Legionella pneumophila* (Legionnaires' disease) and *Legionella micdadei* (Pittsburgh pneumonia agent)[3] *Chlamydia trachomatis*, a known cause of neonatal pneumonitis, may also cause atypical pneumonia in the adult. Of all these agents, the elderly patient is especially predisposed to development of influenza pneumonia and Legionnaires' disease, while the others occur far less commonly.[4]

The presence of an atypical pneumonia should be suspected when certain clinical features are present (Table 7-1). In general, the atypical

**Table 7-1
Differential Features of Typical and
Atypical Pneumonias**

Clinical Features	Typical Pneumonia	Atypical Pneumonia
Onset	Abrupt	Gradual
Fever > 103°F	Common	Less common
Chills	Common	Uncommon
Pleuritic pain	Common	Uncommon
Relative bradycardia	Uncommon	Common
Sputum		
Volume	Abundant	Minimal
Character	Purulent	Thin, mucoid
Gram stain	Many organisms	Few or no organisms
Chest radiograph	Pleural-based consolidation	Perihilar, interstitial infiltrates
Response to betalactam antibiotics	Good	Little or none*

*Except *Legionella micdadei*.

pneumonias have a more insidious onset, frequently with several days of mild prodromal upper respiratory tract symptoms such as coryza, rhinorrhea, and sore throat, as well as other nonspecific systemic complaints such as low-grade fever, malaise, headache, myalgias, and arthralgias.[5] While disease is mild in most patients, the elderly tend to be more severely affected. Certain occupational, environmental, or epidemiologic exposure factors may also suggest an atypical pneumonia. Occasionally, there may be various extrapulmonary findings (eg, rashes, prominent gastrointestinal symptoms) which should make one consider an unusual etiology. Sputum production, though generally scanty, when present will demonstrate polymorphonuclear leukocytes (PMNs) with either no bacteria (ie, "sterile sputum") or no predominant microorganism. The chest roentgenogram frequently reveals an infiltrate which is more extensive than one would expect from the physical findings, and the presence of interstitial infiltrates, especially radiating from the lung hila, should suggest an atypical pneumonia. The presence of pleural-based infiltrates, especially with an associated pleural effusion, is more likely to be due to a typical bacterial pneumonia. Finally, failure of resolution of pneumonia, or more importantly progression of pneumonic disease, while on betalactam agents, should prompt an immediate search for an atypical pneumonia agent.[6]

When an atypical pneumonia occurs in a young adult, the clinical features are usually sufficiently dissimilar from bacterial pneumonia to allow accurate presumptive diagnosis. In the elderly though, even typical pneumonias have an insidious onset, with fever, malaise, and mental status changes being the prominent findings.[7] The febrile response and pulmonary defense mechanism are impaired in the elderly.[8] Physical signs of consolidation may be absent, and the elderly patient may not be able to produce or expectorate the grossly purulent sputum which is characteristic of bacterial pneumonias.[9] The chest film also tends to be more variable and atypical in the older patient, and this problem is further compounded by the high prevalence of underlying chronic obstructive pulmonary disease and congestive heart failure, which will further diminish the diagnostic value of chest radiographs.[10] Thus those features which usually help the clinician to make an early presumptive differentiation between bacterial and atypical pneumonia in the younger patient are obscured in the elderly because of physiologic and pathologic changes attendant on advanced age.

Discernment of the less common atypical pneumonias in the older patient is frequently difficult, and requires a high index of suspicion if an early diagnosis is to be made. The procurement of an acute phase serum early in the disease process is usually warranted to allow later diagnosis of the atypical pneumonia, which because of its infrequency and difficulty to culture, may be the only method of definitive diagnosis. Such diagnosis, though, is purely retrospective and will not aid the patient acutely, but is of epidemiologic value. The diagnosis of certain atypical pneumonias, especially influenza, can generally be presumed if a patient has consistent clinical findings during a known community epidemic.[11]

Although the setting and clinical findings generally allow accurate presumptive diagnosis and thus institution of appropriate therapy, occasionally the clinician will be unable to narrow the etiologic possibilities in a case of atypical pneumonia (Table 7-2). In such a situation, empiric therapy should cover all reasonable diagnostic possibilities, and a parenteral tetracycline (eg, doxycycline) will provide coverage against all the traditional atypical pneumonia agents, as well as *Legionella* and *Chlamydia*.

Table 7-2
Empiric Therapy for Atypical Pneumonias in the Elderly

Pneumonia	Antimicrobial Agent	
	First choice	Second choice
Legionella pneumophila	Erythromycin	Tetracycline
Legionella micdadei	Erythromycin	Tetracycline
Mycoplasma	Tetracycline	Erythromycin
Psittacosis	Tetracycline	Chloremphenicol
Q fever	Tetracycline	Chloremphenicol
Tularemia	Streptomycin	Tetracycline
Chlamydia trachomatis	Tetracycline	Erythromycin

LEGIONELLA PNEUMOPHILA

Legionnaires' disease is caused by *Legionella pneumophila*, a fastidious, pleomorphic gram-negative bacillus first isolated following the Philadelphia epidemic in 1976, though serologic evidence has demonstrated that outbreaks had occurred for many years previously.[12,13] The organism may be found in soil, especially in close association with bodies of water, and is worldwide in distribution. Outbreaks have been associated with exposure to construction sites, where airborne spread is facilitated.[14] The hydrophilic nature of *L pneumophila* is also responsible for the occurrence of outbreaks in association with contaminated air-conditioner cooling towers and hospital shower heads, both of which result in nosocomial Legionnaires' disease.[15] Epidemic outbreaks generally occur in the late summer or early autumn, while sporadic cases occur all year long with slight clustering in the summer season.[16] (Table 7-3).

The precise incidence of community-acquired Legionnaires' disease is not known, since several studies report a wide range of results.[17] Factors responsible for this uncertainty include differences in the population studied, methods used, time of year when the study was done, and the geographical location. A recent report by Yu et al disclosed Legionnaires' disease as the most common pathogen causing community-acquired pneumonia, though this prospective study was apparently done at the time of an outbreak in an endemic area.[18] In general though, most authorities agree that the incidence of Legionnaires' disease is frequently underestimated.[11] Although Legionnaires' disease is responsible for less than 10% of cases of nosocomial pneumonia, higher rates have been noted in association with point source outbreaks.

Table 7-3
Diagnostic Features of Legionnaires' Disease

1. Association with hospitals, hotels, water supplies, or immunosuppression
2. Pneumonitis with multisystemic abnormalities
3. High nonremitting fever with recurrent rigors
4. Nonproductive cough (initially)
5. Relative bradycardia
6. Sputum with polymorphonuclear leukocytes but no organisms; normal flora
7. Rapid progression of nodular or consolidative infiltrates (asymmetrical)
8. Suggestive laboratory studies:
    a. Abnormal liver function tests
    b. Lowered serum phosphorus
    c. Elevated serum creatine phosphokinase levels
    d. No significant cold agglutinin titer
9. Poor response to betalactam agents, aminoglycosides

Legionnaires' disease occurs in all ages, with the median age in epidemics being about 56 years, while nosocomial outbreaks tend to affect an older age group. Predisposing factors have been associated with up to two thirds of cases, and especially includes smokers. Other significant underlying conditions have included neoplasms, renal transplantation, rheumatologic diseases, corticosteroid therapy, cardiac disease, pulmonary disease (including chronic obstructive pulmonary disease), renal disease, diabetes mellitus, and alcohol abuse.[19] Experimental evidence has indicated that alveolar macrophages and the cell-mediated immune system are crucial in the host defense against *L pneumophila*.[20] The age-related attenuation of T cell function in the elderly would theoretically make them more susceptible to this intracellular pathogen.[8] The increased occurrence of Legionnaires' disease in smokers and patients on steroid therapy, which suppress pulmonary alveolar macrophage function and the cell-mediated immune response, would appear to support this. Thus the elderly population is at marked risk for the development of Legionnaires' disease, and clinical studies have shown that those over 60 years of age have a twofold increased risk of acquiring pneumonia.[12]

Infection with *L pneumophila* may present in three different forms: (1) asymptomatic infection, (2) Pontiac fever, and (3) acute pneumonia. Asymptomatic infection, which is detectable only by seroconversion, was found to occur at a rate of 0.8% in one study, though other studies have noted seroprevalence rates up to 50%.[21] Thus asymptomatic infection may be very common. Pontiac fever, a nonpneumonic form of Legionnaires' disease which occurs in epidemics only, is associated with a high attack rate (about 90%), a short incubation period (about 36 hours), and no mortality. The clinical illness is mild and self-limited, usually beginning abruptly with malaise and generalized headache and myalgias, rapidly progressing to fever and chills. Although a dry cough commonly occurs, other pulmonary symptoms are rare. Chest films are always negative, and the acute illness generally lasts no more than five days, though weakness may persist. Pontiac fever is uncommon, and is usually suspected when there is a sudden outbreak of flulike illness which can be traced to a common source, often water-associated. Sporadic cases may occur, but are extremely difficult to differentiate from other self-limited febrile diseases, especially influenza, which would be the most likely diagnosis in the elderly.[22,23]

Pneumonia is the most frequent clinical expression of infection with *L pneumophila*, and may vary from a mild illness not requiring hospitalization to a fulminant, fatal pneumonitis. Although the individual clinical features of Legionnaires' disease are not pathognomonic, the full clinical picture is frequently sufficiently distinct as to suggest the diagnosis. Legionnaires' disease should always be considered in an elderly patient presenting with pneumonia, especially with a history of smoking, emphysema, or chronic bronchitis.[23] Onset is often insidious, with malaise, weakness, headache, or anorexia. Rapidly rising fever follows, associated with chills in about 75% of cases. The high fever is often poorly responsive to antipyretics, and even patients on corticosteroids will manifest high fever. A moderate cough is an early manifestation, and may be productive of small amounts of mucoid or mucopurulent sputum. Mild hemoptysis occurs in 20% to 40% of patients, while pleuritic chest pain is found in about 30% to 40% of cases.[17]

Extrapulmonary symptoms are characteristic of Legionnaires' disease, and most typically include a watery, nonsanguinous diarrhea, occasionally with nausea and emesis. Nonfocal neurologic findings, mainly headache and altered mental status, are common and suggest a diffuse toxic encephalopathy.[24] Physical findings typically include a relative bradycardia in ≥ two thirds of cases, while pulmonary signs vary from a few rales to overt consolidation. The chest roentgenogram, though not pathognomonic for Legionnaires' disease, frequently demon-strates infiltrates which are more extensive than would be predicted from the physical examination, as is common with most of the atypical pneumonias. Early radiographic findings include asymmetrical diffuse patchy infiltrates or poorly marginated rounded densities which typically expand to involve the entire lung or become bilateral in a lobar-segmental pattern. Pleural effusions are unusual, and small when present, while cavitation is rare.[4,25,26]

Laboratory studies in a patient with Legionnaires' disease reveal a number of abnormalities, none of which are pathognomonic and many of which may be due to other underlying conditions prevalent in the elderly. Certain findings in the appropriate clinical setting, however, should alert the clinician to the possibility of Legionnaires' disease and prompt the procurement of more specific diagnostic tests. Gram stain of expectorated sputum or transtracheal aspirate typically demonstrates moderate amounts of PMNs with no organisms. A peripheral leukocytosis is common. Mild proteinuria, microscopic hematuria, and moderate elevations of BUN and serum creatinine are also frequent, as are mild transient elevations of bilirubin, hepatic transaminases, and alkaline phosphatase. Hyponatremia, possibly due to inappropriate secretion of antidiuretic hormone, and hypophosphatemia may occur. Arterial blood gases generally reflect hypoxia and hypercarbia reflective of the severity of disease. Occasionally, cross-reacting mycoplasma serology (complement fixation) has been noted.[4,27]

Confirmation of Legionnaires' disease is most rapidly achieved by direct fluorescent antibody staining of pulmonary secretions or tissue, which will be positive in about half of those with infection. Detection of L pneumophila antigens in sputum or urine may eventually become available, and would greatly expedite the diagnosis. Isolation by culture on charcoal yeast extract agar yields results in two to six days in about 50%, while blood cultures are infrequently positive. A single serologic titer of 1:256 or greater is good presumptive evidence of Legionnaires' disease, though a fourfold increase between acute and convalescent specimens to a titer of 1:128 or greater is more specific. The convalescent specimen should be obtained 4 to 8 weeks after illness onset due to the typically delayed antibody response.[28]

Erythromycin is the drug of choice in the treatment of Legionnaires' disease, and in severe cases, rifampin may be added.[19] Early institution improves survival. In most cases, 4 g/day intravenously (IV) for 1−2 weeks followed by oral therapy for ⩾ 2 weeks is adequate. Relapses are rare and will generally respond to a repeated course. Despite in vitro evidence of a wide susceptibility to several agents, only the tetracyclines, preferably doxycycline, and trimethoprim-sulfamethoxazole (TMP-SMX), have proven useful in clinical settings.[29] In the DRG era, doxycycline (IV) is a more cost effective alternative to erythromycin and is associated with essentially no significant side effects (vs erythromycin with phlebitis, diarrhea, ototoxicity, and hepatotoxicity).[17] Full supportive measures, including nutritional supplements, discontinuance of corticosteroids, and correction of predisposing conditions are also important, especially in those with severe disease. Although most patients respond within two days, not infrequently fever may persist for up to a week. Improvement of the radiographic picture tends to lag. Overall mortality is 15% to 20%, but the prognosis is adversely affected by underlying illness, immunosuppression, advanced age, and delay in initiation of appropriate therapy. Common sequelae include persistent malaise and weakness for several weeks to months, and occasionally retrograde amnesia. Person-to-person spread of *Legionella* has not been documented, but this potential clearly exists.[4,26]

LEGIONELLA MICDADEI

In the wake of Legionnaires' disease, a group of closely related microorganisms, called *Legionella*-like organisms (LLO) have been identified.[30] Several of these organisms are pathogenic for man, but only *Legionella micdadei*, the Pittsburgh pneumonia agent (PPA), has been adequately studied. Pneumonia caused by *L micdadei* was originally described in immunosuppressed patients, especially renal transplant recipients.[31] Subsequently, infections in nonimmunocompromised hosts have been identified, and these may occur concurrently with Legionnaires' disease since both organisms share the same ecological niches.[32,33] Serologic evidence suggests that infection may be more widespread than anticipated.[34] Risk factors include immunosuppression, especially in patients on steroids, smoking, chronic pulmonary disease, malignancy, and alcoholism.[35] Other chronic diseases including heart, renal, hepatic, and diabetic, also predispose the patient to *L micdadei* infection, and virtually all will have some underlying predisposition. Almost 90% of cases are nosocomial, and the mean patient age is about 62 years.

The clinical presentation is similar to that of Legionnaires' disease with sudden onset of high fever, productive cough with dyspnea, and alteration of mental status. Pleuritic chest pain, diarrhea, and abdominal pain occur less frequently. The usual laboratory findings include sputum gram stain with neutrophils but no predominant organism, elevated hepatic enzymes in about three fourths, and hyponetremia is one third of cases. Acid-fastness has been reported. Although the radiographic picture is not distinctive, infiltrates are rapidly progressive, asymmetrical and may be segmental or lobar. The finding of rounded segmental infiltrates have been noted and may be an early clinical clue.[36] Rapid diagnosis may be achieved by direct fluorescent staining of sputum, pleural fluid, or lung tissue, with confirmation by culture from these same specimens. Seroconversion between acute and convalescent samples will yield a retrospective diagnosis.

The Pittsburgh pneumonia agent, unlike *L pneumophila*, does not produce a betalactamase and thus has a wider in vitro susceptibility pattern.[34] Despite this, erythromycin still appears to be the agent of choice, perhaps because of the drug's ability to achieve adequate intracellular levels. The combination of a betalactam agent and an aminoglycoside, commonly used for nosocomial pneumonias, is not effective against *L micdadei*, and a lack of response should suggest the possibility of Pittsburgh pneumonia. Even with appropriate therapy, mortality is about 50%, and is probably related to the high incidence of serious underlying disease especially in the very old. Other *Legionella* species have been reported in elderly patients with pneumonia.[17,36-38]

MYCOPLASMA PNEUMONIA

Mycoplasma pneumoniae, the etiologic agent of primary atypical pneumonia, is the major cause of pneumonia in adolescents and young adults, and has been considered unusual in persons over 40 years of age. Recent reports, however, have emphasized an increasing occurrence in older adults, and more importantly, infection in the elderly may be more severe, including adult respiratory distress syndrome (ARDS). Patients with chronic obstructive pulmonary disease appear to be more susceptible to infection by *M pneumoniae* and also tend to have increased morbidity. Spread of infection is slow, usually requiring close contact with an ill person, and usually occurs in an intrafamilial pattern. Thus, an elderly person living in a setting in prolonged exposure to school-aged children is probably at higher risk for acquiring *M pneumoniae*, though the attack rate is still low because of pre-existing immunity.[39,40]

Clinical mycoplasmal pneumonia is characterized by insidious onset of low-grade fever, headache, and malaise, frequently with a nonexudative pharyngitis, Myalgias, arthralgias, and bullous myringitis otitis may occasionally be noted, but a protracted nonproductive cough becomes the predominant symptom.[41] The chest roentgenogram most commonly reveals a patchy segmental bronchopneumonia or interstitial infiltrate in the lower lung fields, usually unilateral, with extension from the hilar region. Small effusions may occur in up to 25% of cases. Typically, the radiographic findings are discordant with the physical findings. Cold agglutinins develop in over half of cases, especially those with serious illness, by the end of the first week. Although nonspecific, a cold agglutinin titer greater than 1:64 is highly suggestive of *M pneumoniae*, and a rapid bedside test for cold hemagglutinins can be performed by observing agglutination in a 1-mL sample of anticoagulated blood placed in ice, which disassociates again at body temperature.[42] A positive test is indicative of a titer greater than or equal to 1:64. Definitive diagnosis, however, rests on a significant (fourfold) rise in specific antibody titer, usually by complement fixation, or by cultural isolation from sputum, throat swab, or tissue. Both serologic and cultural confirmation will be delayed, so early diagnosis depends heavily on the clinical picture. A single acute complement fixation titer greater than 1:64 is good evidence for infection with *M pneumoniae*, especially with a cold aggultinin titer $\geq$ to 1:64.[3]

Diagnostic difficulties may be encountered when either severe pulmonary disease or extrapulmonary manifestations occur, in which case many clinicians do not consider *M pneumoniae* as a possible cause, resulting in underdiagnosis. The older adult is especially prone to severe disease and the extrapulmonary complications can occur in all age groups.[43] Dermatologic findings attributable to *M pneumoniae* include maculopapular, vesicular, and urticarial rashes, as well as erythema multiforme, which may occur in severe form (Stevens-Johnson syndrome). Neurologic complications, mainly aseptic meningitis, meningoencephalitis, and a mononeuritis or polyneuritis, may occur in up to 10% of cases. Gastrointestinal abnormalities, manifested as anorexia, nausea, vomiting, diarrhea, and elevated hepatic enzymes may be prominent.[3,41] Hemolytic anemia may occur, especially with high cold agglutinin titers. Cardiac involvement is unusual, generally being manifested as ECG evidence of a myocarditis or pericarditis. Any of these extrapulmonary manifestations may occur with minimal or no evidence of respiratory disease; thus a mycoplasmal etiology is frequently not considered. In the older adult, most of these extrapulmonary features would usually be attributed to another cause, including as a complication of one of the many chronic illnesses prevalent in the aged population. Mycoplasmal pneumonia should be considered as a potential pulmonary pathogen in the elderly, especially in those with chronic pulmonary disease or who are not responding to cell wall–active agents. Antibiotics of choice are either erythromycin or a tetracycline, since absence of a cell wall renders beta-lactam agents ineffective.[44] Although recovery is the rule, resolution of symptoms and radiographic abnormalities may be delayed for several weeks.

ZOONOTIC PNEUMONIAS

The zoonotic pneumonias include those atypical pneumonias which are frequently, though not exclusively, associated with animal contact. The three classical organisms, *Coxiella burnetii* (Q fever), *Chlamydia psittaci* (psittacosis or ornithosis), and *Francisella tularensis* (tularemia), and *Yersinia pestis* (plague) are all exceedingly rare, possess definite epidemiologic associations, and harbor no special predilection for the elderly. In the absence of the proper occupational or environmental exposure, these pneumonias would be unusual. The aged population is generally at an overall decreased risk for infection by these agents, though participation of the retired elderly in outdoor leisure activities or in the care of pets should always be sought in the history of a patient with pneumonia. In contrast, *Pasteurella multocida*, which is most frequently associated with local wound infection secondary to cat or dog bites, has been identified as a cause of lower respiratory tract infection with a predilection for the elderly, having a median age of 69 years in one review.[45] Although animal exposure is frequent, up to 15% of cases have no known history of exposure. Individuals with chronic obstructive pulmonary disease may have colonization of the upper respiratory tract by *P multocida*, and pneumonia presumably occurs as a result of spread into the lower respiratory tract.[46]

The clinical picture of *P multocida* pneumonia is variable, usually resembling a typical bacterial pneumonia with fever, malaise, dyspnea, and a productive cough. The chest film generally reveals lobar pneumonia, though multilobar or patchy infiltrates have been noted.[45] Evidence of chronic pulmonary disease will be present in the majority, and the finding of gram-negative bacilli in the sputum smear in this setting may be erroneously interpreted as *Haemophilus influenzae* unless the typical bipolar staining characteristic is noted. Isolation from sputum or occasionally blood is usually not difficult. Penicillin G in high dose for ten to 14 days is the antimicrobial agent of choice, though tetracycline or doxycycline can also be used. Mortality is high, about one third of cases, and is related to the frequent occurrence of major complications, especially empyema or bacteremia with disseminated infection, as well as to the underlying pre-existent pulmonary disease.[45]

Tularemia in man occurs most often as a lymphocutaneous infection following either animal exposure (especially rabbits or hares) or tick or deer fly bites.[47] Thus, trappers, hunters, and campers are especially predisposed. Transmission by ingestion of contaminated water or meat is rare. Tularemic pneumonitis occurs in about 15% of cases, generally by hematogenous spread from the primary focus of infection, and occasionally by direct inhalation.[48] Pneumonia occurs in half of the typhoidal forms of tularemia, and in about 10% to 15% of the more common ulceroglandular syndrome. Tularemia generally begins with the acute onset of fever, chills, fatigue, and prostration, and development of pneumonia is characterized by a nonproductive cough. Radiographic findings usually include patchy infiltrates, occasionally associated with hilar adenopathy.[49] Bloody pleural effusions with a mononuclear pleocytosis may occur. Sputum gram stain and culture are invariably negative, with diagnostic confirmation dependent on serologic studies, especially a fourfold rise in agglutination titer. Streptomycin in a dose of 15–20 mg/kg/day intramuscularly (IM) for seven to ten days is the drug of choice, with close attention to the renal dysfunction prevalent in the older adult. Tetracycline or chloramphenicol, though less effective, are the usual alternative agents. Some reports have stressed the effectiveness of gentamicin and erythromycin.[50,51]

Q fever is an acute systemic rickettsial disease caused by the obligate intracellular bacterium *Coxiella burnetii*. The organism differs significantly from other rickettsial microbes by virtue of a negative Weil-Felix reaction, lack of arthrobud transmission, and absence of rash.[52] Domestic livestock serve as the reservoir of infection and humans acquire the disease by inhalation of airborne pathogens. Disease occurs mainly as an occupational hazard in abattoir workers, ranchers, farmers, veterinarians, and rarely in laboratory workers.[53] Clinically, characteristic features include sudden onset of severe headache, often retrobulbar, with high fever, chills, and myalgias.[54] Relative bradycardia and hepatosplenomegaly may be noted, but skin rashes are rare. Laboratory evidence of hepatitis is common.[52] Pneumonia occurs variably, characterized by minimal pulmonary symptoms but conspicuous multiple rounded, ground-glass infiltrates often in a hilar-fan pattern on chest radiograph.[3,55] Diagnosis is by serology, though a high index of suspicion is usually necessary. Tetracycline or chloramphenicol may be given, though there is no firm evidence that antibiotics alter the clinical course. Erythromycin may be effective. Q fever pneumonitis tends to be benign and self-limited, though full recovery may be prolonged for several weeks, especially in the elderly patient.[55,56]

Chlamydia psittaci is found worldwide in most avian species, including domestic fowl.[57] Disease in humans, referred to either as psittacosis or ornithosis, occurs sporadically and generally requires exposure to birds, though such exposure need not be close or prolonged.[52] Up to 20% of cases are not associated with a known avian source. Although the organism is acquired by inhalation, pulmonary involvement actually occurs by hematogenous spread from the reticuloendothelial cells of the spleen and liver, where initial replication occurs.

Psittacosis is a systemic disease with a variable clinical presentation, but the lung is the most commonly involved site.[58] Onset following a 1- to 2-week incubation period is usually acute, with high fever, chills, and prominent headache and myalgias, especially of the neck and back, though a more insidious course can occur. A persistent nonproductive cough is frequent, but pleuritic pain is unusual. The patient may complain of sore throat, epistaxis, or photophobia, while gastrointestinal (GI) symptoms are less frequent. Common physical findings include tachypnea, relative bradycardia, splenomegaly in up to 70% of cases, and nontender hepatomegaly. An evanescent maculopapular facial rash (Horder's spots) may occasionally be noted.[3,52] Complications include dyspnea and cyanosis in severe cases of pneumonitis, encephalitis, myocarditis, pericarditis, hepatitis, and pancreatitis. Thrombophlebitic problems may be seen during convalescence. The chest radiograph generally reveals patchy reticular infiltrates extending into the lower lung fields from the hilar region, though lobar consolidative changes can occur. The radiographic picture is typically worse than the physical examination would suggest.[58]

The diagnosis of psittacosis should be considered in the patient with an atypical pneumonia who has an avian exposure history, severe headache or myalgias, relative bradycardia, and splenomegaly. Confirmation requires a fourfold rise in specific complement-fixing antibodies to a reciprocal titer of 1:32 or higher, and is the preferred method of diagnosis since isolation by culture is hazardous. Tetracycline generally produces a prompt response, though slow defervescence and relapses are not infrequent. The prognosis with appropriate therapy is excellent, with a mortality rate below 1%.[52]

Although plague is exceedingly rare, an upsurge of cases in the American Southwest has been noted over the past decade.[59] An endemic reservoir persists in small wild mammals, especially wild rodents, and although most cases occur within these endemic regions, travelers through these areas account for up to 5% of cases, and tend to have a higher mortality due to delayed diagnosis.[60] Most cases occur in persons under the age of 20 years. Cats have been implicated in several cases.[61] Bubonic plague accounts for 90% to 95% of cases, typically presenting with high fever, rigors, and regional lymphadenopathy. Pneumonic plague develops in only a minority (less than 5%), but mortality is high.[62] Furthemore, such cases of secondary pneumonic plague can initiate a cycle of airborne primary pneumonic plague. The mitral clinical and radiographic presentations may be subtle, and bloody sputum is common. Diagnosis should be suspected in a person with the appropriate clinical syndrome with an epidemiologic exposure history. Early treatment (within 24 hours) using streptomycin is lifesaving, with tetracycline being an alternative. Strict isolation is required for the pneumonic patient.[62]

CHLAMYDIA TRACHOMATIS

Pneumonitis due to *Chlamydia trachomatis* has long been recognized as a distinctive clinical entity in the newborn, and recent evidence has suggested a causative role for this agent in atypical pneumonia in the adult.[63] Prospective studies of pneumonia frequently demonstrate a substantial number of cases undiagnosable by culture or serology, and *C trachomatis* could conceivably be responsible for a number of these cases. One prospective study of 27 cases of atypical pneumonia over a 1-year period revealed two cases of chlamydial pneumonitis.[64] Tack et al reported on six cases of chlamydial pneumonia, all of whom were compromised hosts.[4] Interestingly, the two elderly patients, who were in their seventies, had chronic bronchitis, with one on steroids, and the other afflicted with diabetes mellitus.

Serologic evidence for community-acquired chlamydial pneumonia in nonimmunocompromised hosts was presented by Komaruff et al.[63] Although the number of reported cases are insufficient to construct a typical clinical picture, the resultant pneumonitis would seem to approximate an atypical pattern. Fever, chills, productive cough, and myalgias have been noted, and the chest radiograph may involve more than one lobe with diffuse, hazy nonsegmental infiltrates. The source of chlamydia is not clear, though chlamydial pharyngitis has been described and could act as the origin.[65] If future studies confirm *C trachomatis* as an etiologic agent of atypical pneumonitis in the adult, the importance and incidence of infection in the elderly needs to be discerned, since therapy with beta-lactam agents is ineffective. Tetracycline/doxycycline would be preferred.

VIRAL PNEUMONIA

Viruses, as primary agents of pneumonia in the nonimmunocompromised host, occur more frequently in the pediatric age group. In adults, only influenza virus has been consistently implicated as a cause of primary viral pneumonia, with adenovirus, respiratory syncytial virus (RSV), parainfluenza virus, and the enteroviruses accounting for a far smaller proportion of cases. The importance of viral respiratory infection is especially evident in the elderly, particularly in regard to influenza, since this patient population bears a disproportionately greater proportion of the associated morbidity and mortality.[66] Furthermore, viral respiratory infections predispose the patient to subsequent secondary bacterial pneumonia.[67]

The viral agents of pneumonia produce an atypical pneumonia syndrome when the lower respiratory tract becomes primarily involved. A prodromal period of upper respiratory tract symptoms frequently precedes the onset of pneumonitis in many cases, and may be prolonged. Extrapulmonary manifestations of infection, such as headache, myalgias, arthralgias, anorexia, weakness, and malaise, are usually prominent with viral illness. The epidemiologic setting, such as the season or occurrence in closed populations, is important in recognition of a viral etiology. Further evidence for a viral pneumonia includes scanty sputum production, and diffuse interstitial infiltrates on the chest radiograph, usually bilateral in distribution, with radiation from the perihilar areas and sparing of the peripheral lung fields.[68]

Influenza, perhaps more than any other infectious disease, has been closely associated with the elderly. The influenza viruses, RNA viruses of the orthomyxovirus group, are separated into three distinct serotypes (A, B, and C) on the basis of nucleoprotein polypeptides. Influenza A is the most virulent, and is the cause of pandemics and major epidemics of influenza.[69] Antigenic variation of the two surface glycoproteins, hemagglutinin and neuraminidase, are responsible for recurring waves of influenza. Minor antigenic variation (antigenic drift), probably due to point mutations, occurs frequently and is responsible for the nearly annual occurrence of winter epidemics. Incomplete immunity to this new stain results in mild disease. Major antigenic variation (antigenic shift) due to genetic recombination occurs only every 10 to 15 years or more, but results in widespread pandemics since the majority of the population bears no immunity.[70] Alterations in the hemagglutinin are probably most important, since this antigen changes frequently and is responsible for viral attachment to respiratory epithelial cells.[71]

The epidemiologic features of influenza A, though characteristic, are highly variable due to the propensity of the virus to undergo antigenic change in an unpredictable fashion.[70] Attack rates and morbidity are highest in the young, who are least immune. However, severe complications and death are more common in those over the age of 65 years.[72] Epidemic influenza occurs annually during the winter months, initially noted by a surge of acute febrile respiratory disease in children, followed by similar illness in adults, and culminating in increased hospitalizations. At this point, excess mortality becomes apparent, which serves as a reliable indicator of the presence of an influenza epidemic in the community.[73] Although patients over the age of 45 years account for only 13% of all influenza isolates, they are responsible for half of all influenza-related hospitalizations and about 95% of all influenza-related deaths.[74] In one prospective study of patients hospitalized with pneumonia and influenza syndrome, there was an overall mortality rate of 12%, with 68% of fatal cases occurring in patients over the age of 65 years.[75] Close to 95% of nonsurvivors had underlying chronic cardiac or pulmonary disease, and the highest mortality was observed in those cardiac patients who also had either diabetes mellitus or pulmonary disease. However, even the otherwise healthy elderly have increased rates of hospitalization and pneumonia following influenza.[76] In the nursing home setting, influenza A can be devastating, with a 25% attack rate and 30% mortality reported in one outbreak.[77]

In most individuals, influenza causes a mild, self-limited upper respiratory tract infection characterized by abrupt onset of fever with chills, nonproductive cough, mild substernal chest pain, frontal headache, and myalgias.[78] Prostration disproportionate to the degree of illness is common, and the presence of ocular symptoms and flushed facies distinguishes influenza from other viral etiologies.[11] The entire clinical course of uncomplicated influenza generally lasts no more than seven days, though the elderly may occasionally have protracted malaise and weakness (postinfluenzal asthenia).

The influenza virus is a primary respiratory tract pathogen which rapidly attacks and causes sloughing of ciliated epithelial cells. This leads to defective mucociliary function with resultant inability to clear secretions, and thus to obstruction of the lower respiratory tract.[67] Abnormal pulmonary function testing, with poor gas exchange and an increase in peripheral airway resistance, has been noted even in those without obvious lower tract involvement, and such defects may be persistent.[79] Thus the elderly patient who may already suffer some degree of age-related pulmonary dysfunction would be particularly predisposed to the respiratory complications of influenza. Indeed, in the elderly, the typical features of influenza may be overshadowed by the effects of hypoxia, eg, confusion, stupor, coma, or heart failure.

The major complication of influenza is pneumonia, and the incidence of pneumonia may increase twofold during major influenza A epidemics.[80] Infection with influenza virus impairs the host's immune system, thus predisposing the individual to bacterial superinfection. Defective alveolar macrophage function has been noted, and this may also have a secondary effect on T cell function, resulting in defective intracellular killing of bacteria and thus predisposing to secondary bacterial invasion.[81,82] Studies of skin test reactivity in patients with influenzalike illness have demonstrated anergy only in those actually infected with influenza.[83] In combination with the age-related T cell dysfunction, the elderly would be especially prone to bacterial superinfection. Defective polymorphonuclear leukocyte phagocytic activity due to an unknown mechanism has also been noted following influenza infection.[84]

Louria et al have described four types of lower respiratory tract involvement with influenza.[85] The most common, accounting for half of cases, is secondary bacterial pneumonia, which is characterized by a classic influenza illness followed by a one- to four-day period of apparent clinical recovery, and then marked by the recrudescence of fever in association with a cough productive of purulent sputum, pleuritic chest pain, and often rigors. Focal consolidation consistent with a bacterial pneumonia will be seen on chest radiographs. Although *Streptococcus pneumoniae* is the most common pathogen, *Staphylococcus aureus*, an otherwise rare pulmonary pathogen, occurs frequently in the postinfluenzal setting.[86] *Haemophilus influenzae* may also be seen. Important risk factors include chronic obstructive pulmonary disease, chronic heart disease, and diabetes mellitus. Thus the elderly, who bear a disproportionate amount of these chronic illnesses, are especially predisposed to postinfluenzal bacterial pneumonia with its attendant high mortality.[87]

A smaller percentage of patients may develop primary influenza pneumonia.[85] Major risk factors are chronic heart disease, especially rheumatic mitral stenosis, as well as chronic pulmonary disease and pregnancy. Clinically, there is progression of fever with nonproductive cough, marked dyspnea, and cyanosis after a week of influenzalike illness. Tachypnea is an important early indication of lower respiratory tract infection in the elderly.[88] The chest film is characteristic of an atypical pneumonia, with diffuse, nodular interstitial infiltrates radiating from the hilar regions. Blood gases reveal severe hypoxia, while many PMNs but no organisms would be evident on sputum gram stain. Sputum viral culture yields influenza A in high titer. Unlike secondary bacterial pneumonia, there is no response to antibiotic therapy, and none should be given in the absence of bacterial superinfection, since premature therapy will select a more resistant bacteria. Therapy of primary influenza pneumonia is supportive, and mortality is very high.[71]

Simultaneous viral and bacterial pneumonia may occur occasionally, and has a highly variable clinical presentation. Patients with chronic pulmonary disease are at risk, and most typically present with persistence of fever and worsening of respiratory status following several days of influenzalike illness. Cough productive of purulent sputum is usual, culture of which will yield both influenza virus and a predominant bacterial pathogen, with the same bacterial etiologic spectrum as for postinfluenzal pneumonia. There may be some response to antibiotic therapy. The fourth and least common form of influenzal involvement of the lower respiratory tract is the "bronchiolitic" form, characterized by the physical findings of pneumonia, but with a chest film devoid of infiltrates.[85] Influenza B, though usually associated with respiratory disease in children, is capable of causing severe illness in adults, though pneumonia is rare.[89] The elderly have been noted to be highly susceptible in both the hospital and institutional setting, with high attack rates but minimal mortality.[90,91]

Vaccination of susceptible individuals at high risk for complications of influenza is effective, resulting in reduced attack rates, an amelioration of the severity of infection, and a decreased incidence of complications. Overall efficacy approximates 75%, though lower response rates have been noted in the elderly.[92,93] Despite their poorer serologic response, reductions in hospitalization rates by 72% and mortality rates by 87% has been demonstrated in the noninstitutionalized vaccinated elderly.[94] The nonvaccinated state has been identified as a risk factor for acquisition of influenza A by the elderly in one study.[95] In a nursing home outbreak of influenza A, recent vaccination afforded a 46.6% efficacy rate, while those residents vaccinated 1 year previously were only minimally protected.[66] The antigen content was doubled in 1981 to boost antibody response in the elderly, and further efforts are required to increase the delivery to susceptible elderly, since no more than 20% of those at risk received the vaccine.[96]

The vaccine should be given annually in the fall to those at high risk, with one subcutaneous dose being sufficient. Three levels of risk have been established: (1) persons with chronic pulmonary or cardiac disease and nursing home residents, (2) health care providers who have extensive contact with high-risk patients, and (3) all healthy persons over the age of 65 years, as well as those under 65 who have chronic disease, ie, diabetes mellitus, renal disease, anemia, immunosuppression, or asthma. Egg allergy is the only contraindication. Minor discomfort at the injection site occurs in about half of vaccine recipients, but systemic side effects develop in fewer than 1% to 2%. Guillain-Barré syndrome occurred only in association with the swine-flu vaccination program of 1976. Vaccination of those over the age of 65 years has been found to be cost-effective.[93,97,98]

Amantidine hydrochloride is effective in both the treatment and chemoprophylaxis of influenza A, preventing widespread parenchymal involvement by an unknown mechanism.[99,100] In the treatment of influenza, early administration (within 48 hours of onset) will diminish severity of illness in half of cases, and should be given for three to five days only. When used prophylactically, amantidine has a 75% to 90% efficacy rate, though this drug is not recommended for general use or as a substitute for vaccination. Amantidine should be used in an individual in whom vaccination is contraindicated (eg, allergy, severe reaction), when the vaccine may be relatively inefficacious (eg, major antigenic change, immunosuppression), as an adjunct in a vaccinated person with an exceedingly high risk for severe complications, or for hospital or institutional staff members to prevent or limit nosocomial outbreak. Administration for only 5 to 7 weeks is required. A susceptible individual may receive vaccine and amantidine simultaneously, with the latter continued for 2 weeks, at which time a protective antibody response should have occurred.[97] Rimantidine, a related compound with rare side effects, may soon become the agent of choice in chemoprophylaxis of influenza A.[101]

Although many viral agents other than influenza A or B may cause acute pneumonia in the adult, only adenovirus has been implicated commonly, and then mainly in the crowded military barracks setting, where extensive spread among a susceptible population is facilitated.[102] Other viruses occasionally responsible for pneumonia in the adult include parainfluenza virus, RSV, enteroviruses, and rhinovirus in the normal host, while varicella zoster virus, cytomegalovirus, and Epstein-Barr virus may cause pneumonitis in the immunocompromised host. Illness caused by these pathogens is usually restricted to the upper respiratory tract, presenting with symptoms typical of the common cold. When primary viral pneumonia occurs, the presentation is that of an atypical pneumonia with diffuse interstitial pulmonary infiltrates. Although diagnosis requires cultural or serologic confirmation, the epidemiologic setting and assocated extrapulmonary findings will often suggest the etiologic agent.

The majority of these noninfluenza respiratory viruses have no special predilection for the elderly, except perhaps for RSV.[103] Although predominantly a pediatric pathogen, bronchopneumonia in the institutionalized elderly due to RSV has been reported, including a concurrent outbreak with influenza A.[104] Severe bronchopneumonia developed in nearly half of the elderly residents of a nursing home who became infected with the RSV in one report.[105] Chronic obstructive pulmonary disease is a major predisposition. The RSV, like the influenza virus, predisposes the patient to subsequent bacterial pneumonia, and the major cause of lower respiratory tract involvement may well be due to secondary bacterial invasion.

REFERENCES

1. Ohar S, Shastri SR, Lenora RAK: Aging and the respiratory system. *Med Clin North Am* 1976;60:1121–1139.
2. Weitekamp MR, Aber RC: Nonbacterial and unusual pneumonias in the elderly. *Geriatrics* 1984;39:87–100.
3. Cunha BA, Quintiliani R: The atypical pneumonias. *Postgrad Med* 1979;66:95–102.
4. Gardner P, Arnow PM: Hospital-acquired pneumonias, in Braunwald E, Isselbacher K, Petersdorf RG, et al (eds): *Harrison's Principles of Internal Medicine*, ed 11. New York, McGraw-Hill Book Co, 1987, pp 470–474.
5. Donowitz GR, Mandell GL: Acute pneumonia, in Mandell GL, Douglas RG Jr, Bennett JE (eds): *Principles and Practice of Infectious Disease*, ed 2.

New York, John Wiley & Sons, 1985, pp 394–404.
6. File TM, Tan JS, Murphy DP: Atypical pneumonia syndrome. *Primary Care* 1981;8: 673–694.
7. Finkelstein MS: Unusual features of infection in the aging. *Geriatrics* 1982; 37:65–78.
8. Toews GB: Determinants of bacterial clearance from the lower respiratory tract. *Semin Respir Infect* 1986;1:68–78.
9. Verghese A, Berk SL: Bacterial pneumonia in the elderly. *Medicine* 1983;62: 271–285.
10. Horton JM, Pankey GA: Pneumonia in the elderly. *Postgrad Med* 1982;71: 114–123.
11. Douglas RG: Influenza: the disease and its complications. *Hosp Pract* 1976;11:43–50.
12. Cunha BA (ed): Legionnaires' disease. *Semin Respir Dis* 1987;2:189–279.
13. Thacker SB, Bennett JV, Tsai TF, et al: An outbreak in 1965 of severe respiratory illness caused by the Legionnaires' disease bacterium. *J Infect Dis* 1978;138:512–519.
14. Storch G, Baine WB, Fraser DW, et al: Sporadic community-acquired Legionnaires' disease in the United States: a case control study. *Ann Intern Med* 1979;90:596–600.
15. Meyer RD: Legionnaires' disease: aspects of nosocomial infection. *Am J Med* 1984;76:657–663.
16. England AC, Fraser DW, Plikaytis BD, et al: Sporadic legionellosis in the United States: the first thousand cases. *Ann Intern Med* 1981;94:164–170.
17. Cotton EM, Strampfer MJ, Cunha BA: *Legionella* and *Mycoplasma* pneumonia—a community hospital experience with atypical pneumonias. *Clin Chest Med* 1987;8:441–453.
18. Yu VL, Kroboth FJ, Shonnard J, et al: Legionnaires' disease: new clinical perspective from a prospective pneumonia study. *Am J Med* 1982;73:357–361.
19. Edelstein PH, Meyer RD: Legionnaires' disease: a review. *Chest* 1984;85: 114–120.
20. Horwitz MA, Silverstein SC: Legionnaires' disease bacterium (*Legionella pneumophila*) multiples intracellularly in human monocytes. *J Clin Invest* 1980;66:441–450.
21. Haley CE, Cohen ML, Halter J, et al: Nosocomial Legionnaires' disease: a continuing common source epidemic at Wadsworth Medical Center. *Ann Intern Med* 1979;90:583–586.
22. Palmer SR, Zamiri I, Ribeiro CD, Gajewska A: Legionnaires' disease cluster and reduction in hospital hot water temperatures. *Br Med J [Clin Res]* 1986;292:1494–1495.
23. Muder RR: Mode of transmission of *Legionella pneumophila*. A critical review. *Arch Intern Med* 1986;146:1607–1612.
24. Johnson JD, Raff MJ, VanArsdal JA: Neurologic manifestations of Legionnaires' disease. *Medicine* 1984;63: 303–310.
25. Power KJ: Intensive care aspects of severe *Legionella* pneumonia. *Anaesthesia* 1986;41:620–622.
26. Swartz MN: Clinical aspects of Legionnaires' disease. *Ann Intern Med* 1979;90:492–495.
27. Grady GF, Gilfillan RF: Relation of *Mycoplasma pneumoniae* seroreactivity, immunosuppression, and chronic disease to Legionnaires' disease. *Ann Intern Med* 1979;90:607–610.

28. Edelstein PH, Meyer RD, Finegold SM: Laboratory diagnosis of Legionnaires' disease. *Am Rev Respir Dis* 1980;121:317–327.
29. Cunha BA, Jonas M: Legionnaires' disease treated with doxycycline. *Lancet* 1981;1:1107.
30. Fraser DW: Bacteria newly recognized as nosocomial pathogens. *Am J Med* 1981;70:432–438.
31. Pasculle AW, Myerowitz RL, Rinaldo CR: New bacterial agent of pneumonia isolated from renal-transplant recipients. *Lancet* 1979;2:58–61.
32. Aronson MD, Komaroff AL, Pasculle AW, et al: *Legionella micdadei* (Pittsburgh pneumonia agent) infection in non-immunosuppressed patients with pneumonia. *Ann Intern Med* 1981;94:485–486.
33. Muder RR, Yu VL, Vickeus RM, et al: Stimultaneous infection with *Legionella pneumophila* and Pittsburgh pneu-monia agent. *Am J Med* 1983;74:609–614.
34. Muder RR, Yu VL, Zuravleff JJ: Pneumonia due to the Pittsburgh pneumonia agent: New clinical perspective with a review of the literature. *Medicine* 1983;62:120–128.
35. Yu VL, Zuravleff JJ, Eder EM, et al: Pittsburgh pneumonia agent may be a common cause of nosocomial pneumonia: seroepidemiologic evidence. *Ann Intern Med* 1982;97:724–726.
36. Gobbo PN, Strampfer MJ, Schoch P, et al: *Legionella micdadei* pneumonia in normal hosts. *Lancet* 1986;2:969.
37. Chunhaswasdikul B, Sukonthaman A, Lind K, Chinachoti T: *Legionella jordanis* pneumonia: a case report. *J Med Assoc Thai* 1986;2:108–114.
38. Cunha BA, Strampfer MJ, Schoch PE, et al: Empyema and *Legionella bozemanii*. *Ann Intern Med* 1986;105:626.
39. Clyde WA: Mycoplasma infections, in Braunwald E, Isselbacher K, Petersdorf RG, et al (eds): *Harrison's Principles of Internal Medicine,* ed 11. New York, McGraw-Hill Book Co, 1987, pp 757–759.
40. **Westerberg SC, Smith CB, Renzitti AD:** *Mycoplasma* infections in patients with chronic obstructive pulmonary disease. *J Infect Dis* 1973;127:491–497.
41. Levine DP, Lerner AM: The clinical spectrum of *Mycoplasma pneumoniae* infections. *Med Clin North Am* 1978;62:961–978.
42. Griffin JP: Rapid screening for cold agglutinins in pneumonia. *Ann Intern Med* 1969;70:701–705.
43. Murray HW, Masur H, Senterfit LB, et al: The protean manifestations of *Mycoplasma pneumoniae* infection in adults. *Am J Med* 1975;58:229–242.
44. Shames JM, George RB, Holliday WB, et al : Comparison of antibiotics in the treatment of mycoplasmal pneumonia. *Arch Intern Med* 1970;125:680–684.
45. Weber DJ, Wolfson JS, Swartz MN, et al: *Pasteurella multocida* infections: reported of 34 cases and review of the literature. *Medicine* 1984;63:133–154.
46. Berk SL, Ortega G, Kasprzyk D, et al: *Pasteurella multocida* pneumonia in an elderly patient. *J Am Geriatr Soc* 1984;32:618–620.
47. Boyce JM: *Francisella tularensis* (tularemia), in: Mandell GL, Douglas RG Jr, Bennett JE (eds): *Principles and Practice of Infectious Diseases*, ed 2. New York, John Wiley & Sons, 1985, pp 1290–1294.
48. Miller RP, Bates JH: Pleuropulmonary tularemia: a review of 29 patients. *Am Rev Respir Dis* 1969;99:31–41.
49. Dennis JM, Bondreau RP: Pleuropulmonary tularemia: its roentgen manifestations. *Radiology* 1957;68:25–30.
50. Mason WL, Egelsbach HT, Little SF, et al: Treatment of tularemia,

including pulmonary tularemia, with gentamicin. *Am Rev Respir Dis* 1980;121:39−45.
51. Westerman EL, McDonald J: Tularemia pneumonia mimicking Legionnaires' disease — isolation of organism on CYE agar and successful treatment with erythromycin. *South Med J* 1983;76:1169−1170.
52. Murray HW, Tuazon C: Atypical pneumonias. *Med Clin North Am* 1980;64:507−527.
53. Brown GL: Q fever. *Br Med J* 1973;2:41−43.
54. Huebner RJ, Jellison WL, Beck MD: Q fever: a review of current knowledge. *Ann Intern Med* 1949;30:495−509.
55. Millar JK: The chest film findings in Q fever: a series of 35 cases. *Clin Radiol* 1978;39:371−375.
56. Sienko DG, Bartlett PC, McGee HB, et al: Q fever. *Arch Intern Med* 1988;148:609-616.
57. Potter ME, Kaufman AF: Psittacosis in humans in the United States, 1975−1977. *J Infect Dis* 1979;140:131−134.
58. Schaffner W, Drutz DJ, Duncan GW, et al: The clinical spectrum of endemic psittacosis. *Arch Intern Med* 1967;119: 433−443.
59. Kaufman AF, Boyce JM, Martone WJ: Trends in human plague in the United States. *J Infect Dis* 1980;41:522−524.
60. Mann JM, Schmid GP, Stoesa PA, et al: Peripatetic plague. *JAMA* 1982;247: 47−48.
61. Werner SB, Weidmer CE, Nelson BC, et al: Primary plague pneumonia contracted from a domestic cat at South Lake Tahoe, Calif. *JAMA* 1984;251:929−931.
62. Butler T, Mahmoud AAF, Warren KS: Algorithms in the diagnosis and management of exotic diseases, XXV. Plague. *J Infect Dis* 1977;136:317−320.
63. Komaroff AL, Aronson MD, Schachter J: *Chlamydia trachomatis* infection in adults with community-acquired pneumonia. *JAMA* 1981;24:1319−1322.
64. Marrie TJ, Haldane EV, Noble MA, et al: Causes of atypical pneumonias results of a one-year prospective study. *Can Med Assoc J* 1981;125:1118−1123.
65. Komaroff AL, Aronson MD, Pass TM, et al: Serologic evidence of chlamydial and mycoplasmal pharyngitis in adults. *Science* 1983;22:927−929.
66. Budnick LD, Stricof RL, Ellis F: An outbreak of influenza A in a nursing home, 1982. *NY State J Med* 1984;84:235−238.
67. Loosli CG: Influenza and the interaction of viruses and bacteria in respiratory infections. *Medicine* 1973;152:369−384.
68. Reichman RC, Dolin R: Viral pneumonias. *Med Clin North Am* 1980;64:491−506.
69. Seneca H: Influenza: epidemiology, etiology, immunization and management. *J Am Geriatr Soc* 1980;28:241−250.
70. Langmuir AD, Schoenbaum SC: The epidemiology of in-fluenza. *Hosp Pract* 1976;11:49−56.
71. Douglas RG, Betts RF: Influenza virus, in Mandell GL, Douglas RG Jr, Bennett JE (eds): *Principles and Practice of Infectious Disease*, ed 2. New York, John Wiley & Sons, 1985, pp 846−866.
72. Glezen WP: Serious morbidity and mortality associated with influenza epidemics. *Epidemiol Rev* 1982;4:25−44.
73. Glezen WP, Payne AA, Snyder DN, et al: Mortality and influenza. *J Infect Dis* 1982;146:313−321.

74. Couch RB, Cate TR: Managing influenza in older patients. *Geriatrics* 1983;38:61–74.
75. Barker WH, Mullooly JP: Pneumonia and influenza deaths during epidemics implications for prevention. *Arch Intern Med* 1982;142:85–89.
76. Barker WH, Mullooly JP: Impact of epidemic type A influenza in a defined adult population. *Am J Epidemiol* 1980; 112:798–811.
77. Goodman RA, Orenstein WA, Munro TF, et al: Impact of influenza A in a nursing home. *JAMA* 1982;247:1451–1453.
78. Blumenfeld HL, Kilbourne ED, Louria DB, et al: Studies on influenza in the pandemic of 1957–1958. I. An epidemio-logic, clinical and serological investigation of an intrahospital epidemic, with a note on vaccination efficacy. *J Clin Invest* 1959;38:199–212.
79. Hall WJ, Douglas RG, Hyde RW, et al: Pulmonary mechanics after complicated influenza A infection. *Am Rev Respir Dis* 1976;113:141–147.
80. Foy HM, Cooney MK, Allan I, et al: Rates of pneumonia during influenza epidemics in Seattle, 1964 to 1975. *JAMA* 1978;241:253–258.
81. Warshauer D, Goldstein E, Akers T, et al: Effect of influenza viral infection on the ingestion and killing of bacteria by alveolar macrophages. *Am Rev Respir Dis* 1977;115:269–277.
82. Gardner ID: Suppression of antibacterial immunity by infection with influenza virus. *J Infect Dis* 1981;144:225–231.
83. Reed WP, Olds JW, Kisch AL: Decreased skin-test reactivity associated with influenza. *J Infect Dis* 1972;125:398–402.
84. Larson HE, Blades R: Impairment of human polymorpho-nuclear leukocyte function by influenza virus. 1976; *Lancet* 1:283.
85. Louria DB, Blumenfield HL, Ellis JT, et al: Studies on influenza in the pandemic of 1957–1958. II. Pulmonary complications of influenza. *J Clin Invest* 1959;38:213–265.
86. Schwarzmann SW, Adler JL, Sullivan RJ, et al: Bacterial pneumonia during the Hong Kong influenza epidemic of 1968–1969. *Arch Intern Med* 1971;127:1037–1041.
87. Alling DW, Blackwelder WC, Stuart-Harris CH: A study of excess mortality during influenza epidemics in the United States, 1968–1976. *Am J Epidemiol* 1981;113:30–43.
88. McFadden JP, Price RC, Eastwood HD, et al: Raised respiratory rate in elderly patients: a valuable physical sign. *Br Med J* 1982;284:626–627.
89. Baine WB, Luby JP, Martin SM: Severe illness with influenza B. *Am J Med* 1980;68:181–189.
90. Van Voris LP, Belshe RB, Shaffer JL: Nosocomial influenza B virus in the elderly. *Ann Intern Med* 1982;96:153–158.
91. Hall WN, Goodman RA, Noble GR, et al: An outbreak of influenza B in an elderly population. *J Infect Dis* 1981;144: 297–302.
92. Patriarca PA, Weber JA, Parker RA, et al: Efficacy of influenza vaccine in nursing homes. Reduction in illness and complications during an influenza A (H3N2) epidemic. *JAMA* 1985; 253:1136–1139.
93. Immunization Practices Advisory Committee. 1986–1987 Update on vaccine and antiviral agent available for control of influenza. *MMWR* 1986;35:1–9.
94. Barker WH, Mullooly JP: Influenza vaccination of elderly persons: reduction in pneumonia and influenza hospitalizations and deaths. *JAMA* 1980;244:2547–2549.
95. Mathur U, Bentley DW, Hall CB, et al: Influenza A/Brazil/78 (H1N1) infection in the elderly. *Am Rev Respir Dis* 1981;123: 633–635.

96. Ruben FL: Prevention of influenza in the elderly. *J Am Geriatr Soc* 1982;30:577–580.
97. Centers for Disease Control: Prevention and control of influenza. *MMWR* 1984;33:253–260, 265–266.
98. Riddiough MA, Sisk JE, Bell JC: Influenza vaccination: cost-effectiveness and public policy. *JAMA* 1983;249:3189–3195.
99. Van Voris LP, Betts RF, Hayden FG, et al: Successful treatment of naturally occurring influenza A/USSR/77 H1N1. *JAMA* 1981;245:1128–1131.
100. Dolin R, Reichamn RC, Madore HP, et al: A controlled trial of amantidine and rimantidine in the prophylaxis of influenza A infection. *N Engl J Med* 1982;307:580–584.
101. Patriarca PA, Kater NA, Kendal AP, et al: Safety of prolonged administration of rimantidine hydrochloride in the prophylaxis of influenza virus infections in nursing homes. *Antimicrob Agents Chemother* 1984;26:101–103.
102. Dudding BA, Wagner SC, Zeller JA, et al: Fatal pneumonia associated with adenovirus type 7 in three military trainees. *N Engl J Med* 1972;286:1289–1292.
103. Dolin R: Common viral respiratory infections, in Braunwald E, isselbacher K, Petersdorf RG, et al (eds): *Harrison's Principles of Internal Medicine*, ed 11. New York, McGraw-Hill Book Co, 1987, pp 677–681.
104. Mathur U, Bentley DW, Hall CB: Concurrent respiratory syncytial virus and influenza A infections in the institutionalized elderly and chronically ill. *Ann Intern Med* 1980;93:49–52.
105. Garrie DG, Gray J: Outbreak of respiratory syncytial virus infection in the elderly. *Br Med J* 1980;281:1253–1254.

8

Community-Acquired Pneumonia

Martin C. McHenry

Despite substantial progress, pneumonia continues to be a major public health problem, and a diagnostic and therapeutic pitfall for practicing physicians. More than 3 million cases occur in the United States each year.[1] Infections of lung increase in frequency as age advances and mortality rises correspondingly.[2-9] Pneumonia and influenza together constitute the fourth most common cause of death among the elderly.[10] Diagnosis is difficult because pneumonia often presents insidiously in the aged with a minimum of symptoms and signs, or it may masquerade as other pulmonary or extrapulmonary diseases.[6,11-19]

Organisms causing pneumonia in patients in the geriatric age group are often different from those causing the disease in younger persons.[20] Elderly patients are more likely than younger persons to experience unfavorable reactions to antimicrobial drugs.[21-24] Furthermore, geriatric patients are more at risk than younger persons for delay in resolution of pneumonia, empyema, bacteremia, and extrapulmonary complications.[6,8,9,17,25] Mortality and various complications increase when institution of appropriate therapy is delayed.[6-8]

Organisms causing pneumonia appear to be considerably different for patients with infections acquired in the community than for patients with infections contracted in the hospital.[26,27] This chapter is concerned with community-acquired pneumonia in elderly patients.

EARLY DESCRIPTIONS OF THE PROBLEM

Evidence of pneumonia has been found in Egyptian mummies of great antiquity, and in the writings of Hippocrates,[3] but our modern understanding of the condition began with the clinical and pathologic descriptions of Laennec in 1819.[3,28] In 1835 and 1836, Hourmann and Dechambre[29-33] published accounts of clinical and pathologic studies of pneumonia in elderly patients. Disease would often present insidiously with a paucity of signs and symptoms referable to the lungs. Sudden and unexpected death developed in some persons and pneumonia was first diagnosed at autopsy. Many years later, in the section on lobar pneumonia in a famous textbook of medicine, Osler provided a memorable description of the disease in the aged: "The disease may be latent and set in without chill; the cough and expectoration are slight, the physical signs ill-defined and changeable, and the constitutional symptoms out of all proportion to the extent of the local lesion."[34]

In 1946, Zeman and Wallach[6] reported a study of pneumonia in 166 patients over 60 years of age. The pneumococcus was the most frequent pathogen, but the cause was undetermined in a sizeable proportion of cases. Most patients were treated with a sulfonamide and some received penicillin G. The overall mortality was 20% and was considerably higher than the mortality in younger patients. There was a high incidence of underlying diseases of the heart, lungs, and CNS, nutritional deficiencies, and diabetes mellitus. These conditions often dominated the clinical picture, obscured the diagnosis of pneumonia, and limited the chances for survival. Complications such as recurrent pneumonia, pleural empyema, purulent meningitis, and bacterial endocarditis were not uncommon, and involvement of multiple pulmonary lobes was present in a majority of fatal cases.

Zeman and Wallach[6] described the unusual features of pneumonia in the aged. In some patients, pneumonia was unsuspected during life and discovered only at autopsy; in others, recognition was delayed by an afebrile clinical course or an insidious illness; and in still others, extrapulmonary manifestations directed attention initially away from the lungs. Especially misleading were signs and symptoms referred to the abdomen, an "apoplectiform" illness resembling a cerebrovascular accident, or a toxic psychosis making patients unmanageable. Equally challenging were stoical patients who did not complain and continued their usual activity until they collapsed and died; the authors noted that pneumonia was not an uncommon cause of sudden death in the elderly.[6,35] Physical signs were often unreliable or misleading, even when there was extensive pulmonary involvement. At times, the chest x-ray film findings were normal initially when clinical examination strongly suggested pneumonia, but when they were repeated at a later time, the diagnosis was confirmed.

In the years that elapsed since the study of Zeman and Wallach, many studies of pneumonia have been reported, but surprising few were concerned with the disease in the elderly per se. However, workers called attention to an increasing number of older patients with chronic diseases who required hospitalization for treatment of community-acquired pneumonia. The pneumococcus continued to be the most commonly identified etiologic organism,[36-57] but there was an increasing proportion of cases attributed to other pathogens.[20,46,47,58]

HOST ALTERATIONS PREDISPOSING TO PNEUMONIA

Limited information is available concerning factors which render the aged susceptible to pneumonia, and it is difficult to separate changes caused by aging per se from those due to the effects of associated disease.[59-61] Colonization of the oropharynx by pathogenic bacteria increases with age,[62,63] especially with a decline in an elderly person's mobility and with increasing debility.[63] Since most bacterial pneumonias begin with inhalation or aspiration into the lung of organisms present in the upper respiratory tract, this alteration of the oropharyngeal flora in the elderly may be an important first step in the pathogenesis of pneumonia.[64-66]

There is a decline in the efficiency of elimination of foreign material by the bronchi with increasing age,[59] and aged persons have a significantly slower mucociliary clearance than do younger adults.[67,68] Pulmonary function declines with age due to loss of elastic tissue surrounding alveoli and alveolar ducts, the increased anteriorposterior diameter of the chest, and the weakening of the respiratory muscles.[69,70] Weakness of the respiratory muscles may interfere with the efficiency of the cough reflex. A number of factors may predispose aged patients to aspiration, including disordered patterns of breathing, reduced levels of consciousness due to drugs or diseases of the CNS, and impairment of the lower esophageal sphincter.[69-71]

Function of T lymphocytes declines with increasing age, and antibody responses to new antigens are diminished.[60,72] Although the numbers of polymorphonuclear leukocytes (PMNs) in peripheral blood do not decrease with age,[73,74] bone marrow reserves of neutrophils may be diminished.[75] Conditions which occur with increased frequency in the aged may either predispose to or limit survival for pneumonia; included in this category are chronic obstructive pulmonary disease, congestive heart failure, diabetes mellitus, renal failure, and chronic alcoholism.[36,76-81] Epidemics of influenza increase both the rate of pneumonia and the mortality of the disease in the elderly.[82-88] Infection with the influenza virus enhances the ability of pathogenic bacteria to colonize the oropharynx, disrupts normal mucociliary transport, depresses surfactant levels, and decreases the phagocytic and bactericidal capacities of the pulmonary alveolar macrophage.[89,90] Influenza vaccine appears to reduce both pneumonia and associated deaths among elderly patients.[91]

FREQUENCY OF ETIOLOGIC AGENTS

Table 8-1 lists 24 studies of community-acquired pneumonia in adults reported since 1948. These studies were conducted prospectively or retrospectively in large municipal or university teaching hospitals at various times. Different criteria were employed for admission to the hospital, for inclusion in the studies, and for designation of etiology. The proportion of patients aged 60 years or more (when specified) ranged from 20% to 100%. *Streptococcus pneumoniae* was the most common pathogen, but the incidence varied from approximately 5% to 80%, reflecting, at least in part, variations in criteria used for assignment of etiology.

Although not shown in Table 8-1, there was also marked variation in the incidence of pathogens other than *S pneumoniae*. For example, pathogens second in frequency to the pneumococcus in one study were *Legionella* organisms,[54] in other studies were enteric gram-negative bacilli and *Staphylococcus aureus*,[46,47] and in still others were *Haemophilus influenzae*.[16,40,55] Viral infections other than influenza appeared to be uncommon causes of pneumonia in civilian adults.[46] *Mycoplasma pneumoniae* was not a common cause of pulmonary infection in the aged. Pneumonia of uncertain etiology varied in different studies from virtually none to more than 50%. In most studies, cultures for anaerobic bacteria[92] were not routinely utilized; when they are, anaerobes become an important cause of community-acquired pneumonia in the elderly.[93]

Many patients with pneumonia who seek care in major teaching hospitals are treated as outpatients.[45,51,92] Only the ones with the most serious illness are hospitalized, and published studies are concerned primarily with these individuals. Elderly patients with mild illness who respond to outpatient therapy have not been studied in great detail; they may well have a different spectrum of pathogens responsible for pnuemonia, perhaps with an even higher frequency of infection due to *S pneumoniae*.[51]

PNEUMOCOCCAL PNEUMONIA

Pneumococcal pneumonia occurs on an annual basis 1 to 2 times for each 1000 persons in the United States[94-98]; the risk of the disease in the elderly is considerably higher, ranging from 14 to 46 cases per 1000 persons each year.[98,99] Although antibiotics have caused a significant reduction of deaths from pneumococcal pneumonia, the incidence of the disease has not been altered appreciably by their availability.[9,97] Dowling and Lepper[7] reported an overall mortality of 30.5% in patients with untreated pneumococcal pneumonia; this compared with a fatality of 16.9% in patients treated with specific serum, 12.3% for those treated

Table 8-1
Studies of Community-Acquired Pneumonia in Civilian Adults

Reference	Location and Date(s) of Study	No. of Patients	Sex* M	Sex* F	Age Range (yr) (No. of Elderly)	Pneumococcal Etiology
Humphrey et al [36]	London, 1942–1944	351			12–70	79.2%†
Crofton et al [37]	London, 10/1/49–9/30/50	110	61	49	8–86 (mean=45.5)	26.4%†
Grist et al [38]	Glasgow, 10/50–3/51	129			13–84	65%†
McCallum [39]	Montreal, 7/1/55–6/30/56	231	133	98	20–80 (≥61=38.5%)	15.7%†
Bath et al [40]	Edinburgh, 1960–1962	156	70%	30%	12–90 (≥60=48.7%)	30.8%†
Oswald et al [41]	London, 1949–1958	1330	861	469	<4 – >75 (≥65=20.8%)	31%‡ (20%sole pathogen) 17.1%§
Mufson et al [42]	Washington, DC, 10/61–5/64	427	68%	32%	10–99 (≥60=24.6%)	(bacteremic)
Schwartzman et al [43]	Atlanta, 12/22/68–1/11/69	238			Median=52	48.2%∥
Bisno et al [44]	Memphis, 12/18/68–1/21/69	106	49	57	"Peak incidence in 6th and 7th decades"	21.7%†
Fekety et al [45]	Baltimore, 10/28/65–5/31/66	100			11–100	62%†
Sullivan et al [46]	Atlanta, 7/1/67–6/30/68	292			Mean=54	62%¶
Dorff et al [47]	Milwaukee, 10/1/69–3/30/70	148	96	52	14–94 (mean=57)	53%†
Fiala [48]	Philadelphia, 10/1/66–4/10/67	193	113	80	Mean=50.9	55%†
Burns et al [49]	Sydney, Australia, 1972	222*	67%	33%	<40 – >65 >65=35%	47%–67%**

Reference	Location and Date(s) of Study	No. of Patients	Sex* M	Sex* F	Age Range (yr) (No. of Elderly)	Pneumococcal Etiology
Moore et al [50]	Baltimore, 9/1/71 – 5/31/72	154	96	58	21 – 86 (mean = 50)*	40.3%[†]
White et al [51]	Bristol, 1/74 – 3/80	210	138	72	12 – 100 (mean = 54)	11.5%[†]
Sulkava & Pettersson [52]	Helsinki, Finland, 1976	198	122	76	15 – 91 (mean = 57.5)	4.5%[†]
Boerner & Zwadyk [53]	Durham, N C, 1-year period	89				36%[†]
MacFarlane et al [54]	Nottingham, 7/17/80 – 8/13/81	127	92	35	13 – 79 (mean = 51)	76%[†]
Klimek et al [55]	Hartford, 1981	204			"Majority over 50 years"	36%[†]
Fick & Reynolds [57]	New Haven 1/69 – 1/72 1/79 – 1/82	935 1175				46%[†] 21%[†]
Garb et al [58]	Springfield, Mass, 1/71 – 11/76	70			> 65	34.3%[†]
Ebright & Rytel [20]	Milwaukee, 1973	160			20 – > 65 (≥ 65 = 31%)	34.8%[†]
Gleckman [16]	Worcester, Mass	58			"Elderly"	40%[††]

* M = male; F = female.
† Percentage of total number of patients with pneumonia in study.
‡ Percentage of patients with pneumonia from whom sputum specimens were obtained for cultures.
§ Percentage of patients with pneumonia from whom blood cultures were obtained.
‖ Percentage of patients with bacterial pneumonia.
¶ Percentage of patients with pneumonia in whom an etiologic diagnosis was made.
# Number includes both community-acquired and nosocomial pneumonias.
** Percentage of patients with bronchopneumonia and lobar pneumonia, respectively.
†† Percentage of patients in whom an adequate sputum specimen was obtained before antimicrobial drug therapy.

with a sulfonamide, and 5.1% for patients treated with antibiotics. For patients 60 years or older who received no specific therapy, the mortality was 59%; this compared with a fatality of 48% in patients treated with specific serum, 32% in patients treated with a sulfonamide, and 16% in patients treated with antibiotics. Many other workers have substantiated the high case fatality rates from pneumococcal pneumonia among the elderly.[2,3,5,8,9,96,99]

In patients treated with antibiotics, other important factors associated with increased mortality of pneumococcal pneumonia are concomitant debilitating disease, multilobar involvement, bacteremia, leukopenia, and infections due to type I and III pneumococcus.[8] Bacteremia occurs in from 15% to 25% of patients with pneumococcal pneumonia and is associated with an overall mortality of 18% to 35%, but in geriatric patients the mortality may be considerably higher.[100] Death from bacteremic pneumococcal pneumonia often occurs before antimicrobial drug therapy can alter the course of the disease,[9] and treatment in an intensive care unit does not improve survival.[101] Case fatality rates of bacteremic pneumococcal pneumonia appear to be as high in persons from average American communities as they are in inner-city populations where patients use large municipal teaching hospitals.[102,103]

Studies of pneumococcal pneumonia in the preantibiotic era were largely confined to patients with lobar pneumonia.[3] Traditionally, pneumococcal pneumonia was characterized by an explosive onset, a protracted shaking chill, pleuritic chest pain, dyspnea, productive cough, purulent or rusty sputum, prostration, and lobar consolidation. This classic form of the full-blown clinical syndrome appears to be uncommon today.[104] The majority of patients hospitalized for pneumococcal pneumonia have a roentgenographic pattern of bronchopneumonia rather than the classic lobar pattern.[105] Incomplete consolidation on chest films is seen more frequently in elderly persons than in younger patients.[106] In the antibiotic era, pneumococcal pneumonia is best viewed as a disease process with a broad spectrum of clinical and radiologic presentations and severity.[104,105,107]

Patients with chronic cardiopulmonary disease, diabetes mellitus, chronic alcoholism, hepatic cirrhosis, or disorders of humoral immunity appear to be at increased risk for pneumococcal pneumonia. Patients who have required hospitalization for pneumonia in the preceding 5 years also appear to be at increased risk.[108] Elderly persons are more susceptible than younger persons to delay in resolution of pneumococcal pneumonia,[25] empyema, bacteremia, extrapulmonary complications,[6,8,9,17] and recurrent disease.[109]

Compared with younger patients, elderly persons with pneumococcal disease more frequently have a limited febrile response to infection,[7,16,99,110] a delay in diagnosis or therapy, and a higher risk of death.[110] The disease often presents insidiously and frequently is accompanied by dehydration.[111] Older patients report rigors and pleuritic chest pain less frequently than younger patients.[100] Elevated temperature (when present) and tachypnea[112] are among the most important clinical clues.[16] Not infrequently, CNS signs, such as confusion or stupor, may predominate; or pneumonia may initially be mistaken for congestive heart failure. With an unclear history, lack of fever, and pre-existing respiratory and cardiac disease, the geriatric patient with pneumococcal pneumonia appears to be at greater risk than younger patients for receiving a wrong diagnosis on admission to the hospital.[100,110]

There is considerable controversy as to criteria for definitive microbiologic diagnosis of pneumococcal pneumonia. Some investigators accept only positive cultures of blood or pleural fluid as evidence of the disease, but this leads to underdiagnosis. A minority of patients with pneumococcal pneumonia have bacteremia, and pleural empyema occurs infrequently. Many physicians rely on cultures of expectorated sputum for etiologic diagnosis. Expectorated sputum is inevitably contaminated by the normal flora of the nasopharynx. Since pneumococci may be inhabitants of the nasopharynx in from 5% to 70% of normal persons, recovery of S pneumoniae from sputum cultures is not, of itself, firm evidence of pneumococcal infection.[113]

Studies have shown that sputum cultures are frequently negative in patients with bacteremic pneumococcal pneumonia,[48,51] or they may reveal potential pathogens other than those causing the pneumonia.[51] For example, in a retrospective analysis of 51 patients with unquestionable bacteremic pneumococcal pneumonia, Barrett-Connor[113] found that 45% of cultures of sputum or nasopharyngeal aspirates, obtained before any antimicrobial drug therapy, failed to yield pneumococci; in 27% of specimens, an additional potential pathogen was isolated. Failure to recover pneumococci may be due to submission of an inadequate specimen, uneven distribution of the pathogens in sputum, delays in transportation and processing of specimens,[113-115] or failure to detect organisms when they are present in cultures.[116] Studies reveal that physicians themselves rarely participate in collection of sputum from patients, that the responsibility is frequently relegated to inexperienced personnel, and that material unsuitable for study is frequently submitted to the laboratory after considerable delay.[115,117]

Recovery of pneumococci may be enhanced when sputum specimens are collected by experienced persons, inoculated into appropriate media without delay, and special precautions are undertaken to detect the organisms in cultures.[116,118] Microscopic examination of specimens from patients with penumonia may differentiate saliva from sputum.[115] Specimens containing many buccal squamous epithelial cells (>25/low power field) are heavily contaminated with saliva,[119] and are unsuitable for culture.[115] Specimens containing numerous PMNs and few, if any, squamous epithelial cells, are representative of lower respiratory secretions and are suitable for culture. Microscopic examination of gram smears of sputum may detect pathogens which otherwise might be missed in cultures. The yield of pathogens in sputum cultures appears to be increased when technicians are aware of their presence in the smear.[120]

In an effort to overcome contamination of sputum with oropharyngeal secretions, transthoracic needle aspiration of the lung[121] or transtracheal aspiration has been utilized for diagnosis of pneumonia.[122-126] Neither of these procedures is without risk, and they are not ordinarily required in community-acquired pneumonia. A relatively low yield of positive cultures is encountered with transthoracic needle aspiration,[127] and transtracheal aspiration may yield false-positive results in some patients.[122-124] False-positive results from transtracheal aspiration may be caused by the presence of pathogens in the trancheobronchial tree in patients with chronic bronchitis in the absence of pneumonia,[128,129] misdirection of the transtracheal catheter during insertion, or aspiration of oral secretions during the procedure.[119,130,131] Specimens of sputum obtained by bronchoscopy are also subject to contamination by oropharyngeal bacteria, which are introduced during the passage of the instrument.[127] A method has been devised, utilizing a double catheter brush system and a distal occluding plug, to reduce such contamination at bronchoscopy.[132,133] Flatauer et al suggested that the gram stain of bronchoscopically obtained pulmonary secretions gave better clinical correlation than culture of the same specimen.[134]

Whenever possible, a gram-stained smear of expectorated sputum should be obtained from patients with community-acquired pneumonia. A positive gram smear in pneumococcal pneumonia reveals numerous PMNs and a preponderance of lancet-shaped gram-positive diplococci. This type of smear is indicative of pneumococcal etiology, regardless of culture results and can be used as a basis for therapy.[53,135] Unfortunately, gram smears may be negative in some cases of pneumococcal pneumonia.[135] At times they may be difficult to evaluate because of the presence of oropharyngeal bacteria morphologically resembling pneumococci. A Quelling test with omniserum is a simple, inexpensive, and rapid means of identifying pneumococci in such sputum smears.[136,137]

Counterimmunoelectrophoresis (CIE) has been used as a method for diagnosis of pneumococcal pneumonia. It is a rapid diagnostic test for detection of pneumococcal polysaccharide antigens in serum, urine, and sputum. Prior treatment with antimicrobial drugs may rapidly eliminate viable pneumococci from sites of infection, but may not interfere with antigen detection. When antigen is sought in both serum and concentrated urine, a diagnosis may be established in between 50% to 75% of cases of bacteremic pneumococcal pneumonia.[138] The rate of identification is lower in nonbacteremic cases. During antibiotic therapy, concentration of antigen in the circulation declines progressively, but it may persist for 2 weeks or longer. There appears to be a correlation between fatality and antigenemia. Delayed resolution of pneumonia has been observed in patients with prolonged antigenemia.[139]

Counterimmunoelectrophoresis of sputum appears to be a sensitive diagnostic test in pneumococcal pneumonia, and may be positive in some cases in which sputum cultures are negative.[140-143] However, it may be no more sensitive than the gram-stained smear of sputum,[142] and it may be positive with pneumococcal colonization of the tracheobronchial tree in the absence of pneumonia (ie, bronchitis).[140,142] Kalin and Lindberg[144] found that for rapid diagnosis direct gram stain and CIE on sputum were about equally effective, but they were complementary; the two tests together were associated with a higher diagnostic yield than either test alone. Downes and Ellner[145] stated that CIE should not be used to replace the gram stain or culture of sputum. However, they noted that the detection of pneumococcal polysaccharide in sputum by this rapid and relatively simple method can assist physicians in the evaluation of sputum culture results. Coagglutination is another rapid method for identification of pneumococcal antigen in sputum, and it appears to be more sensitive than CIE[146]; but experience in pneumococcal pneumonia is limited.

Most pneumococci are exquisitely sensitive to penicillin G; the minimum inhibitory concentration (MIC) of the drug for these stains is less than or equal to 0.06 µg/mL.[147] Isolates of pneumococci relatively resistant to penicillin G, with MICs ranging from 0.1 to 1.0 µg/mL, have been identified in many parts of the world.[148] These MICs are well below clinically achievable concentrations of penicillin G in most areas of the body, but infections at sites where penicillin penetrates poorly, such as the meninges, may not respond to penicillin G therapy in ordinary dosage. Isolates of pneumococci requiring more than 1 µg/mL of penicillin G for inhibition of growth are unequivocally resistant and will not respond to penicillin G therapy regardless of dosage; these organisms are frequently resistant to multiple antibiotics, but vancomycin is consistently effective. The incidence of relatively resistant pneumococci in the United States is very low; infection due to highly resistant strains has not been a problem in this country. However, it is now recommended that in vitro susceptibility tests be done immediately on all pneumococci isolated from blood or CSF.[147]

In recent years, a polyvalent vaccine of pneumococcal capsular polysaccharides has become available for clinical use in the United States. Although there is unequivocal evidence from randomized controlled trials that the pneumococcal vaccine is effective in young men, demonstration of efficacy in the elderly has not been established and is a matter of controversy.[149-151] Pneumonia in elderly patients caused by serotypes of *S pneumoniae* not represented in the vaccine has been a problem in some areas of the United States.[152-153] Because of the continuing high mortality of pneumococcal pneumonia in elderly patients, even in those who are treated with appropriate antibiotics,[9] it seems reasonable to utilize the vaccine at least until new data become available.[151]

NONPNEUMOCOCCAL PNEUMONIA

The incidence of community-acquired pneumonia due to gram-negative bacilli, such as *Klebsiella pneumoniae* and *Escherichia coli*, appears to be increased in the elderly, especially in those who reside in nursing homes,[47,58] but not exclusively in persons in this category.[20] Many of the reported victims of this disease are medically indigent persons from inner-city populations with a high incidence of associated illness, including chronic alcoholism, chronic obstructive pulmonary disease and bronchitis, congestive heart failure, diabetes mellitus, and chronic renal insufficiency.[20,46,47,154] The rising incidence of pneumonia due to these pathogens cannot be fully explained on the basis of predisposing antibiotic therapy, although it may be a factor in some patients.[58] A number of patients with gram-negative bacillary pneumonia have disease of the CNS or other conditions conducive to aspiration of oropharyngeal secretions; abnormal colonization of the oropharynx of these persons appears to represent the prelude to a potentially lethal event.

In some patients with gram-negative bacillary pneumonia, the roentgenographic findings may be characterized by diffuse alveolar infiltrates, rapid progression to cavitation, and the development of abscesses or empyema.[155] However, in most patients the radiologic and clinical expressions of the disease are not sufficiently distinctive to differentiate this type of pneumonia from other serious pulmonary infections. Frequently, early presumptive etiologic diagnosis depends on gram-stained smears of fresh sputum specimens which show a predominance of gram-negative bacilli and an abundance of PMNs.[26,27,156] Some physicians recommend a combination of antibiotics including an aminoglycoside for therapy.[157] Even with appropriate treatment, mortality is high.

In some areas in the United States and other countries, *Haemophilus influenzae* has emerged as an important cause of community-acquired pneumonia in adults.[46,158-168] The incidence appears to be rising, and in some locations, *H influenzae* appears to be second only to the pneumococcus as a cause of acute pulmonary infection in the elderly.[168,169] The organism has a propensity to cause pulmonary infection in patients with chronic obstructive lung disease, chronic alcoholism, diabetes mellitus, or defects of humoral immunity. Most victims have at least one serious underlying disease. The clinical presentation with fever, cough, and sputum production differs little from other types of bacterial pneumonia.[158] Illness due to typeable strains of *H influenzae* may be associated with a more acute onset and higher incidence of bacteremia than that caused by nontypeable strains.[164] Most patients with *H influenzae* pneumonia present with a roentgenographic pattern of bronchopneumonia, but a sizeable proportion may have lobar disease.[158,166] There may be a wide variety of nonspecific clinical and radiologic manifestations, but an early pleural reaction is an important feature in at least one half of the cases.[158,160,165]

Most cases of pneumonia due to *H influenzae* in elderly patients now appear to be caused by nontypeable strains[163,164] and bacteremia occurs infrequently.[17] *Haemophilus influenzae* may be an inhabitant of the normal flora of the nasopharynx,[165] and may colonize the tracheobronchial tree of patients with chronic bronchitis in the absence of pneumonia.[128,129] Consequently, diagnosis of pneumonia on the basis of cultures of expectorated sputum or transtracheal aspirates may not always be reliable.[165] Conversely, stringent criteria requiring positive blood or pleural fluid cultures for definitive diagnosis result in marked underestimation of the frequency of the disease.[166] Observation of a predominance of tiny, pleomorphic, gram-negative coccobacilli on the smear of an adequate specimen of sputum is an important diagnostic finding, and facilitates institution of appropriate initial therapy.[17,157,158,162,163,165] At times, when the gram-stained smear of sputum shows a predominance of organisms compatible with *H influenzae*, the pathogen fails to grow in cultures,[157] probably due to the well-recognized difficulties in isolating this organism from sputum.[157,167] Care must be taken to avoid overdecolorization of the gram smears because *Haemophilus* organisms may be mistaken for pneumococci.[158,165]

Patients with pneumonia caused by betalactamase-producing strains of *H influenzae* have been reported in whom treatment with penicillin G and ampicillin failed to eradicate the disease.[161] However, recent studies from some areas of the United States indicate that most nontypeable strains of *H influenzae* are susceptible to penicillin G and ampicillin; treatment with ampicillin appears to be quite effective.[161,163] Some workers have described the efficacy of cefamandole therapy for *H influenzae* pneumonia.[168,169,171] Smith et al[165] stated that the significance of antibiotic resistance of the organisms in pneumonia is far less than it is in septicemia and meningitis. These authorities noted that "inappropriate" antibiotics often appear to be effective for treatment of *H influenzae* pneumonia for reasons that are not entirely clear.[165]

Legionnaires' disease is estimated to cause from 1% to 4% of community-acquired pneumonias in the United States, and most cases occur in middle-aged or elderly adults.[172] The disease may occur sporadically or in epidemics in the community.[173,176] About 73% of cases occur between the months of June and October,[173] in contrast to pneumococcal pneumonia which develops most frequently in the late winter or early spring.[3] During the 2 weeks before onset of disease, a sizeable proportion of patients have a recent history of overnight travel, have been a hospital visitor, have lived near or been exposed to a construction site or excavation, or have attended a convention.[173] Male sex, cigarette smoking, and alcohol consumption also appear to be risk factors.[172] The case fatality ratio is significantly higher for patients 50 years or older than for younger persons, for persons with chronic bronchitis and emphysema, and for those who are immunocompromised.[172-174]

Certain clinical clues which may heighten suspicion of Legionnaires' disease include high fever, recurrent shaking chills, and relative bradycardia; neurologic symptoms suggesting an encephalopathy; watery diarrhea; and lack of response to treatment with penicillins, cephalosporins, and aminoglycosides. Roentgenographic findings may consist initially of patchy areas of bronchopneumonia or poorly marginated nodular densities[177,178]; in the absence of appropriate therapy, these may progress rapidly to lobar or multilobar consolidation. Although clinical and radiologic clues may be helpful, in many patients Legionnaires' disease may be quite difficult to differentiate from other types of community-acquired pneumonia,[179] and microbiologic studies are essential.[180-182] Even prompt response to erythromycin therapy may not be definitive, because pneumococcal or mycoplasmal pneumonia may also respond to this drug.

The gram smear of sputum characteristically shows inflammatory cells and a paucity of bacteria.[174,180] In order to obtain the highest diagnostic yield in Legionnaires' disease, authorities recommend a group of tests, including the direct immunofluorescent antibody (DFA) test of respiratory tract secretions, pleural fluid, or lung; indirect immunofluorescent antibody (IFA) studies; and cultures of respiratory secretions, pleural fluid, blood, or diseased lung.[180,181] A positive DFA test on respiratory secretions is a rapid, specific diagnostic method, but it is not especially sensitive. Therefore a true positive FTA test is diagnostic, but a negative one does not exclude Legionnaires' disease. Culture of respiratory secretions on selective media now appears to be the most sensitive way to make the diagnosis.[180,181] Buffered charcol yeast extract agar with both α-ketoglutarate and antimicrobial drugs added makes it possible to isolate *Legionella pneumophila* and some other species from expectorated sputum.[182] Serologic testing by the IFA method depends on demonstration of a fourfold or greater rise in titer, which requires a matter of weeks and does not occur in all patients.[180] However, one group of investigators found that antibody titers were elevated in 27% of cases of Legionnaires' disease within 1 week of onset of pneumonia.[181] IFA antibody tests might therefore be useful in early diagnosis in some patients. Tests for soluble antigen in the urine may be useful in establishing an early diagnosis, but are not as yet generally available.[182]

Aspiration of oropharyngeal secretions appears to be a common mechanism for development of pneumonia in the elderly.[93,168,183] Predisposing factors are reduced levels of consciousness with impaired gag or cough reflexes, defective swallowing, or incompetent cardioesophageal sphincters.[168,183] When aspiration takes place in the community, pulmonary infection is most likely to be due to oropharyngeal anaerobic bacteria.[77] The clinical course of anaerobic pneumonia may be similar to that of pneumococcal pneumonia with regard to fever, leukocyte count, and early radiologic abnormalities.[184] The response to appropriate antimicrobial drug therapy may be similar, especially when initiated early in the course of illness before cavitation occurs.[184] Anaerobic pneumonia is often an indolent illness; chills and bacteremia are uncommon.[92] The presence of carious teeth, peridontal disease, or gingivitis and malodorous sputum should lead to suspicion of the diagnosis[92] but is not present in all cases.[184,185] Gram smears of expectorated sputum may show the characteristic changes described by Gopalakrishna and Lerner: abundant PMNs or necrotic debris and a profusion of bacteria (gram-positive cocci, pleomorphic gram-negative bacilli, and even spirochetes).[185]

In patients with anaerobic pneumonia, infiltrates typically involve dependent areas of the lungs. If aspiration occurred when the patient was upright, the basilar segments of the lower lobes are most likely to be affected; if (as is more likely) the patient was in a recumbent position, the posterior segments of the upper lobes, the superior segments of the lower lobes, or both areas, are likely to be involved. The illness is deceptive and, without prompt diagnosis and treatment, may progress to cavitary lung abscess and empyema. Treatment of these conditions is more difficult and prolonged than is therapy for uncomplicated pneumonia.

The organisms most frequently responsible for anaerobic pneumonia are anaerobic streptococci, *Fusobacterium nucleatum*, and *Bacteroides melaninogenicus*.[92] These and other anaerobes causing pneumonia have usually been susceptible to penicillin G. However, in recent years some strains of *B melaninogenicus* and other oral anaerobes have emerged resistant to penicillin G; failures of therapy with this drug have been noted in some instances.[186] Clindamycin appears to be effective for treatment of anaerobic pneumonia which fails to respond to penicillin G therapy. Experience with treatment of anaerobic pulmonary infections with metronidazole has been disappointing and cannot be recommended.[187,188]

Although less common than pneumococci or gram-negative bacteria as a cause of community-acquired pneumonia in the elderly,[46,47] pneumonia due to *Staphylococcus aureus* nevertheless is an infection to consider because mortality is quite high.[189] It may be a complication of bacteremia from sources of infection elsewhere in the body, but in the elderly it most commonly arises primarily in the lungs, often as a sequela to influenza.[43,82,85] At greatest risk for death are patients with chronic cardiopulmonary or other debilitating diseases. The development of pneumatoceles or spontaneous pneumothorax during the course of pneumonia is strongly suggestive of *S aureus* pneumonia,[26,27] but this occurs infrequently in the elderly where the clinical and radiologic presentation is quite variable. Lung abscesses and empyema develop in some patients. Bacteremia is uncommon in primary staphylococcal pneumonia, occurring in less than 20% of the cases. Microscopic examination of sputum specimens may be helpful; in typical cases, there are numerous PMNs and a predominance of gram-positive cocci in clumps or clusters, and some of the organisms may be engulfed by leukocytes. Most strains of *S aureus* likely to cause pneumonia today are resistant to penicillin G, but many are susceptible to semisynthetic penicillinase-resistant penicillins such as methicillin, nafcillin, or oxacillin. Vancomycin appears to be the drug of choice for infection due to methicillin-resistant staphylococci. Pleural empyema, if present, requires drainage. Because of extensive tissue destruction and abscess formation, a protracted period of antibiotic therapy (4–6 weeks or more) may be required to cure staphylococcal pneumonia.

Respiratory syncytial and parainfluenza viruses appear to be common causes of pneumonia and other respiratory disorders in infants and young children, but these highly contagious viruses may cause pneumonia in elderly patients,[190,191] and outbreaks have been described in extended care facilities.[192] Recently, investigators[193] have suggested that the diagnosis of viral pneumonia be improved by routinely testing sputum specimens for viruses.

Pneumonia is the major complication of influenza virus infection and may be due either to the virus itself [82] or to secondary infection with *Streptococcus pneumoniae, Staphylococcus aureus,* or other bacterial pathogens.[43,82,83,85] At great risk are elderly patients with chronic cardiac or pulmonary diseases. It may develop several days to a week after the onset of typical influenza, often after a brief period of apparent improvement. It is heralded by dyspnea and cyanosis and frequently pursues a rapidly lethal course. For this reason, routine annual immunization with influenza vaccine is strongly recommended for the elderly and other high-risk groups, but, regrettably, less than 20% of high-risk patients are immunized each year.[194] Amantidine hydrochloride also may be useful as prophylaxis against influenza A in those who are at high risk and may be beneficial for treatment of uncomplicated influenza A if initiated within 48 hours of the onset of symptoms. There is no evidence at present that it is effective or ineffective for treatment of influenzal pneumonia.

Mycoplasma pneumoniae appears to be an uncommon cause of pneumonia in the elderly but occasionally cases occur and may be severe.[195]

Branhamella catarrhalis (formerly *Neisseria catarrhalis*) has been identified as a cause of community-acquired pneumonia in a number of elderly patients in recent years.[195-198] Gram-negative diplococci are frequently seen in sputum smears. Some strains produce a betalactamase and may be resistant to penicillin G.[199,200] Most strains appear to be susceptible to cephalosporins, erythromycin, trimethoprim-sulfamethoxazole, and tetracycline and are resistant to clindamycin.[199,200]

DIAGNOSIS AND THERAPY

Early diagnosis and prompt institution of appropriate antimicrobial drug therapy are essential to minimize morbidity and mortality from pneumonia in the elderly. The disease may have protean manifestations and may masquerade under the guise of a variety of pulmonary or extrapulmonary disorders. In the lungs, it may be mistaken for bronchitis, chronic obstructive pulmonary disease, congestive heart failure, pulmonary embolism, atelectasis, aspiration of gastric contents, pulmonary neoplasm, and the adult respiratory distress syndrome.[19,201] Outside the lungs, manifestations such as mental confusion, hypotension, azotemia, or ileus may predominate, and the physician has to have a high index of suspicion. The absence of fever, or even cough, does not exclude the diagnosis.

Once a clinical diagnosis of pneumonia is established on chest film, the physician must determine the identity of the causative organism. Perhaps the single most important procedure in pursuing an early diagnosis is the examination of an acceptable specimen of sputum. When elderly patients are weak and unable to cough, or when they are confused, obtunded, or uncooperative, it may not be possible to obtain an adequate specimen of expectorated sputum; it may then be necessary to obtain material by nasotracheal or transtracheal aspiration, endotracheal intubation, or even by bronchoscopy. However, in many elderly patients with community-acquired pneumonia, just a little effort by the physician to get the patient to cough up a good specimen will remove the need for an invasive procedure.

Sputum specimens should be taken promptly to the laboratory where they can be gram-stained in a few minutes and inoculated into appropriate culture media without delay. The smear should be examined by the responsible physician and other competent observers. Microscopic examination of the smear will confirm that the specimen did originate in the lungs rather than the oropharynx, and may also provide clues to the microbial etiology of the pulmonary infection. Two or three blood cultures should be obtained before institution of therapy, especially in patients with moderate or severe illness requiring hospitalization. In the event that pleural effusion is present, thoracentesis should be performed;

cultures should be obtained and smears of the pleural fluid should be examined before institution of therapy. Counterimmunoelectrophoresis (CIE), latex agglutination, or coagglutination on serum, concentrated urine, sputum, or pleural fluid may rapidly provide early evidence of the presence of antigens of *Streptococcus pneumoniae* or other pulmonary pathogens. Serologic tests may be helpful in the diagnosis of Legionnaire's disease.

In elderly patients, it is often necessary to initiate antimicrobial drug therapy for pneumonia on the basis of a presumptive etiologic diagnosis after appropriate microbiologic studies have been started, but before the causal agent has been definitively identified or its in vitro susceptibility has been determined. Frequently the gram smear of sputum or other clinical clues may be helpful in establishing an accurate presumptive etiologic diagnosis. Table 8-2 lists the drugs I currently prefer for initial therapy of pneumonia based on the presumed cause of the infection. When the elderly patient with pneumonia appears to be seriously ill and the gram-stained smear of sputum is not definitive, a combination of a third-generation cephalosporin (cefotaxime, ceftizoxime, ceftriaxone, or cefoperazone) and erythromycin will provide broad coverage against the usual pathogens. Definitive antimicrobial drug therapy is determined subsequently from the results of microbiologic studies and the patient's response to initial therapy.

Table 8-2
Currently Preferred Antimicrobial Drugs for Initial Presumptive Therapy of Community-Acquired Pneumonia in the Elderly*

Presumptive Etiologic Organism	First Choice	Second Choice
Streptococcus pneumoniae	Penicillin G or V	Erythromycin; a first-generation cephalosporin[†]; chloramphenicol; vancomycin; clindamycin
Klebsiella pneumoniae	A third-generation cephalosporin[‡] ± an aminoglycoside	An aminoglycoside[§] and piperacillin; chloramphenicol; trimethoprim-sulfamethoxazole
Escherichia coli	A third-generation cephalosporin[‡] ± an aminoglycoside	An aminoglycoside[‡] and piperacillin; chloramphenicol; trimethoprim-sulfamethoxazole

Presumptive Etiologic Organism	First Choice	Second Choice
Haemophilus influenzae	A third-generation cephalosporin‡ or cefuroxime	Chloramphenicol; trimethoprim-sulfamethoxazole; ampicillin
Legionella pneumophila and other *Legionella* sp	Erythromycin	Rifampin; doxycycline
Anaerobic pneumonia due to anaerobic *Streptococcus, Bacteroides melaninogenicus, Fusobacterium nucleatum*, and related pathogens	Penicillin G or clindamycin	Cefoxitin; chloramphenicol
Staphylococcus aureus		
Nonpenicillinase-producing	Penicillin G	A first-generation cephalosporin†; vancomycin
Penicillinase-producing	Methicillin, oxacillin, or nafcillin	A first-generation cephalosporin†; vancomycin
Methicillin-resistant	Vancomycin	Trimethoprim-sulfamethoxazole
Branhamella catarrhalis	A first-generation cephalosporin†	Erythromycin; trimethoprim-sulfamethoxazole
Mycoplasma pneumoniae	Erythromycin	A tetracycline

* Definitive antimicrobial therapy is determined subsequently from the results of microbiological data and the patient's response to initial therapy.
† Cefazolin, cephalothin, cephradine, or cephapirin.
‡ Cefotaxime, ceftizoxime, ceftriaxone, cefoperazone, or ceftazidime.
§ Gentamicin, tobramycin, amikacin, or netilmicin.

REFERENCES

1. *Acute Conditions. Incidence and Associated Disability, United States July 1977 – June 1978*, Series 10, No. 132. US Dept of Health, Education, and Welfare publication No. (PHS) 79-1560, Hyattsville, MD, National Center for Health Statistics, 1979.
2. Tilghman EC, Finland M: Clinical significance of bacteremia in pneumococcic pneumonia. *Arch Intern Med* 1937;59:602–609.
3. Heffron R: Pneumonia with special reference to pneumococcus lobar pneumonia. Cambridge, Mass, Harvard University Press, 1979.
4. Stahle DC: A clinical analysis of fifteen thousand cases of pneumonia. An evaluation of the effectiveness of various therapeutic agents. *JAMA* 1942;116:440–447.
5. Flippin HF, Schwartz L, Domm AH: Modern treatment of pneumococcic pneumonia. *JAMA* 143;121:230–237.

6. Zeman FD, Wallach K: Pneumonia in the aged. An analysis of one hundred sixty-six cases of its occurrence in patients sixty years old and over. *Arch Intern Med* 1946;77:678–699.
7. Dowling HF, Lepper MH: The effect of antibiotics (penicillin, aureomycin, and terramycin) on the fatality rate and incidence of complications in pneumococcic pneumonia. A comparison with other methods of therapy. *Am J Med Sci* 1951;222:396–403.
8. Van Metre TE Jr: Pneumococcal pneumonia treated with antibiotics. The prognostic significance of certain clinical findings. *N Engl J Med* 1954;251:1048–1052.
9. Austrian R, Gold J: Pneumococcal bacteremia with especial reference to bacteremic pneumococcal pneumonia. *Ann Intern Med* 1964;60:759–776.
10. Kovar MD: Health of the elderly and use of health services. *Public Health Rep* 1977;92:9–19.
11. Woodford-Williams E: Diagnosis and management of pneumonia in the aged. *Br Med J* 1966;1:467–470.
12. Austrian R: Pneumonia in later years. *J Am Geriatr Soc* 1981; 29:481–489.
13. Hill CD, Stamm WE: Pneumonia in the elderly: the fatal complication. *Geriatrics* 1982;37:40–50.
14. Horton JM, Pankey GA: Pneumonia in the elderly. A growing problem demanding special handling. *Postgrad Med* 1982;71: 114–123.
15. Esposito AL: Bacterial pneumonia in the elderly, in Pennington JE (ed): *Respiratory Infections: Diagnosis and Management.* New York, Raven Press, 1983, pp 159–169.
16. Gleckman RA: Community-acquired pneumonia, in Gleckman RA, Gantz NM (eds): *Infections in the Elderly.* Boston, Little Broen & Co, 1983,pp 73-89.
17. Verghese A, Berk SL: Bacterial pneumonia in the elderly. *Medicine* 1983;62:271–285.
18. Berk SL: Bacterial pneumonia in the elderly: The observations of Sir William Osler in retrospect. *J Am Geriatr Soc* 1984; 32:683–685.
19. Gleckman RA, Roth RM: Community-acquired bacterial pneumonia in the elderly. *Pharmacotherapy* 1984;4:81–88.
20. Ebright JR, Rytel MW: Bacterial pneumonia in the elderly. *J Am Geriatr Soc* 1980;28:220–223.
21. Cluff LE, Caranasos GJ, Stewart RB: *Clinical Problems with Drugs.* Philadelphia, WB Saunders Co, 1975.
22. Vestal RE: Drug use in the elderly: a review of problems and special considerations. *Drugs* 1978;16:358–382.
23. Moellering RC Jr: Factors influencing the clinical use of antimicrobial agents in elderly patients. *Geriatrics* 1978;33: 83–91.
24. Triggs EJ, Nation RL: Pharmacokinetics in the aged. *J Pharmacokinet Biopharm* 1975;3:387–418.
25. Jay SJ, Johanson WG, Pierce AK: The radiographic resolution of *Streptococcus pneumoniae* pneumonia. *N Engl J Med* 1975; 293:798–801.
26. McHenry MC, Alfidi RJ, Deodhar SD, et al: Hospital-acquired pneumonia. *Med Clin North Am* 1974; 58:565–580.
27. McHenry MC: The infectious pneumonias. *Hosp Pract* 1980; 15:41–52.
28. Garrison FH: *An Introduction to the History of Medicine,* ed 4. Philadelphia, WB Saunders Co, 1929.
29. Hourmann M, Dechambre R: Recherches cliniques pour servir à l'historie des maladies des vieillards. Maladies des organes de la respiration. *Arch Gen Med Paris 2º Ser* 1835;8:405–427.

30. Hourmann M, Dechambre R: Recherches cliniques pour servir à l'historie des maladies des vieillards. Respiration chez les vieillards. *Arch Gen Med* 1835;9:338 – 357.
31. Hourmann M, Dechambre R: Recherches cliniques pour servir à l'historie des maladies des vieillards. Pneumonie des vieillards. I. partie — Caractères anatomiques. *Arch Gen Med* 1836; 10:269 – 296.
32. Hourmann M, Dechambre R: Recherches cliniques pour servir à l'historie des maladies des vieillards. Pneumonie des vieillards. II. partie — Etiologie et symptomatologie. *Arch Gen Med* 1836;12:27 – 51.
33. Hourmann M, Dechambre R: Recherches cliniques pour servir à l'historie des maladies des vieillards. Pneumonie des vieillards. II. partie — Symptomatologie. Symptômes généraux. *Arch Gen Med* 1836;12:164 – 194.
34. Osler W, quoted in Harvey AM, McKusick VA (eds): *Osler's Textbook Revisited.* New York, Appleton-Century-Crofts, 1967.
35. Helpern M, Rabson SM: Sudden and unexpected natural death — general considerations and statistics. *N Y State J Med* 1945;45:1197 – 1201.
36. Humphrey JH, Joules H, Van der Walt ED: Pneumonia in North West London 1942-1944: Bacterial pneumonias. *Thorax* 1948;3:112-121.
37. Crofton JW, Fawcett JW, James DG, et al: Pneumonia in West London, 1949 – 1950. *Br Med J* 1951; 2:1368 – 1374.
38. Grist NR, Landsman JB, Anderson T, et al: Studies in the aetiology of pneumonia in Glasgow 1950 – 1951. *Lancet* 1952;1:640 – 646.
39. McCallum L: Respiratory infections at the Montreal General Hospital July 1, 1955 – June 30, 1956. *Can Med Assoc J* 1958;78:323 – 325.
40. Bath JCL, Boissard GPB, Calder MA, et al: Pneumonia in hospital practice in Edinburgh 1960 – 1962. *Br J Dis Chest* 1964;58:1 – 16.
41. Oswald NC, Simon G, Shooter RA: Pneumonia in hospital practice. *Br J Dis Chest* 1961;55:109 – 118.
42. Mufson MA, Chang V, Gill V, et al: The role of viruses, mycoplasmas and bacteria in acute pneumonia in civilian adults. *Am J Epidemiol* 1967;86: 526 – 544.
43. Schwarzmann SW, Adler JL, Sullivan RJ Jr, et al: Bacterial pneumonia during the Hong Kong influenza epidemic of 1968 – 1969. Experience in a city-country hospital. *Arch Intern Med* 1971;127:1037 – 1041.
44. Bisno AL, Griffin JP, Van Epps KA, et al: Pneumonia and Hong Kong influenza: a prospective study of the 1968 – 1969 epidemic. *Am J Med Sci* 1971; 261:251 – 263.
45. Fekety FR Jr, Caldwell J, Gump D, et al: Bacteria, viruses, and mycoplasmas in acute pneumonia in adults. *Am Rev Respir Dis* 1971;104:499 – 507.
46. Sullivan RJ Jr, Dowdle WR, Marine WM, et al: Adult pneumonia in a general hospital. *Arch Intern Med* 1972;129:935 – 942.
47. Dorff GJ, Rytel MW, Farmer SG, et al: Etiologies and characteristic features of pneumonias in a municipal hospital. *Am J Med Sci* 1973;266: 349 – 358.
48. Fiala M: A study of the combined role of viruses, mycoplasmas and bacteria in adult pneumonia. *Am J Med Sci* 1969; 257:44 – 51.
49. Burns MW, Devitt L, Bryant DH: Pneumonia in a city hospital. *Med J Aust* 1976;2:787 – 791.
50. Moore MA, Merson MH, Charache P, et al: The characteristics and mortality of outpatient pneumonia. *Johns Hopkins Med J* 1977;140:9 – 14.
51. White RJ, Blainey AD, Harrison KJ, et al: Causes of pneumonia presenting to a district general hospital. *Thorax* 1981;36:566 – 570.

52. Sulkava R, Pettersson T: Outcome of patients admitted to the hospital with suspected pneumonia. *Ann Clin Res* 1980;12:59–63.
53. Boerner DF, Zwadyk P: The value of the sputum Gram's stain in community-acquired pneumonia. *JAMA* 1982;247:642–645.
54. MacFarlane JT, Finch RG, Ward MJ, et al: Hospital study of adult community-acquired pneumonia. *Lancet* 1982;2:255–258.
55. Klimek JJ, Ajemian E, Fontecchio S, et al: Community-acquired bacterial pneumonia requiring admission to hospital. *Am J Infect Control* 1983;11: 79–82.
56. Ponka A, Sarna S: Differential diagnosis of viral, myco-plasmal, and bacteraemic pneumococcal pneumonias on admission to hospital. *Eur J Respir Dis* 1983;64:360–368.
57. Fick RB Jr, Reynolds HY: Changing spectrum of pneumonia — News media creation or clinical reality? *Am J Med* 1983; 74:1–8.
58. Garb JL, Brown RB, Garb JR, et al: Differences in etiology of pneumonias in nursing home and community patients. *JAMA* 1978;240:2169–2172.
59. Gardner ID: The effect of aging on susceptibility to infection. *Rev Infect Dis* 1980;2:801–810.
60. Phair JP: Host defense in the aged, in Gleckman RA, Gantz NM (eds): *Infections in the Elderly*. Boston, Little Brown & Co, 1983, pp 1–12.
61. Esposito AL, Pennington JE: The pathogenesis of bacterial pneumonia, in Gleckman RA, Gantz NM (ed): *Infections in the Elderly*. Boston, Little Brown & Co, 1983, pp 53–62.
62. Phair JP, Kauffman CA, Bjornson A: Investigation of host defense mechanisms in the aged as determinants of nosocomial colonization and pneumonia. *J Reticuloendothel Soc* 1978;23:397–405.
63. Valenti WM, Trudell RG, Bentley DW: Factors predisposing to oropharyngeal colonization with gram-negative bacilli in the aged. *N Engl J Med* 1978; 298:1108–1111.
64. Johanson WG, Pierce AK, Sanford JP: Changing pharyngeal bacterial flora of hospitalized patients. Emergence of gram-negative bacilli. *N Engl J Med* 1969;281:1137–1140.
65. Johanson WG Jr, Higuchi JH, Chaudhuri TR, et al: Bacterial adherence to epithelial cells in bacillary colonization of the respiratory tract. *Am Rev Respir Dis* 1980;121:55–63.
66. Woods DE, Straus DC, Johanson WG Jr, et al: Role of fibronectin in the prevention of adherence of *Pseudomonas aeruginosa* to buccal cells. *J Infect Dis* 1981;143:784–790.
67. Goodman RM, Yergin BM, Landa JF, et al: Relationship of smoking history and pulmonary function tests to tracheal mucous velocity in non-smokers, young smokers, ex-smokers, and patients with chronic bronchitis. *Am Rev Respir Dis* 1978; 117:205–214.
68. Puchelle E, Zahm JM, Bertrand A: Influence of age on bronchial mucociliary transport. *Scand J Respir Dis* 1979; 60:307–313.
69. Dhar S, Shastri SR, Lenora RAK: Aging and the respiratory system. *Med Clin North Am* 1976;60:1121–1139.
70. Brandstetter RD, Kazemi H: Aging and the respiratory system. *Med Clin North Am* 1983;67:419–431.
71. Huxley EJ, Viroslav J, Gray WR, et al: Pharyngeal aspiration in normal adults and patients with depressed consciousness. *Am J Med* 1978;64:564–568.
72. Price GB, Makinodan T: Immunologic deficiencies in senescence — I. Characterization of intrinsic deficiencies. *J Immunol* 1972;108: 403–412.

73. Polednak AP: Age changes in differential leukocyte count among female adults. *Hum Biol* 1979;50:301–311.
74. Jernigan JA, Gudat JC, Blake JL, et al: Reference values for blood findings in relatively fit elderly persons. *J Am Geriatr Soc* 1980;28:308–314.
75. Timaffy M: A comparative study of bone marrow function in young and old individuals. *Gerontol Clin* 1962;4:13–18.
76. Johanson WG Jr, Pierce AK, Sanford JP, et al: Nosocomial respiratory infections with gram-negative bacilli: the significance of colonization of the respiratory tract. *Ann Intern Med* 1972;77:701–706.
77. Lorber G, Swenson RM: Bacteriology of aspiration pneumonia: a prospective study of community- and hospital-acquired cases. *Ann Intern Med* 1974;81:329-331.
78. Smith FE, Palmer DL: Alcoholism, infection, and altered host defenses: a review of clinical and experimental observations. *J Chronic Dis* 1976;29:35–49.
79. Mackowiak PA, Martin RM, Jones SR, et al: Pharyngeal colonization by gram-negative bacilli in aspiration-prone persons. *Arch Intern Med* 1978;138:1224–1227.
80. Mackowiak PA, Martin RM, Smith JW: The role of bacterial interference in the increased prevalence of oropharyngeal gram-negative bacilli among alcoholics and diabetics. *Am Rev Respir Dis* 1979;120:589–593.
81. Palmer DL: Microbiology of pneumonia in the patient at risk. *Am J Med* 1984;76(5A):53–60.
82. Louria DB, Blumenfeld HL, Ellis JT, et al: Studies on influenza in the pandemic of 1957–1958. II. Pulmonary complications of influenza. *J Clin Invest* 1959;38:213–265.
83. Martin CM, Kunin CM, Gottlieb LS, et al: Asian influenza A in Boston, 1957–1958. II. Severe staphylococcal pneumonia complicating influenza. *Arch Intern Med* 1959;103:532–542.
84. Eickhoff TC, Sherman IL, Serfling RE: Observations on excess mortality associated with epidemic influenza. *JAMA* 1961;176:776–782.
85. Petersdorf RG, Fusco JJ, Harter DH, et al: Pulmonary infections complicating Asian influenza. *Arch Intern Med* 1959;103:262–272.
86. Foy HM, Cooney MK, Allan I, et al: Rates of pneumonia during influenza epidemics in Seattle, 1964–1975. *JAMA* 1979;241:253–258.
87. Barker WH, Mullooly JP: Pneumonia and influenza deaths during epidemics. Implications for prevention. *Arch Intern Med* 1982;142:85–89.
88. Alling DW, Blackwelder WC, Stuart-Harris CH: A study of excess mortality during influenza epidemics in the United States, 1968–1976. *Am J Epidemiol* 1981;113:30–43.
89. Jakab GJ: Mechanisms of virus-induced bacterial superinfections of the lung. *Clin Chest Med* 1981;2:59–66.
90. Reynolds HY: Normal and defective respiratory host defenses, in Pennington JE (ed): *Respiratory Infections: Diagnosis and Management.* New York, Raven Press Books, 1983, pp 1–23.
91. Barker WH, Mullooly JP: Influenza vaccination of elderly persons. Reduction in pneumonia and influenza hospitalizations and deaths. *JAMA* 1980;244:2547–2549.
92. Bartlett JG, Fiengold SM: Anaerobic infections of the lung and pleural space. *Am Rev Respir Dis* 1974;110:56–77.
93. Gleckman R, Blagg N, Hilbert D: Community-acquired pneumonia in the elderly: The changing microbiology. *Intern Med Specialist* 1982;3:47–53.

94. Page MI, Lunn JS: Pneumococcal serotypes associated with acute pneumonia. *Am J Epidemiol* 1973;98:255–261.
95. Wood WB Jr: Pneumococcal pneumonia, in Beeson PB, McDermott W (eds): *Cecil's Textbook of Medicine*, ed 13. Philadelphia, WB Saunders Co, 1971, pp 494–507.
96. Mufson MA, Kruss DM, Wasil RE, et al: Capsular types and outcome of bacteremic pneumococcal disease in the antibiotic era. *Arch Intern Med* 1974;134:505–510.
97. Austrian R: Pneumococcal infection. *Prev Med* 1974;3:443–445.
98. Valenti WM, Jenzer M, Bentley DW: Type-specific pneumococcal respiratory disease in the elderly and chronically ill. *Am Rev Respir Dis* 1978;117:233–238.
99. Mufson MA: Pneumococcal infection. *JAMA* 1981;246:1942–1948.
100. Esposito AL: Community-acquired bacteremic pneumococcal pneumonia. Effect of age on manifestations and outcome. *Arch Intern Med* 1984;144:945–948.
101. Hook EW III, Horton CA, Schaberg DR: Failure of intensive care support to influence mortality from pneumococcal bacteremia. *JAMA* 1983;249:1055–1057.
102. Mufson MA, Oley G: Pneumococcal disease in a medium-sized community in the United States. *JAMA* 1982;248: 1486–1489.
103. Dee TH, Berger CS: Pneumococcal disease in a Wisconsin community hospital. *Wis Med J* 1982;81:29–31.
104. Artabane TA, Jones FL Jr: Pneumococcal pneumonia revisited: an analysis of thirty-one bacteremic cases. *Bull Geisinger Med Center* 1974;26:37–44.
105. Ort S, Ryan JL, Barden G, et al: Pneumococcal pneumonia in hospitalized patients. Clinical and radiological presentations. *JAMA* 1983;249:214–218.
106. Ziskind MM, Schwarz MI, George RB, et al: Incomplete consolidation in pneumococcal lobar pneumonia complicating pulmonary emphysema. *Ann Intern Med* 1970;72:835–839.
107. Kantor HG: The many radiologic facies of pneumococcal pneumonia. *Am J Radiol* 1981;137:1213–1220.
108. Fedson DS, Baldwin JA: Previous hospital care as a risk factor for pneumonia. Implications for immunization with pneumococcal vaccine. *JAMA* 1982;248:1989–1995.
109. Winterbauer RH, Bedon GA, Ball WC Jr: Recurrent pneumonia predisposing illness and clinical patterns in 158 patients. *Ann Intern Med* 1969;70:689–700.
110. Finkelstein MS, Petkun WM, Freedman ML, et al: Pneumococcal bacteremia in adults: age-dependent differences in presentation and outcome. *J Am Geriatr Soc* 1983;31:19–27.
111. Finkelstein MS: Unusual features of infections in the aging. *Geriatrics* 1982;37: 65–78.
112. McFadden JP, Price RC, Eastwood HD, et al: Raised respiratory rate in elderly patients: A valuable physical sign. *Br Med J* 1982;1:626–627.
113. Barrett-Connor E: The nonvalue of sputum culture in the diagnosis of pneumococcal pneumonia. *Am Rev Respir Dis* 1971;103:845–848.
114. Jefferson H, Dalton HP, Escobar MR, et al: Transportation delay and the microbiological quality of clinical specimens. *Am J Clin Pathol* 1975;64:689–693.
115. Washington JA II: Noninvasive diagnostic techniques for lower respiratory infections, in Pennington JE (ed): *Respiratory Infections: Diagnosis and Management.* New York, Raven Press, 1983, pp 41–54.

116. Drew WL: Value of sputum culture in diagnosis of pneumococcal pneumonia. *J Clin Microbiol* 1977;6:62–65.
117. Jacobson JT, Burke JP, Jacobson JA: Ordering patterns, collection, transport, and screening of sputum cultures in a community hospital: evaluation of methods to improve results. *Infect Control* 1981;2:307–311.
118. Thorsteinsson SB, Musher DM, Fagan T: The diagnostic value of sputum culture in acute pneumonia. *JAMA* 1975; 233:894–895.
119. Geckler RW, Gremillion DH, McAllister CK, et al: Microscopic and bacteriological comparison of paired sputa and transtracheal aspirates. *J Clin Microbiol* 1977;6:396–399.
120. Heineman HS, Chawla JK, Lofton WM: Misinformation from sputum cultures without microscopic examination. *J Clin Microbiol* 1977; 6:518–527.
121. Bullowa JGM: The reliability of sputum typing and its relation to serum therapy. *JAMA* 1935;105:1512–1518.
122. Tempest B, Morgan R, Davidson M, et al: The value of respiratory tract bacteriology in pneumococcal pneumonia among Navajo Indians. *Am Rev Respir Dis* 1974;109:577–578.
123. Davidson M, Tempest B, Palmer DL: Bacteriologic diagnosis of acute pneumonia. Comparison of sputum, transtracheal aspirates, and lung aspirates. *JAMA* 1976;235:158–163.
124. Bartlett JG: Diagnostic accuracy of transtracheal aspiration bacteriologic studies. *Am Rev Respir Dis* 1977;115:777–782.
125. Berk SL, Holtsclaw SA, Kahn A, et al: Transtracheal aspiration in the severely ill elderly patient with bacterial pneumonia. *J Am Geriatr Soc* 1981;29:228–231.
126. Berk SL, Wiener SL, Eisner LB, et al: Mixed *Streptococcus pneumoniae* and gram-negative bacillary pneumonia in the elderly. *South Med J* 1981;74:144–146.
127. Bartlett JG: Bacteriological diagnosis of pulmonary infections, in Sackner MA (ed): *Diagnostic Techniques in Pulmonary Diseases*. New York, Marcel Dekker Inc, 1980, pp. 707-745.
128. Bjerkestrand G, Digranes A, Schreiner A: Bacteriological findings in transtracheal aspirates from patients with chronic bronchitis and bronchiectosis. A preliminary report. *Scand J Respir Dis* 1975;56:201–207.
129. Berman SJ, Mathison DA, Stevenson DD, et al: Transtracheal aspiration studies in asthmatic patients in relapse with "infective" asthma and in subjects without respiratory disease. *J Allergy Clin Immunol* 1975;56:206–214.
130. Irwin RS, Demers RR, Pratter MR, et al: Evaluation of methylene blue and squamous epithelial cells as oropharyngeal markers: A means of identifying oropharyngeal contamination during transtracheal aspiration. *J Infect Dis* 1980;141:165–171.
131. Haas H, Morris JF, Samson S, et al: Bacterial flora of the respiratory tract in chronic bronchitis: comparison of transtracheal, fiberbronchoscopic and oropharyngeal sampling method. *Am Rev Respir Dis* 1977;116:41–47.
132. Wimberley NW, Bass JB Jr, Boyd DW, et al: Use of a bronchoscopic protected catheter brush for the diagnosis of pulmonary infections. *Chest* 1982;81:556–562.
133. Wallace RJ Jr: (Another) New technique for an old disease. The protected brush catheter and bacterial pneumonia. *Chest* 1982;81:532–533.
134. Flatauer FE, Chabalko JJ, Wolinsky E: Fiberoptic bronchoscopy in bacteriologic assessment of lower respiratory tract secretions. Importance of a microscopic examination. *JAMA* 1980;244:2427–2429.

135. Rein MF, Gwaltney JM Jr, O'Brien WM, et al: Accuracy of Gram's stain in identifying pneumococci in sputum. *JAMA* 1978;239:2671–2673.
136. Merrill CW, Gwaltney JM Jr, Hendley JO, et al: Rapid identification of pneumococci. Gram stain vs. the Quellung reaction. *N Engl J Med* 1973;288:510–512.
137. Austrian R: The Quellung reaction, a neglected microbiologic technique. *Mt Sinai J Med* 1976;43:699–709.
138. Anhalt JP, Kenny GE, Rytel MW: Detection of microbial antigens by counter immunoelectrophoresis Cumitech 8. Washington, American Society for Microbiology, 1978.
139. Coonrod JD, Drennan DP: Pneumococcal pneumonia: Capsular polysaccharide antigenemia and antibody responses. *Ann Intern Med* 1976;84:254–260.
140. Leach RP, Coonrod JD: Detection of pneumococcal antigens in the sputum in pneumococcal pneumonia. *Am Rev Respir Dis* 1977;116:847–851.
141. Spencer RC, Savage MA: Use of counter and rocket immunoelectrophoresis in acute respiratory infections due to *Streptococcus pneumoniae*. *J Clin Pathol* 1976;29:187–190.
142. Schmid RE, Anhalt JP, Wold AD, et al: Sputum counterimmunoelectrophoresis in the diagnosis of pneumococcal pneumonia. *Am Rev Respir Dis* 1979;119:345–348.
143. Telenti A, Leiva PS: Persistence of pneumococcal antigens in sputum after treatment of pneumonia. *Scand J Infect Dis* 1984;16:323–324.
144. Kalin M, Lindberg AA: Diagnosis of pneumococcal pneumonia: a comparison between microscopic examination of expectorate, antigen detection, and cultural procedures. *Scand J Infect Dis* 1983;15:247–255.
 Downes BA, Ellner PD: Comparison of sputum counterimmunoelectrophoresis and culture in diagnosis of pneumococcal pneumonia. *J Clin Microbiol* 1979;10:662–665.
146. Guzzetta P, Toews GB, Robertson KJ, et al: Rapid diagnosis of community-acquired bacterial pneumonia. *Am Rev Respir Dis* 1983;128:461–464.
147. Thornsberry C, Swenson JM: Antimicrobial susceptibility tests for *Streptococcus pneumoniae*. *Lab Med* 1980;11:83–86.
148. Ward J: Antibiotic resistant *Streptococcus pneumoniae*, Clinical and epidemiologic aspects. *Rev Infect Dis* 1981;3:254–266.
149. Austrian R: A reassessment of pneumococcal vaccine. *N Engl J Med* 1984;310:651–653.
150. Hirschmann JV, Lipsky BA: Pneumococcal vaccine in the United States. A critical analysis. *JAMA* 1981;246:1428–1432.
151. Schwartz JS: Pneumococcal vaccine: Clinical efficacy and effectiveness. *Ann Intern Med* 1982; 96:208–220.
152. Bentley DW, Ha K, Mamot K, et al: Pneumococcal vaccine in the institutionalized elderly: Design of a nonrandomized trial and preliminary results. *Rev Infect Dis* 1981;3(suppl): S71–S81.
153. Shlaes DM, Mandell R, Bass S, et al: Bacteremia caused by *Streptococcus pneumoniae* of nonvaccine serotypes. *Am Rev Respir Dis* 1982;126:712–713.
154. Tillotson JR, Lerner AM: Pneumonias caused by gram-negative bacilli. *Medicine* 1966;45:65–76.
155. Unger JD, Rose HD, Unger GF: Gram-negative pneumonia. *Radiology* 1973;107:283–291.
156. Swartz MN: Pneumonias: Usual and unusual etiologies. *Ala J Med Sci* 1975;12:369–377.

157. Crane LR, Lerner AM: Gram-negative bacillary pneumonias, in Pennington JE (ed): *Respiratory Infections: Diagnosis and Management*. New York, Raven Press, 1983, pp 227–250.
158. Levin DC, Schwarz MI, Matthay RA, et al: Bacteremic *Haemophilus influenzae* pneumonia in adults. A report of 24 cases and a review of the literature. *Am J Med* 1977;62:219–224.
159. Everett ED, Rahm AE Jr, Adaniya R, et al: *Haemophilus influenzae* pneumonia in adults. *JAMA* 1977;238:319–321.
160. Wallace RJ Jr, Musher DM, Martin RR: *Haemophilus influenzae* pneumonia in adults. *Am J Med* 1978;64:87–93.
161. Stratton CW, Hawley HB, Horsman TA, et al: *Haemophilus influenzae* pneumonia in adults. Report of five cases caused by ampicillin-resistant strains. *Am Rev Respir Dis* 1980;121:595–598.
162. Wallace RJ Jr, Musher DM, Septimus EJ, et al: *Haemophilus influenzae* infections in adults: Characterization of strains by serotypes, biotypes, and ß-lactamase production. *J Infect Dis* 1981;144:101–106.
163. Berk SL, Holtsclaw SA, Wiener SL, et al: Nontypeable *Haemophilus influenzae* in the elderly. *Arch Intern Med* 1982;142:537–539.
164. Musher DM, Kubitschek KR, Crennan J, et al: Pneumonia and acute febrile tracheobronchitis due to *Haemophilus influenzae*. *Ann Intern Med* 1983;99:444–450.
165. Smith AL, Pappas P, Plorde J: *Haemophilus influenzae* pneumonia in Pennington JE (ed): *Respiratory Infections. Diagnosis and Management*, New York, Raven Press, 1983, pp 269–281.
166. Hirschmann JV, Everett ED: *Haemophilus influenzae* infections in adults: report of nine cases and a review of the literature. *Medicine* 1979;58:80–94.
167. Douglas RM, Devitt L: Pneumonia in New Guinea 1. Bacteriological findings in 632 adults with particular reference to *Haemophilus influenzae*. *Med J Aust* 1973;1:42–49.
168. Smith JK, Wiener SL: Life threatening infections in the elderly. The pneumonias. *Drug Ther* 1978; 3:19–36.
169. Gleckman RA, Esposito AL: Bacterial pneumonia in the elderly: a reappraisal of conventional therapy, with a note on cefamandole. *J Am Geriatr Soc* 1979;27: 345–347.
170. Burns MW, Devitt L, Bryant DH: Why do sputum cultures fail to yield pathogens? *Med J Aust* 1973;2:768–769.
171. Lauermann M, Barz M, Tally F: Cefamandole in the treatment of *Haemophilus influenzae* and other pneumonias and lung abscess. *Curr Ther Res* 1979;25:573–583.
172. Cordes LG, Fraser DW: Legionellosis: Legionnaires' disease; Pontiac fever. *Med Clin North Am* 1980;64:395–416.
173. England AC III, Fraser DW, Plikaytis DB, et al: Sporadic legionellosis in the United States: The first thousand cases. *Ann Intern Med* 1981;94:164–170.
174. Edelstein PH, Meyer RD: Legionnaires' disease. A review. *Chest* 1984;85:114–120.
175. Helms CM, Wintermeyer LA, Zeitler RR, et al: An outbreak of community-acquired Legionnaires' disease pneumonia. *Am J Public Health* 1984;74:835–836.
176. Helms CM, Viner JP, Weisenburger DD, et al: Sporadic Legionnaires' disease: Clinical observations on 87 nosocomial and community-acquired cases. *Am J Med Sci* 1984;288:2–12.

177. Dietrich PA, Johnson RD, Fairbank JT, et al: The chest radiograph in Legionnaires' disease. *Radiology* 1978;127: 577–582.
178. Kirby BD, Peck H, Meyer RD: Radiographic features of Legionnaires' disease. *Chest* 1979;76: 562–565.
179. Yu VL, Kroboth FJ, Shonnard J, et al: Legionnaires' disease: New clinical perspective from a prospective pneumonia study. *Am J Med* 1982;73:357–361.
180. Edelstein PH, Meyor RD, Finegold SM: Laboratory diagnosis of Legionnaires' disease. *Am Rev Respir Dis* 1980;121: 317–327.
181. Zuravleff JJ, Yu VL, Shonnard JW, et al: Diagnosis of Legionnaires' disease. An update of laboratory methods with new emphasis on isolation by culture. *JAMA* 1983;250: 1981–1985.
182. Edelstein PH: State of the art lecture: Laboratory diagnosis of Legionnaires' disease, in Thornsberry C, Balows A, Feely JC, et al (eds): *Legionnella, Proceedings of the Second International Symposium*. Washington, American Society for Microbiology, 1984, pp 3–5.
183. Zavala DC: The threat of aspiration pneumonia in the aged. *Geriatrics* 1977;32:46–51.
184. Bartlett JG: Anaerobic bacterial pneumonitis. *Am Rev Respir Dis* 1979;119:19–23.
185. Gopalakrishna KV, Lerner PI: Primary lung abscess: analysis of 66 cases. *Cleve Clin Q* 1975;42:3–13.
186. Levison ME, Mangura CT, Lorber B, et al: Clindamycin compared with penicillin for the treatment of anaerobic lung abscess. *Ann Intern Med* 1983;98:466–471.
187. Sanders CV, Hanna BJ, Lewis AC: Metronidazole in the treatment of anaerobic infections. *Am Rev Respir Dis* 1979; 120:337–343.
188. Perlino CA: Metronidazole vs. clindamycin in the treatment of anaerobic pulmonary infection. Failure of metronidazole therapy. *Arch Intern Med* 1981;141:1424–1427.
189. Tuazon CV: Gram-positive pneumonias. *Med Clin North Am* 1980;64:343–361.
190. Respiratory syncytial virus infection in the elderly 1976–82. *Br Med J* 1983;287:1618–1619.
191. Parainfluenza infection in the elderly 1976–82. *Br Med J* 1983;287:1619.
192. Parainfluenza outbreaks in extended-care facilities — United States. *MMWR* 1978;27:475–476.
193. Kimball AM, Foy HM, Cooney MK, et al: Isolation of respiratory syncytial and influenza viruses from sputum of patients hospitalized with pneumonia. *J Infect Dis* 1983;147:181–183.
194. Glezen WP: Viral pneumonia as a cause and result of hospitalization. *J Infect Dis* 1983;147:765–770.
195. Dean NL: Mycoplasmal pneumonias in the community hospital. The "unusual" manifestations become common. *Clin Chest Med* 1981;2:121–131.
196. Srinivasan G, Raff MJ, Templeton WC, et al: *Branhamella catarrhalis* pneumonia. Report of two cases and review of the literature. *Am Rev Respir Dis* 1981;123:533–535.
197. Louie MH, Gabay EL, Mathisen GE, et al: *Branhamella catarrhalis* pneumonia. *West J Med* 1983;138:47–49.
198. Diamond LA, Lorber B: *Branhamella catarrhalis* pneumonia immunoglobulin abnormalities: a new association. *Am Rev Respir Dis* 1984;129:876–878.

199. Doern GV, Siebers KG, Hallick LM, et al: Antibiotic susceptibility of betalactamase-producing strains of *Branhamella (Neisseria) catarrhalis. Antimicrob Agent Chemother* 1980;17:24–29.
200. Ahmad F, McLeod DT, Croughman MJ, et al: Antimicrobial susceptibility of *Branhamella catarrhalis* isolates from bronchopulmonary infections. *Antimicrob Agents Chemother* 1984;26:424–425.
201. Mostow SR: Pneumonias acquired outside the hospital: Recognition and treatment. *Med Clin North Am* 1974;58: 555–564.

9

Nosocomial Pneumonia

Michael R. Weitekamp
Robert C. Aber

Pneumonia accounts for 10% to 20% of all nosocomial infections.[1,2] Although it ranks third among the sites of nosocomial infection, pneumonia is more likely to cause or contribute to death than the more common urinary tract or surgical wound infections.[3]

The incidence of nosocomial pneumonia among all age groups ranges from five to 90 cases per 1000 patients admitted to or discharged from acute care hospitals per year in the United States. In 1983, hospitals that participated in the National Nosocomial Infections Study (NNIS 1983) with the Centers for Disease Control (CDC) reported an overall lower respiratory tract infection rate of 5.5/1000 patients discharged[4] The Study of the Efficacy of Nosocomial Infection Control (SENIC) conducted by CDC reported a nosocomial pneumonia infection rate of 9/1000 patients hospitalized.[2]

The SENIC project also reported that surgical patients were 3.9 times more likely to develop nosocomial pneumonia (definite or probable) than nonsurgical patients. Surgical patients experienced 74% of all nosocomial pneumonias.

The SENIC data identified several risk factors for nosocomial pneumonia. Intrinsic patient risk (based on underlying diagnoses and surgical procedures), thoracoabdominal incisions, and duration of the operative procedure are major risk factors, whereas, increasing age, male sex, and duration of postoperative hospitalization are less strongly associated with nosocomial pneumonia.

Garibaldi et al[5] reported that in addition to intrinsic risk, thoracoabdominal location of the incision, and longer duration of the operative procedure, a history of cigarette smoking, and a longer preoperative hospitalization were also major risk factors for nosocomial infection.

Gross et al[6] reported on the decade-specific risk of nosocomial infections, and found a relatively constant infection rate of 10/1000 patients discharged from birth to the end of the fifth decade. Thereafter the rate rose logarithmically and peaked at more than 100 infections per 1000 patients after 70 years. Sixty-four percent of all nosocomial infections occurred in patients more than 60 years old, whereas only 23% of all patients included in the study fell into this age group. The nosocomial pneumonia infection rate was 2/1000 patients from birth until the sixth decade, and thereafter rose dramatically to 16.9/1000 in the eighth decade and beyond. These rates were not adjusted for duration of hospitalization or for other risk factors described above.

The pathogenesis of most nosocomial pneumonias is by aspiration of oropharyngeal secretions and microorganisms into the lower airways, in conjunction with varying degrees of impairment of normal respiratory host defense mechanisms. Less common pathogenetic mechanisms are airborne, hematogenous or contiguous spread, and activation of endogenous infection in situ. It is difficult to determine precisely the reasons why the risk of nosocomial infections, including pneumonia, increases with age, but age-related changes in the immune response, the structural and functional integrity of organs and tissues, and nutrition have been documented.[7] Also, the frequency of selected invasive devices and procedures probably increases with age.

ETIOLOGIC AGENTS

A variety of organisms may cause pneumonia in the hospitalized, elderly patient, and can be divided into those likely to have been acquired in the hospital and those endogenous to the patient which have become reactivated in the hospital.

Most cases of nosocomial pneumonia in the elderly are caused by aerobic Gram-negative bacilli.[8] Local microbial ecology varies geographically and will dictate which genus and species (spp) predominates. Even within a hospital, pathogens may vary from one nursing unit to the next. Variations in antibiotic prescribing and infection control practices undoubtedly account for some of these differences. In a 1-year prospective surveillance of male patients admitted to an acute care geriatric ward in London, Andrews et al[9] found a higher frequency of gram-negative bacillary infection in those who acquired pneumonia in the community rather than in the hospital. The authors suggested that this may be due to the very judicious use of antibiotics in that particular hospital as compared with more liberal use in the community. This pattern has not been reported from hospitals in the United States. Summary data from the NNIS 1983 give the following distribution for Gram-negative rods as the cause of lower respiratory tract infection: *Pseudomonas aeruginosa* (15.1%), *Klebsiella* spp (12.8%), *Enterobacter* spp (10.0%), *Escherichia coli* (9.1%), *Serratia* spp (5.6%), and *Proteus* spp (4.4%).[4]

Other gram-negative organisms may also cause pneumonia in the elderly hospitalized patient. *Haemophilus influenzae* is increasingly recognized as a cause of both community- and hospital-acquired pneumonia in patients over the age of 50 years, especially in those who are alcoholic or have chronic obstructive pulmonary disease. Deficient serum opsonizing activity for *H influenzae* has been identified in some patients.[10] *Branhamella catarrhalis* (formerly *Neisseria catarrhalis*) has been reported as a pulmonary pathogen in elderly, debilitated patients.[11] Twenty-five cases of pneumonia in mechanically ventilated patients due to *Acinetobacter calcoaceticus* were reported by Glew et al; most were elderly and mortality was 44%.[12]

Gram-positive infections are usually caused by *Staphylococcus aureus* and *Streptococcus* spp. *S aureus* accounted for 12.8% of the lower respiratory tract infections in NNIS 1983. Although reported as causing 1.1% of the lower respiratory tract infection in NNIS 1983, coagulase-negative staphylococci commonly contaminate sputum cultures and their role in geriatric nosocomial pneumonia is not convincing. *Streptococcus pneumoniae* was isolated by transtracheal aspiration in seven of 35 patients (20%) in a recent study of nosocomial pneumonia in the elderly.[13] Verghese et al[14] reported seven cases of fatal necrotizing nosocomial pneumonia in elderly patients due to *S agalactiae* (group B streptococcus). Historically viewed as a cause of neonatal sepsis and meningitis, the group B streptococcus is increasingly recognized as an aggressive pathogen in the elderly and diabetic patient.[15] A protracted outbreak of serious infections, including pneumonia, caused by a single serotype of *S pyogenes* (group A streptococcus) has been reported in a nursing home.[16] Enterococcal (group D streptococcus) colonization, bacteremia, and nosocomial pneumonia have been associated with the use of broad spectrum cephalosporins.[17,18]

The role of anaerobic organisms in nosocomial infection has not been fully defined; expectorated sputum is an inappropriate specimen for anaerobic culture and transtracheal aspiration (TTA) is not routinely performed by most physicians. In a report on TTA in 32 severely ill, elderly patients with pneumonia, 18 infections were acquired in hospital or nursing homes and anaerobic organisms were not important pathogens.[19] However, anaerobic pleuropulmonary infections have been associated with bronchogenic carcinoma, periodontal disease, and aspiration, conditions likely to be found in an elderly population.

Although the incidence of tuberculosis in the United States is declining, the proportion of elderly patients infected is increasing. Most cases result from reactivation of dormant infection and may first become evident during hospitalization for an unrelated problem. Stead recently reported an epidemic of tuberculosis among elderly residents of a nursing home where both patient-to-patient and patient-to-staff transmission were documented.[20]

Both *Legionella pneumophila* and *L micdadei* are well-recognized causes of nosocomial pneumonia in the elderly and immunosuppressed.[21,22] Knowledge of the ecology and epidemiology of these organisms is incomplete and the incidence of infection varies geographically. Our hospital, in central Pennsylvania, has been culturing for *Legionella* spp for over 3 years; with a large elderly and immunosuppressed patient population (including both renal and heart transplant recipients), we have yet to diagnose nosocomial legionellosis.

Candida and *Aspergillus* are the most common fungi causing nosocomial pneumonia, but generally, only in severely immunocompromised patients with rapidly fatal underlying diseases. *Candida* spp are often recovered from respiratory cultures in elderly, debilitated patients, especially in those who have received antibiotics; however, a diagnosis of *Candida* pneumonia cannot reliably be made without demonstrating tissue invasion, or by positive blood or pleural fluid cultures. Clusters of *Aspergillus* pneumonia in immunocompromised patients have been associated with hospital construction and renovation.

The impact of nosocomial viral infection on the elderly is still being defined.[23] Valenti et al in Rochester, New York, reported that 25% of 142 nosocomial lower respiratory tract infections detected between December 1, 1977 and April 30, 1979 were caused by viruses.[24] Among adults on the psychiatry, medicine, and surgery services, influenza virus and rhinovirus caused exogenously acquired respiratory tract infections, whereas members of the *Herpesvirus* group caused reactivated disease. Nosocomial acquisition of influenza viruses A and B, and respiratory syncytial virus has been documented in the elderly.[25]

Although extremely unusual as causes of nosocomial pneumonia, parasites such as *Pneumocystis carinii*, *Toxoplasma gondii*, and *Strongyloides stercoralis* occur occasionally in severely immunocompromised hosts, usually due to reactivation of latent infection.

Mycoplasmas and *Chlamydia* are not recognized nosocomial pathogens in the elderly. However, a role for these organisms in hospital-acquired infection may emerge with improved methods for detection.

DIAGNOSIS AND DIFFERENTIAL DIAGNOSIS

Generally, the elderly patient with nosocomial pneumonia presents with a combination of the following: fever, increased pulmonary secretions or sputum, pleuritic chest pain, cough, hypoxemia, leukocytosis with a left shift, or evidence of parenchymal disease on chest film or physical examination. However, as is true with most infections in the elderly, insidious and atypical signs and symptoms may occasionally obscure or delay diagnosis; fever may be absent and cough reflexes blunted, total WBC count may be low (left shift usually persists), and agitation, confusion, lethargy, or coma may be the first manifestation of sepsis or hypoxia. Pre-existing abnormalities on the chest film may obscure the evaluation of a new infiltrate; old granulomatous disease, atelectasis, congestive heart failure, bronchiectasis, pulmonary fibrosis, pneumoconiosis, neoplasia, and postpneumonectomy and radiation changes are some examples.

Acute, noninfectious conditions such as pulmonary edema, contusion or hemorrhage, pleural effusion, pulmonary embolism with infarction, allergic drug or blood product reaction, and chemical pneumonitis may also mimic pneumonia on the chest film. Furthermore, no particular pattern of infiltrate can reliably predict either the presence of pneumonia or the microbiologic cause. For instance, diffuse, bilateral infiltrates are characteristic of viral pneumonia, yet may be seen in pneumonia caused by bacteria such as *H influenzae* and *S aureus*, in pneumonia which develops while on a mechanical ventilator, and with such noninfectious problems as chemical aspiration pneumonitis, vasculitis, adult respiratory distress syndrome (ARDS), and congestive heart failure. Cavitation on the chest film may be seen with nosocomial pneumonia due to Gram-negative aerobes, anaerobes, *Legionella* spp, type 3 pneumococcus, *S aureus*, fungi, *Nocardia* spp, *Mycobacterium* spp, and others, as well as with noninfectious processes such as carcinoma, vasculitis, and infarction.

An accurate microbiologic diagnosis in nosocomial pneumonia has important therapeutic implications. One need only to scan the variety of organisms shown in Tables 9-1 and 9-2 to realize that an empiric

Table 9-1
Microorganisms Causing Nosocomial Pneumonia in the Elderly — Acquired in the Hospital

Organism	Most Common	Uncommon
Bacteria	Klebsiella	Acinetobacter
	Pseudomonas	Flavobacterium
	Enterobacter	Haemophilus
	Escherichia	Branhamella
	Proteus	Anaerobes
	Serratia	Legionella
	Staphylococcus	Mycobacterium
	Streptococcus	Nocardia

Organism	Most Common	Uncommon
Fungi	Candida	Torulopsis
	Aspergillus	Rhizopus
		Mucor
Viruses	Influenza	Rhinovirus
	Parainfluenza	Adenovirus
	Respiratory Syncytial Virus	
Chlamydia		
Mycoplasma		

Table 9-2
Microorganisms Causing Nosocomial Pneumonia in the Elderly — Activated or Reactivated in the Hospital

Bacteria	Mycobacterium
	Staphylococcus
	Streptococcus
	Haemophilus
	Nocardia
Fungi	Histoplasma
	Coccidioides
	Aspergillus
	Cryptococcus
Parasites	Pneumocystis
	Toxoplasma
	Strongyloides
Viruses	Herpes Simplex
	Herpes Zoster
	Cytomegalovirus

approach to the therapy of this infection is hazardous. Culture of sputum or pulmonary secretions is the most commonly employed means to determine the etiology of nosocomial pneumonia. Sputum is usually obtained by spontaneous expectoration, nasotracheal or orotracheal suction, or suction via an existing endotracheal tube. Contamination of these specimens with oropharyngeal flora is inevitable. The oropharynx of the seriously ill, hospitalized patient is colonized with both "normal throat flora" (*Streptococcus* spp, *Neisseria* spp, *Haemophilus* spp, and anaerobes) and such hospital-acquired pathogens as aerobic Gram-negative rods (*Enterobacteriaceae* and *Pseudomonas* spp) and *S aureus*. Consequently, culture of such sputum specimens usually results in the growth of several organisms and is poorly predictive of the actual cause of the patient's pneumonia.

The clinician reviewing sputum culture results faces the dilemma of separating colonizing flora from infecting pathogens. Attempts to improve the predictive value of sputum cultures have been made. Murray and Washington reported a system of screening sputum for oropharyngeal contamination prior to culture.[26] A portion of the submitted specimen is placed on a glass slide and stained with methylene blue. The presence of more than ten epithelial cells per low power microscopic field (X 10 objective) suggests significant oropharyngeal contamination and that specimen should not be processed for culture and sensitivity testing because the results will be misleading to the physician. Sputum which contains fewer than ten epithelial cells per low power field and more than 25 polymorphonuclear leukocytes (PMNs) is more likely to yield culture results that predict the actual cause of pneumonia. By no means foolproof, such screening improves the utility of expectorated sputum cultures and results in cost savings by minimizing the laboratory evaluation of unsatisfactory specimens. Specimens submitted from patients who either are, or recently have been intubated, and from patients with chronic bronchitis, will often contain numerous PMNs, few epithelial cells, and still yield culture results which reflect tracheobronchial colonization rather than pneumonia. Differentiating between diffuse lung injury and infection in a patient with ARDS can also be quite difficult.[27]

Microscopic examination of a properly prepared sputum Gram's stain is invaluable as a diagnostic tool and should be part of any evaluation of a patient with suspected pneumonia. The Gram's stain often provides an early presumptive diagnosis and aids in the interpretation of subsequent culture results. Depending on the clinical setting and the sophistication of the laboratory support available, additional information can be obtained from sputum examination. Acid-fast staining and culture for the detection of *Mycobacterium* spp and *Nocardia* spp is available in most hospitals. Silver staining and fungal culture may be indicated in some patients. *Legionella* spp can now be identified by modified silver staining, direct immunofluorescent antibody technique, or culture on selective media. Sputum cytology, normally utilized to detect malignancy, will occasionally suggest pneumonia caused by a member of the *Herpesvirus* genus when characteristic viral inclusion bodies are present in alveolar lining cells. Recent advances in monoclonal antibody technology offer the promise of direct fluorescent antibody tests for detecting most microorganisms in clinical specimens.

More invasive methods for sampling lower respiratory tract secretions include use of fiberoptic bronchoscopy (FOB) and transtracheal aspiration. Distinguishing between purulent tracheitis and early pneumonia in the intubated patient can be quite difficult; FOB may assist by allowing a visual assessment of the airways beyond a purulent trachea. A recently developed technique using a protective sleeve over a brush offers the possibility of deep sampling of pulmonary secretions while minimizing contamination with oropharyngeal flora, but has been disappointing in clinical trials.[28] A group of French investigators feel that combining this technique with quantitative microbiology may improve its specificity.[29]

Transtracheal aspiration involves needle puncture and catheter placement directly into the trachea through the cricothyroid membrane. It requires a cooperative patient, an experienced physician, and carries the attendant risks of inducing hypoxia, cardiac arrhythmia, bleeding, and subcutaneous emphysema. Berk et al feel that TTA can be a safe and useful procedure in evaluating pneumonia, even in the severely ill elderly patient.[19] In patients with chronic bronchitis or in those recently extubated, colonization of the tracheobronchial tree may obscure culture results even from a TTA specimen.

Biopsy of lung tissue to obtain a specimen uncontaminated by the upper airways is usually reserved for immunocompromised patients and critically ill patients in whom less invasive procedures have failed to provide a diagnosis. Biopsy techniques include open biopsy via a limited thoracotomy, transbronchial biopsy through a fiberoptic bronchoscope (specimen likely to still be contaminated), and the use of a percutaneous cutting needle.

Pleural fluid accumulation and empyema formation may be seen in patients with nosocomial pneumonia. Diagnostic thoracentesis may provide valuable microbiologic information; a pleural fluid pH less than 7.2 or a positive fluid Gram's stain or culture should prompt consideration of chest tube placement.

The value of blood cultures should not be overlooked in the patient evaluation. Nosocomial pneumonia is often a necrotizing infection accompanied by bacteremia.

MANAGEMENT

The management of the elderly patient with nosocomial pneumonia is, in principle, similar to the management of any patient with nosocomial pneumonia except for the following: (1) There may be irreversible multiple-organ failure in association with the pneumonia; (2) there may be important ethical considerations in deciding how aggressive to be; (3) the pharmacology and pharmacokinetics of specific drugs may be different in this age group; and (4) although the pneumonia per se may be curable from a microbiologic point of view, organ-system changes related to age will probably not improve, and hence therapeutic goals and expectations must be realistic.

Hypoxemia should be corrected by administering oxygen in the least invasive and most comfortable manner. A nasal cannula or face mask may suffice, but endotracheal intubation or tracheostomy may be necessary. Positive end-expiratory pressure, if used, must be titrated to optimize the balance between oxygenation and cardiac output. Since many elderly patients have chronic obstructive lung disease, arterial blood gases may be an important part of initial management to document an adequate PO_2 without a rise in PCO_2. The presence of substantial coronary artery atherosclerosis or ischemic heart disease make prompt correction of hypoxemia even more important.

Intravascular volume must be optimized, but rapid, large volume shifts are not well tolerated by most elderly patients. Underlying coronary artery or ischemic heart disease is common, and fluid challenge may result in left heart failure with worsening hypoxemia.

Removal or drainage of pulmonary secretions may also reduce hypoxemia, but a recent clinical trial did not find any benefit in the resolution of pneumonia from postural drainage, percussion, and vibration combined with intermittent positive pressure breathing (IPPD).[30] The number of patients studied was small so that significant differences may not have been detected. If cough is not present, insufficient to clear secretions, or not possible, endotracheal suctioning may be used to remove secretions. Fiberoptic bronchoscopy may be used to remove tenacious mucus or plugs, and foreign bodies. Rarely, bronchial lavage is attempted to remove secretions. Changes in body position of the patient, rather than maintenance of the usual recumbent position, may promote drainage of secretions and prevent pooling in dependent bronchopulmonary segment(s).

Respiratory host defense mechanisms should be restored whenever possible. This includes discontinuing or tapering immunosuppressive drugs and corticosteroids, minimizing the concentration of inspired oxygen, correction of anatomical or neurologic abnormalities of the glottis, and minimizing the use of antitussive agents, such as narcotics and CNS depressants.

Closed chest drainage of infected pleural fluid (empyema) should be implemented in most cases of nosocomial pneumonia unless the amount of fluid is small and the microorganism is very susceptible to antimicrobial agents.

Treatment of fever associated with nosocomial pneumonia is a controversial subject and depends more on the hemodynamic or metabolic consequences of the fever than on the infection itself.

Antimicrobial therapy for nosocomial pneumonia is best considered in two phases: (1) *empiric therapy* based on the index of suspicion that the patient has pneumonia, the results of a Gram's stain of respiratory secretions or pleural fluid (if available), and the clinical and epidemiologic setting in which the pneumonia has developed prior to identification of a specific etiologic agent and its antimicrobial susceptibilities; and (2) *specific therapy* based on recovering a putative etiologic agent(s) and determining antimicrobial susceptibilities.

Empiric antimicrobial therapy requires considerable clinical judgement and experience, as well as knowledge about prevalent microorganisms and antimicrobial susceptibility patterns in the hospital, the pharmacology of antimicrobial agents in elderly patients, potential drug-drug interactions, and existing risk factors for adverse reactions to therapy. Since the majority of nosocomial pneumonias, including those in the elderly, are caused by aspiration of oropharyngeal flora containing aerobic Gram-positive and Gram-negative bacteria as well as some oral anaerobes, empiric therapy with a cephalosporin and an aminoglycoside is reasonable. Single-drug therapy, even with the newer broad spectrum penicillins and cephalosporins, is risky in the empiric treatment of nosocomial pneumonias because of the prevalence of multiple resistant bacteria in the hospital and the high mortality associated with nosocomial pneumonia. Appropriate clinical trials may eventually prove single-drug empiric therapy effective and safe in this setting, but such do not exist at present. A convincing gram stain of respiratory secretions or pleural fluid may permit initiation of more specific empiric antimicrobial therapy.

Specific antimicrobial therapy for nosocomial pneumonia is based on: (1) recovering the putative etiologic agents or agents from respiratory secretions, pleural fluid, or blood; (2) determining or anticipating the antimicrobial susceptibilities of these agents; and (3) selecting an appropriate antimicrobial agent or agents based on desired microbiologic and pharmacologic properties to deliver effective, yet safe, treatment. It has not been established that after the etiologic agent has been identified, more than one effective antimicrobial agent increases the response rate of nosocomial pneumonia in any particular patient population or for any specific microorganism, but many experts recommend two-drug antibiotic therapy for additive or potentiating effects since the mortality from nosocomial pneumonia remains high.

It is probably quite safe to assume that all patients over 65 years of age have some reduction of glomerular filtration rate, and hence doses and dosing intervals of antimicrobial agents dependent on renal excretion must be modified accordingly.

Many elderly patients are receiving concomitant drugs, and the potential for drug-drug interactions with antimicrobial agents must be considered in selecting an appropriate specific agent for therapy.

Anticipation and careful observation during antimicrobial therapy remain essential elements in good patient care.

PREVENTION

The epidemiologic tenet that infection only occurs when there is a pathogen, a mode of transmission, and a susceptible host, provides a logical framework in which to view preventive measures for nosocomial pneumonia in the elderly.

Control of Pathogens

The hospital will never be a sterile environment and attempts to make it so are impractical and expensive. Whereas no one will argue the aesthetic appeal of clean walls, floors, and exposed surfaces, studies have suggested that the inanimate environment plays a relatively minor role in nosocomial infection rates.[31] Routine environmental culturing is not cost-effective and cannot be justified. Limited environmental culturing may be indicated during the investigation of an epidemic; *Legionella* spp and *Aspergillus* spp are pulmonary pathogens which have been traced to environmental sources. Potted plants are known to harbor *Pseudomonas* spp, *Aeromonas* spp, *Bacillus* spp, and other potential pathogens, and should not be placed in the rooms of immunocompromised patients. During the 1960s and 1970s numerous epidemics of necrotizing Gram-negative pneumonia were traced to contaminated respiratory support devices such as ventilators, aerosolizers, and nebulizers. With the establishment of procedures for the maintenance and decontamination of this equipment, a dramatic decrease in epidemic nosocomial pneumonia was effected. The CDC has published recent guidelines for the prevention of nosocomial pneumonia which incorporate these procedures and serve as an important reference for anyone involved in the care of hospitalized patients requiring such devices.[32]

With the recognition that oropharyngeal carriage of pathogenic organisms and subsequent aspiration accounts for most nosocomial pneumonia, several attempts have been made to interrupt this process with the use of aerosolized antibiotics.[33,34] Such measures have consistently led to colonization and subsequent infection with more resistant organisms and have been abandoned. Research into the mechanisms of bacterial adherence to epithelial cells may someday provide clinicians with the means to prevent colonization. Treatment of existing tracheobronchial infection and aggressive pulmonary therapy are important preventive measures in the perioperative management of the elderly patient.

An effective personnel health program which encourages the reporting of employee illnesses will minimize the risk of introduction and spread of potential pneumonic pathogens such as *herpes simplex*, *herpes zoster* (shingles, chickenpox), group A streptococcus, and influenza viruses.

Limiting Transmission

Handwashing between patient contacts is the single most important measure for interrupting the transmission of microorganisms. Yet, health professionals are notoriously unreliable in utilizing this simple procedure. Although the use of antibacterial soaps reduces the number of microorganisms on the hands to a greater degree than does the use of plain soap and water, the "major concern . . . regarding handwashing should not be what agent to use, but how to motivate all hospital employees to wash at the appropriate times, using established washing techniques and agents."[35]

Eliminating transmission via aspiration in elderly patients is impossible, but physicians can minimize the risk by the judicious use of sedating medication, avoiding overdistention of the stomach with feedings, and keeping the head of the bed elevated.

An active infection control program (ideally, one full-time infection control practitioner [ICP] for each 250 beds) can be instrumental in reducing the incidence of nosocomial infections.[36] Surveillance of hospital-acquired infection as provided by the ICP is the foundation for interventive and preventive measures, and is mandated by the Joint Commission for Accreditation of Hospitals (JCAH). Inservice of new employees and the continuing education of existing personnel in infection control policy and procedure are important duties of the ICP. The ICP should also be active in ongoing review of hospital policies related to infection control in order to keep them current. Updated isolation procedures to limit transmission of infection in the hospital have recently been published by the CDC.[37]

Altering Host Susceptibility

Physicians who care for adult and geriatric patients have not adopted the concept of immunization in the prevention of disease as readily as pediatricians. Immunization against the influenza viruses is safe, effective, and underutilized. Likewise, the polyvalent pneumococcal vaccine has been shown to be effective, and yet only a small proportion of elderly patients have actually received it.[38] Promising research into immunization against pathogenic Gram-negative bacilli is progressing.[39] Primary care physicians must take a leading role to assure that these technologic advances are properly utilized to the benefit of their patients.

Modern antibiotic therapy has improved survival in bacterial infections, but is truly a double-edged sword. Excessive use has altered the bacterial flora in our hospitals and community, and fostered the emergence of increasingly resistant strains. Infection with resistant bacteria as well as fungi infection can almost always be linked to the use of broad spectrum antibiotic therapy. More subtle and yet, perhaps, equally important are the adverse effects which antibiotics may exert on host defenses.[40] Physicians need to be aware of these risks and more prudent in their use of antibiotics. Such practices as prescribing antibiotics for the common cold, treating asymptomatic bacteriuria in the elderly, and using broad spectrum and multiple antibiotics when a single narrow spectrum agent is indicated are to be discouraged.

Nutritional supplementation to enhance host immunity, therapy of underlying diseases such as diabetes, congestive heart failure, and obstructive lung disease, and the interdiction of smoking are all likely to reduce susceptibility of the elderly patient to pneumonia.

REFERENCES

1. Gardner P, Arnow PM: Hospital-acquired pneumonias, in Braunwald E, Isselbacher K, Petersdorf RG, et al (eds): *Harrison's Principles of Internal Medicine*, ed 11. New York, McGraw-Hill Book Co, 1987, pp 470–474.
2. Haley RW, Hooton TM, Culver DH, et al: Nosocomial in-fections in U.S. hospitals, 1975–1976. Estimated frequency by selected characteristics of patients. *Am J Med* 1981;70:947–959.
3. Gross RA, Neu HC, VanAntwerpen C, et al: Deaths from nosocomial infections — experience in a university and a community hospital. *Am J Med* 1980; 68:219–223.
4. Centers for Disease Control: Nosocomial infection surveillance, 1983, in *CDC Surveillance Summaries* 1984;33(No.22S):9SS–21SS.
5. Garibaldi RA, Britt MR, Coleman ML, et al : Risk factors for nosocomial pneumonia. *Am J Med* 1981;70:677–680.
6. Gross PA, Rapuano C, Adrignolo A, et al: Nosocomial infections: decade-specific risk. *Infect Control* 1983;4:145–147.
7. Gardner I: The effect of aging on susceptibility to infection. *Rev Infect Dis* 1980;2:801–810.
8. Niederman MS, Fein AM: Pneumonia in the elderly. *Clin Geriatr Med* 1986;2:241–268.
9. Andrews J, Chandrasekaran P, McSwiggan D: Lower respiratory tract infections in an acute geriatric male ward: A one year prospective surveillance. *Gerontology* 1984;30: 290–296.
10. Musher DM, Kubitschek KR, Crennan J, et al : Pneumonia and acute febrile tracheobronchitis due to *Haemophilus influenzae*. *Ann Intern Med* 1983;99:444–450.
11. West M, Berk SL, Smith JK: *Branhamella catarrhalis* pneumonia. *South Med J* 1985;75:1021.
12. Glew RH, Moellering RC, Kunz LJ: Infections with *Acinetobacter calcoaceticus* (*Herellea vaginicola*): Clinical and laboratory studies. *Medicine* 1977;56:79–97.
13. Berk SL, Gallemore GM, Smith JK: Nosocomial pneumococcal pneumonia in the elderly. *J Am Geriatr Soc* 1981;29:319–321.
14. Verghese A, Berk SL, Boelen LJ, et al: Group B streptococcal pneumonia in the elderly. *Arch Intern Med* 1982;142:1642–1645.
15. Lerner PI, Gopalakrishna KV, Wolinsky E, et al: Group B streptococcal bacteremia in adults: Analysis of 32 cases and review of the literature. *Medicine* 1977;56:457–473.
16. Ruben FL, Norden CW, Heisler B, et al: An outbreak of *Streptococcus pyogenes* infections in a nursing home. *Ann Intern Med* 1984;101:494–496.

17. Craven DE, Kunches LM, Kilinsky V, et al: Risk factors for pneumonia and fatality in patients receiving continuous mechanical ventilation. *Am Rev Respir Dis* 1986;133:792–796.
18. Yu VL: Enterococcal superinfection and colonization after therapy with moxalactam, a new broad-spectrum antibiotic. *Ann Intern Med* 1981;94:784–785.
19. Berk SL, Holtsclaw SA, Kahn A, et al: Transtracheal aspiration in the severely ill elderly patient with bacterial pneumonia. *J Am Geriatr Soc* 1981;29:228–231.
20. Stead WW: Tuberculosis among elderly persons. An outbreak in a nursing home. *Ann Intern Med* 1981;94:606–610.
21. Kirby BD, Snyder KM, Myer RD, et al: Legionnaires disease: report of 65 nosocomial acquired cases and review of the literature. *Medicine* 1980;59:185–205.
22. Muder RR, Yu VL, Zuraleff JJ: Pneumonia due to Pittsburgh pneumonia agent: new clinical perspective with review of the literature. *Medicine* 1983;62:120–128.
23. Glezen WP: Viral pneumonia as a cause and result of hospitalization. *J Infect Dis* 1983;147:765–770.
24. Valenti WM, Menegus MA, Hall CB, et al: Nosocomial viral infections — I. Epidemiology and significance. *Infect Control* 1980;1:33–37.
25. Harris AA, Levin S, Trenholme GM: Selected aspects of nosocomial infections in the 1980s. *Am J Med* 1984;77(1B):3–10.
26. Murray PR, Washington JA: Microscopic and bacteriologic analysis of expectorated sputum. *Mayo Clin Proc* 1975;50:339–344.
27. Andrews CP, Coalson JJ, Smith JD, et al: Diagnosis of nosocomial bacterial pneumonia in acute, diffuse lung injury. *Chest* 1981;80:254–258.
28. Wimberley NW, Bass JB, Boyd BW, et al: Use of a bronchoscopic protected catheter brush for the diagnosis of pulmonary infections. *Chest* 1982;81:556–562.
29. Chastre J, Viau F, Brun P, et al: Prospective evaluation of the protected specimen brush for the diagnosis of pulmonary infections in ventilated patients. *Am Rev Respir Dis* 1984;130:924–929.
30. Graham, WGB, Bradley DA: Efficacy of chest physiotherapy and intermittent positive breathing in the resolution of pneumonia. *N Engl J Med* 1978;299:624–627.
31. Maki DG, Alvarado CJ, Hassemer CA, et al: Relation of the inanimate hospital environment to endemic nosocomial infection. *N Engl J Med* 1982;307:1562–1566.
32. Simmons BP, Wong ES: Guideline for prevention of nosocomial pneumonia. *Infect Control* 1982; 3:327–333.
33. Feeley TW, duMoulin GC, Hedley-Whyte J, et al: Aerosol polymyxin and pneumonia in seriously ill patients. *N Engl J Med* 1975;293:471–475.
34. Klastersky J, Huysmans E, Weerts D, et al: Endotracheally administered gentamicin for the prevention of infections of the respiratory tract in patients with tracheostomy: A double-blind study. *Chest* 1974;65:650–654.
35. Edberg SC: Handwashing as an adjunct to infection control: An evaluation. *Asepsis* 1981;2:3.
36. Haley RW, Culver DH, White JW, et al: The efficacy of infection surveillance and control programs in preventing nosocomial infections in U.S. hospitals. *Am J Epidemiol* 1985;121:182–205.
37. Garner JS, Simmons BP: CDC guideline for isolation precautions in hospitals. *Infect Control* 1983;4:245–325.

38. Austrian R: Pneumonococcal pneumonia: Diagnostic, epidemiologic, theraupeutic and prophylactic considerations. *Chest* 1986;90:738–743.
39. Braude AI, Ziegler EJ, McCutchan JA, et al: Immunization against nosocomial infection. *Am J Med* 1981;70:463–466.
40. Hauser WE, Remington JS: Effect of antibiotics on the immune response. *Am J Med* 1982;72:711–716.

10

Endocarditis

Carol A. Kauffman
Robert Fekety

Infective endocarditis is a disease of increasing importance to physicians caring for the elderly. The disease was uncommonly noted in those over age 60 years in the preantibiotic era.[1,2] Several reviews on endocarditis in the elderly from the 1940s and 1950s emphasized that the disease was more common than previously thought,[3,4] but still elderly patients accounted for only 3% to 19% of all cases of endocarditis in these two decades.[5,6] In recent years, there has been a dramatic rise in the number of patients over 60 years of age with endocarditis[7,8]; a recent survey of endocarditis in the 1970s found that 55% of patients were over age 60.[9]

The reasons for this increase are not entirely clear but could relate to increasing age of the population overall, to increased longevity of persons with valvular heart disease, and to increased hospitalization of the elderly population with subsequent risk for nosocomially acquired bacteremia and endocarditis.[10] Not only is endocarditis becoming more common in the elderly, but mortality is excessively high in the elderly population. This is especially true of certain types of endocarditis, such as that due to the staphylococcus.[11]

The clinical features of endocarditis have changed over the last 40 years, as has the epidemiology of the disease.[12,13] It is now uncommon to see patients with many of the "classic" signs of subacute bacterial endocarditis.[14] How much this change in the clinical picture is due to the increasing age of patients with endocarditis compared with changes in microbiology, underlying cardiac conditions, and earlier use of diagnostic tests is not clear. No recent study has directly compared young and elderly patients in regard to the clinical manifestations of endocarditis in order to assess the role of age in clinical presentation.

This review focuses on various aspects of endocarditis of special interest to those caring for elderly patients. Underlying conditions, microbiologic aspects and clinical features are discussed as well as diagnostic and therapeutic modalities appropriate for use in the elderly patient with endocarditis.

PREDISPOSING FACTORS

Although classically rheumatic heart disease has been the major underlying pathologic feature predisposing to the development of endocarditis, this has never been as prominent a factor in elderly persons as in younger patients.[3,4,15] Arteriosclerotic or degenerative changes in the valves are the most common underlying pathologic findings in elderly persons dying with endocarditis.[3,4,15] Aortic valve calcification is common, and in many patients is associated with a congenitally bicuspid valve.[15] Mitral valve prolapse and calcified mitral annulus fibrosus also are found as underlying pathologic conditions, especially in elderly women with endocarditis.[15-17] In many instances (19%—37% in various series), no underlying valvular pathology could be identified in elderly patients dying with endocarditis.[15,18]

Overall, the aortic and mitral valves appear to be equally likely to be involved[3,19]; some series show more aortic valve endocarditis[15,18] and others show a preponderance of mitral valve endocarditis.[11,20] Tricuspid valve involvement is uncommonly noted except in patients with coexisting left-sided endocarditis or in those with central catheter-related infections.[3,4,21]

In recent years, an increasing number of elderly patients with endocarditis have acquired this infection in the hospital setting.[10,11,21] Robbins et al found that 15 of their 56 patients (27%) acquired endocarditis in the hospital.[21] Intravenous (IV) catheter-related septicemia was the preceding event in most of these patients, followed by genitourinary (GV) tract procedures. As might be expected, *Staphylococcus aureus* was the most common nosocomially acquired pathogen, followed by enterococci and fungi.[21] In a review of 14 cases of nosocomially acquired endocarditis, Friedland et al found that the mean age was 62 years, the organisms responsible were primarily *S aureus* and enterococci, and at least half of the cases could have been prevented if standard infection control practices had been followed.[10]

MICROBIOLOGY

The importance of various microorganisms causing endocarditis has changed over the last 40 years, not only in the elderly but in all patients with endocarditis.[12] Viridans streptococci have decreased as a cause of endocarditis while staphylococci, gram-negative bacilli, and fungi have increased.[12,13,22] Organisms such as the pneumococcus, group A streptococcus, and the gonococcus now rarely cause endocarditis.[13]

Especially prominent has been the rise in the number of cases of endocarditis due to *S aureus*. Among the elderly, this trend is well documented. Thus, in recent reviews of endocarditis in the elderly, 21% to 29% of cases are due to *S aureus*,[15,21] compared with 0% to 10% in the 1940s and 1950s.[4,23] There are many reasons for the overall increase in cases of *S aureus* endocarditis, especially the increase in IV drug abuse,[12,24] but among the elderly the striking feature is the number of times *S aureus* is acquired as a nosocomial infection, most often related to an indwelling IV catheter.[10,21]

Viridans streptococci, although less common than in the 1940s and 1950s when they caused over 57% of cases of endocarditis in the elderly,[23] still account for about 35% of cases in the elderly.[21,25] *Streptococcus bovis*, only recently routinely separated from viridans streptococci,[26] is an important cause of endocarditis in the elderly because of its association with carcinoma of the colon and other colonic disease prevalent in the elderly.[25,27,28]

Group D enterococci have been important causes of endocarditis in the elderly throughout the last 40 years, accounting for 10% to 20% of cases in most series.[21,23,29] Most of those cases are in elderly men and many are related to GU tract obstruction and manipulation. There is a predilection for aortic valve involvement in these patients, with the murmur of aortic regurgitation characteristically not being detected until after several days of hospitalization.[30]

Although uncommon, gram-negative bacillary endocarditis has increased in recent years.[31] In the elderly, the occurrence of gram-negative bacillary endocarditis may be related to preceding GU tract infection. However, a more important reason for the increase in endocarditis due to gram-negative bacilli, as well as *Staphylococcus epidermidis* and fungi, is the increased use of prosthetic devices to correct cardiac valvular defects.[32]

CLINICAL FEATURES

It is now uncommon to see a patient with a 3- to 4-month history of fevers, night sweats, and weight loss, who on physical examination has splenomegaly, clubbing, a murmur, and a myriad of cutaneous and mucous membrane embolic-vasculitic lesions. If one waits for these classic signs of subacute bacterial endocarditis to become manifest, many patients with endocarditis will be missed. Several reviews dealing with endocarditis in the elderly have emphasized the subtle clinical findings and absence of classic manifestations of disease in the elderly.[19,20,33]

Whether, in fact, the more subtle manifestations of infection alluded to reflect the elderly person's inability to respond to infection as vigorously as a younger person or whether they merely reflect the changes in the clinical patterns of endocarditis seen across all age groups is not clear.

Fever is almost always noted in patients with endocarditis[13,34] although frequently the elderly patient is not aware of the presence of fever prior to admission.[11,19] Most large series of patients with endocarditis show a variable number of patients (usually less than 5%) who remain afebrile throughout their illness.[34,35] Almost always these patients are elderly, but little other data are given regarding the presence of renal failure, length of illness, or how assiduously an elevated temperature was sought. Thus, although rarely the elderly patient with endocarditis may be afebrile, most often fever is present when sought.

Murmurs are present in most patients with endocarditis.[13,20,21,33,34] However, in cases involving the tricuspid valve, murmurs are frequently not heard early in the course of the illness.[13,24] Likewise, acute staphylococcal endocarditis frequently presents without a murmur, which may appear days to weeks later.[11,13] Elderly persons with endocarditis usually do have a murmur but often this is not changed from the "flow" murmur they may have had for years.[25,34] Even an innocent-sounding murmur in an elderly person with a fever has to raise the diagnostic possibility of endocarditis. Recent data show that it is uncommon to hear a changing murmur in patients with endocarditis, be they elderly or young.[13,36]

Central nervous system complaints are seen in 20% to 40% of patients with endocarditis, and frequently they are the initial manifestation of the infection.[34,37-39] Symptoms vary from those of confusion and behavioral changes to those of a major stroke or frank meningitis. The incidence of neurologic symptoms in the elderly appears to be about the same as in other age groups.[19,21,29] However, the major diagnostic pitfall in the elderly is ascribing the neurologic symptoms to vascular disease without considering endocarditis. Fever, especially when a murmur is present, in an elderly patient with a stroke certainly should raise the suspicion of endocarditis and lead to appropriate diagnostic studies.

Musculoskeletal manifestations of endocarditis are common, occurring in 25% to 40% of the patients with endocarditis.[40,41] Arthralgias, myalgias, arthritis, and low back pain are most commonly noted and many times are the initial manifestations of the illness.[40,41] There is no evidence that these symptoms are more common in the elderly patient with endocarditis than in the younger patient with this infection. Musculoskeletal complaints unrelated to endocarditis are very common in elderly individuals. As was noted with neurologic symptoms, musculoskeletal symptoms may actually draw the attention of the physician away from the diagnosis of endocarditis in elderly patients.

Cutaneous and mucous membrane findings, such as petechiae, Roth's spots, Janeway's lesions, Osler's nodes, and splinter hemorrhages, immediately make one think of endocarditis. However, these signs are less commonly seen now than 40 years ago, probably because it is rare for a patient to have infection continuing undiagnosed for several months.[9,13,34,35] Petechiae, both cutaneous and conjunctival, remain the most common skin manifestation noted in patients with endocarditis. Most data indicate these occur as often in elderly patients as in younger patients.[19,21,36]

DIAGNOSIS

When endocarditis is suspected, culture of the blood is the appropriate diagnostic test to be undertaken. Usually two to three sets of blood cultures (each set with an aerobic and an anaerobic bottle) are adequate to detect the organisms causing endocarditis.[42,43] If blood is drawn at different times, persistent bacteremia, frequently an indicator of intravascular infection, can be documented. If only one set of blood cultures is performed, there will be insufficient data available on which to base a secure diagnosis of endocarditis.[44] If the patient has been treated with antibiotics prior to culture of the blood, more cultures over a longer period of time will probably be required to document bacteremia.[45] In this situation, the use of newer blood culture media with resins to inactivate residual antimicrobials may be helpful.[46]

Reports from the 1930s and 1940s emphasized the large number of elderly patients in whom endocarditis was diagnosed only at necropsy (from 58% to 87%).[18,33] Culturing of blood, which was not a routine procedure in those decades, had not been done in most of these cases.[18,33] The common practice of culturing the blood in any febrile elderly patient in hospital should lead to the diagnosis of endocarditis, even if this diagnostic possibility was not entertained on admission; this should lead to many fewer patients dying of undiagnosed endocarditis. Indeed, currently the percentage of cases of endocarditis in the elderly diagnosed only at necropsy is about 10%.[21]

Other tests are merely adjunctive in the diagnosis of endocarditis. A high sedimentation rate, the presence of antiglobulins (rheumatoid factor), anemia, and hematuria help support the diagnosis of endocarditis, but clearly are not specific.

Likewise, although echocardiographic evidence of valvular vegetations may be helpful in evaluating blood culture results, in predicting prognosis, and in determining the need for surgery,[47,48] echocardiography remains only an adjunctive test. The sensitivity of the procedure for detecting vegetations appears to be between 40% to 50% for the M-mode method and between 40% and 60% for the two-dimensional method.[49] In

Table 10-1
Antibiotic Regimens Recommended for Treating Endocarditis in Elderly Persons with Normal Renal Function

Organism	Preferred Regimen	Alternate Regimen (especially for Penicillin-allergic patients)
Penicillin-susceptible (MIC <0.1 µg/mL) α- or viridans streptococcus, *Streptococcus mutans*, or *S sanguis*	*Penicillin G 2 million units q4h IV for 3–4 weeks*; or penicillin as above, plus 0.5 g q12h IM for the first 2 wk. Some experts stop the penicillin as well after 2 wk if the response has been good. Others continue with oral penicillin V (1g q6h) during the third and fourth wk if the patient is reliable and adequate serum bactericidal activity is achieved while on oral therapy	Cefazol in sodium 1.0g q4h hydrochloride vancomycin 0.5g q6h or 1g q12h IV; or erythromycin 2–4g IV or vancomycin hydrochloride 2.0g IV daily plus streptomycin
Streptococcus bovis	Same as for penicillin-susceptible viridans streptococcus	Same as for penicillin-susceptible viridans streptococcus
Streptococcus faecalis (enterococcus), or viridans streptococcus isolates only moderately susceptible to penicillin G (MIC ≥0.1 µg/mL)	*Penicillin G 3 million units q4h IV*, or *ampicillin 3g q6h or 2g q4h IV, plus gentamicin sulfate 1.0 mg/kg q8h IV for 6 wk*. Peak serum gentamicin level need not be > 5 µg/mL. Streptomycin 1.0g q12h IM is preferred to gentamicin if the organism is not high-level resistant to streptomycin (MIC > 2000 µg/mL). *Use an aminoglycoside in every patient.* If ototoxicity develops, it can be discontinued after 4 wk, but IV penicillin or ampicillin should be continued for another 2 wk	Vancomycin hydrochloride 0.5g q6h or 1.0g q12h IV plus gentamicin or streptomycin as at left, for 4–6 wk. Monitor renal function, eighth nerve function, and serum antibiotic concentrations carefully. Nonenterococcal, moderately susceptible streptococci can be treated with cefazolin plus an aminoglycoside

Organism	Preferred Regimen	Alternate Regimen (especially for Penicillin-allergic patients)
Staphylococcus aureus		
a. Nonpenicillinase-producing	*Penicillin G 3–4 million units q4h IV for 4–6 wk*	Vancomycin hydrochloride 0.5g q6h or 1g q12h IV for 4–6 wk
b. Penicillinase-producing, methicillin-sensitive	*Oxacillin sodium or nafcillin sodium 2g q4h IV for 4–6 wk;* no advantage to routine use of aminoglycosides as well	Vancomycin hydrochloride 0.5g q6h or 1g q12h IV for 4–6 wk
c. Methicillin-resistant; these are also resistant to nafcillin and oxacillin and often to aminoglycosides, clindamycin and erythromycin, as well	*Vancomycin hydrochloride 0.5g q6h or 1.0g q12h IV for 4–6 wk.* Give vancomycin over at least 60 min. Refractory cases may require addition of rifampin or an aminoglycoside, or both	Trimethoprim-sulfamethoxazole, 4 ampule (80 mg trimethoprim per ampule) q12h IV for 4–6 wk
Staphylococcus epidermidis (prosthetic valve, penicillin-resistant)	*Vancomycin hydrochloride 0.5g q6h, or 1.0g q12h IV plus rifampin 300 mg q8h orally, and/or gentamicin sulfate 1 mg/kg q8h IV for 6 wk.* The most reliable regimen involves simultaneous use of all three drugs, but this is very toxic, especially in elderly patients. Consider surgery if bacteremia cannot be terminated or recurs	None reported. Trimethoprim-sulfamethoxazole as above may be useful in some patients, based on susceptibility test results. May be necessary to add rifampin and gentamicin, as at left
Haemophilus parainfluenzae, H aphrophilus, or *H influenzae*	*Ampicillin 3g q4h IV plus gentamicin sulfate 1.5 mg/kg q8h IV for 4–6 wk*	Cefuroxime or cefotaxime IV; dosage based on susceptibility test results.
Pseudomonas aeruginosa	*Ticarcillin 3–5g or piperacillin sodium 3–5g q4h IV plus tobramycin 1.5–2.0 mg/kg q8h IV for 6–8 wk;* monitor serum aminoglycoside levels carefully	Antipseudomonal cephalosporins (based on susceptibility tests) plus tobramycin as at left. Other aminoglycosides can also be used instead of tobramycin. Anticipate occasional cross-allergic reactions if patient has had immediate reactions to penicillins.

Table 10-1 (con't)
Antibiotic Regimens Recommended for Treating Endocarditis in Elderly Persons with Normal Renal Function

Organism	Preferred Regimen	Alternate Regimen (especially for Penicillin-allergic patients)
Other organisms, such as *Enterobacteriaceae*, anaerobes, or unusual organisms	Therapy is frequently unsuccessful, and must be guided by the results of quantitative susceptibility tests and measurement of serum bactericidal activity. Metronidazole is the only reliably bactericidal antibiotic for *Bacteroides fragilis*	
Empiric therapy of acute endocarditis prior to obtaining culture results, and without other clues to the nature of the infecting organism	Nafcillin, oxacillin, or vancomycin IV plus gentamicin or tobramycin IV until the nature of the infecting organism is known	
Fungal endocarditis	Amphotericin B IV with gradually increasing doses to 0.5 – 1.0 mg/kg/d, plus surgical replacement of the valve as soon as feasible	
Culture-negative endocarditis	Treat as for *Streptococcus faecalis* endocarditis, as above; obtain serologic tests for rickettsial (Q fever) and *Chlamydia psittaci* endocarditis	Tetracycline for suspected rickettsial or chlamydial endocarditis

a population with a high prevalence of thickened, fibrotic valves, echocardiographic evaluation for the presence of vegetations may be more difficult.

PROGNOSIS

The mortality rate for elderly patients with endocarditis has remained quite high over the last 40 years in spite of the introduction of effective antimicrobial therapy. In early studies, failure to obtain blood cultures and to make the diagnosis of endocarditis led to mortality rates as high as 72% in some series.[33] However, even recent surveys have noted mortality rates as high as 45% in elderly persons with endocarditis.[21] Increasing age clearly is a predictor of a poor prognosis in endocarditis.[8,9,34] In Robbins' study from the 1970s, higher mortality was associated with the presence of acute myocardial infarction, neurologic complications, and *S aureus* as the infecting agent.[21] Indeed, the mortality from *S aureus* endocarditis in the elderly was 89% in one series.[11] This differs markedly from the experience with viridans streptococcal endocarditis in a similar elderly population, in which no patients died.[36] Many times, underlying illnesses, especially in patients with nosocomially acquired endocarditis, are responsible for the dismal outcome in the elderly patient with endocarditis.

TREATMENT

Since the mortality rate in endocarditis in the elderly is much higher than in young persons, treatment directed against the specific infecting organism should begin as soon as possible. In cases where the diagnosis was delayed because of an atypical presentation, or if the patient has already suffered complications of the disesase, the prompt institution of bactericidal therapy may be decisive. If the organism has been isolated and presumptively identified, therapy should be instituted, and can be guided by the recommendations in Table 10-1. A bactericidal regimen is essential and must be continued until the endocardial lesion has been sterilized. Parenteral therapy is always preferred initially. If the organism has been identified as a streptococcus but not yet speciated, initial therapy should be one of those recommended for *Streptococcus faecalis*. Therapy can be tailored to the specific organism after it has been speciated and its susceptibility to antimicrobials has been characterized. It should be kept in mind that endocarditis is one of the few infections where reported clinical experience may be more valuable than in vitro susceptibility test results.

Except for the need to be more concerned about the toxicity of certain antimicrobials, the regimens used to treat endocarditis in the elderly do not differ from those in younger patients. Regimens not requiring the use of aminoglycosides are preferred in the elderly. However, the enterococcus almost always requires use of an aminoglycoside as part of the regimen to achieve bactericidal therapy even when the laboratory reports the organism as being resistant to aminoglycosides by in vitro susceptibility tests.[50] When elderly patients require aminoglycoside therapy, they should be informed of the potential toxicity of these antibiotics for the auditory and vestibular systems and for the kidneys, and should be told that the onset of the ototoxicity may be delayed until after therapy has been discontinued. When aminoglycosides are used, renal function should be monitored regularly (at least 3 times per week), and peak-and-trough concentrations of the aminoglycosides should be measured to insure that adequate and "safe" concentrations of drug are being achieved. A peak concentration of less than 5 µg/mL and a trough of 1−2 µg/mL are desirable with gentamicin or tobramycin. Patients should be told to report hearing loss, dysacusis, tinnitus, or ataxia promptly, and hearing should be monitored with high-frequency tuning forks or other bedside tests of eighth nerve function on a regular basis. Serial audiometric and caloric tests are not practical in most hospitals, but the former may be useful to provide a baseline against which to evaluate changes should symptoms appear. In many patients, symptoms of eighth nerve toxicity may disappear even though therapy with the aminoglycoside is continued; this is especially true with streptomycin. The physician should be reluctant to discontinue any antimicrobial used in the treatment of infective endocarditis unless an alternate regimen that will be bactericidal can be substituted.

When staphylococci are implicated, the organism should be considered a penicillinase producer and therefore resistant to penicillin G, penicillin V, ampicillin, amoxicillin, piperacillin, azlocillin, ticarcillin, mezlocillin, and carbenicillin until bactericidal susceptibility tests on the patient's organism prove otherwise. Thus patients with staphylococcal endocarditis should be treated initially with nafcillin, oxacillin, or vancomycin, as shown in Table 10-1. It is rare for staphylococcal endocarditis on a native valve in an elderly person to be caused by a methicillin-, oxacillin-, and nafcillin-resistant organism, but such isolates need to be considered in patients with hospital-acquired staphylococcal endocarditis.

The need for replacement of a valve destroyed by endocarditis may develop in elderly patients, especially those with staphylococcal infection of the aortic valve. The patient should be seen by a cardiac surgeon as soon as the diagnosis has been established. Early emergent surgery (prior to the cure of the infection) is successful surprisingly often, although published results suggest even better results can be obtained if prosthetic valve surgery can be delayed until the signs of infection have resolved or blood cultures have become sterile.[51] When surgery is performed before the infection has been cured, patients should be treated with an appropriate antibiotic regimen postoperatively until they have had a total of at least 4 to 6 weeks of bactericidal therapy.

The treatment of *S epidermidis* endocarditis is frequently unsuccessful, especially when betalactam antibiotics such as nafcillin or cephalosporins are used; frequently, subpopulations of this organism are resistant to these antimicrobials and can be detected only if large inocula are used in susceptibility testing.[51] This problem is especially difficult and important when patients have prosthetic valve infection.

Patients with prosthetic valve endocarditis frequently require unusual and/or toxic antimicrobial regimens. These are usually selected on the basis of quantitative bactericidal susceptibility tests on the infecting organism. In addition, they frequently require replacement of the infected valve because of persistent bacteremia or sepsis. Such patients should have a careful search for occult abscesses in their spleen, liver, kidneys, extremities, or brain before concluding that the valve is the focus of the persistent bacteremia.

Even though prosthetic valve endocarditis frequently requires surgical removal for a cure, most patients should have a vigorous attempt at optimal and curative antibiotic therapy before surgery is performed since some of them may be cured medically. This usually involves 6 weeks of therapy. Another approach to this problem in patients without hemodynamic or embolic indications for valve replacement is to discontinue the antibiotics for two to three days after 2 weeks of apparently successful antibiotic therapy. If there is a prompt bacteriologic and clinical relapse, antibiotics should be resumed and the patient should be prepared for surgery as soon as possible. If no early relapse occurs, then the antibiotic regimen can be resumed and continued to complete therapy.[52]

Measurement of peak or trough serum inhibitory titers and serum bactericidal titers, or so-called Schlichter tests, against the infecting organism can be helpful in the management of patients with endocarditis. Although not all experts agree on this issue, our experience suggests these tests can be helpful. Peak serum bactericidal titers are of greatest predictive value and use with streptococcal or staphylococcal endocarditis. Where there is no foreign body such as a prosthetic valve, the infection can usually be cured if the peak serum bactericidal titer is consistently 1:8 or greater. It is also desirable to have a trough serum bactericidal titer of at least 1:2. Of course, the patient may die of a complication even though the infection has been cured. Regimens producing lesser degrees of serum bactericidal activity can also be successful, but are much less likely to be so.

It is key to use a standardized test with an inoculum of 10^5 colony forming units (CFU)/mL and a 99.9% bactericidal end point for performance of these tests.[53] In dealing with gram-negative endocarditis with resistant organisms such as *Pseudomonas aeruginosa*, the value of the Schlichter test is much less certain. Our limited personal experience with such organisms suggests that a peak serum bactericidal titer of at least 1:64 is desirable, as well as a trough of 1:8. It is frequently impossible to achieve these levels without having to resort to toxic antimicrobial regimens. Thus the need for surgery in these patients can be anticipated if serum bactericidal titer test results are discouraging, and the clinical response is also poor or delayed.

PROPHYLAXIS

Since elderly patients may be subjected to many procedures resulting in transient bacteremia, they are at greater risk than others of developing a fatal form of endocarditis, especially if they have a prosthetic valve. Chemoprophylaxis for high-risk elderly patients should be considered, according to recommended guidelines, when they undergo these procedures.[54]

REFERENCES

1. Blumer G: Subacute bacterial endocarditis. *Medicine* 1923;2:105–170.
2. Kelson SR, White PD: Notes on 250 cases of subacute bacterial (streptococcal) endocarditis studied and treated between 1927 and 1939. *Ann Intern Med* 1945;22:40–60.
3. Bayles T, Lewis WH: Subacute bacterial endocarditis in older people. *Ann Intern Med* 1940;13:2154–2163.
4. Wallach JB, Glass M, Lukash L, et al: Bacterial endocarditis in the aged. *Ann Intern Med* 1955;42:1206–1213.
5. Cates JE, Christie RV: Subacute bacterial endocarditis. A review of 442 patients treated in 14 centres appointed by the Penicillin Trials Committee of the Medical Research Council. *Q J Med* 1951;20:93–130.
6. Friedberg CK, Goldman HM, Field LE: Study of bacterial endocarditis. Comparisons in ninety-five cases. *Arch Intern Med* 1961;107:6–15.
7. Lowes JA, Williams G, Tabaqchali S, et al: Ten years of infective endocarditis at St. Bartholomew's Hospital: Analysis of clinical features and treatment in relation to prognosis and mortality. *Lancet* 1980;1:133–136.
8. Uwaydah MM, Weinberg AN: Bacterial endocarditis — A changing pattern. *N Engl J Med* 1965;273:1231–1235.
9. von Reyn CF, Levy BS, Arbeit RD, et al: Infective endocarditis: An analysis based on strict case definitions. *Ann Intern Med* 1981;94:505–518.
10. Friedland G, von Reyn CF, Levy B, et al: Nosocomial endocarditis. *Infect Control* 1984;5:284–288.
11. Watanakunakorn C, Tan JS: Diagnostic difficulties of staphylococcal endocarditis in geriatric patients. *Geriatrics* 1973;28:168–173.
12. Sussman JI, Baron EJ, Tenenbaum MJ, et al: Viridans streptococcal endocarditis: Clinical, microbiological, and echocardiographic correlations. *J In-*

fect Dis 1986;154:597–603.
13. Weinstein L, Rubin RH: Infective endocarditis — 1973. Prog Cardiovasc Dis 1973;16:239–271.
14. Kerr A: Subacute Bacterial Endocarditis. Springfield, Ill, Charles C Thomas Publisher, 1955.
15. Thell R, Martin FH, Edwards JE: Bacterial endocarditis in subjects 60 years of age and older. Circulation 1975;51:174–182.
16. Baddour LM, Bisno AL: Infectious endocarditis complicating mitral valve prolapse: Epidemiologic, clinical, and microbiologic aspects. Rev Infect Dis 1986;8:117–137.
17. Burnside JW, DeSanctis RW: Bacterial endocarditis on calcification of the mitral annulus fibrosus. Ann Intern Med 1972;76:615–618.
18. Traut EF, Carter JB, Gumbiner SH, et al: Bacterial endocarditis in the elderly. Geriatrics 1949;4:205–210.
19. Habte-Gabr E, January LE, Smith IM: Bacterial endocarditis: The need for early diagnosis. Geriatrics 1973;28:164–170.
20. Anderson HJ, Staffurth JS: Subacute bacterial endocarditis in the elderly. Lancet 1955;2:1055–1058.
21. Robbins N, DeMaria A, Miller MH: Infective endocarditis in the elderly. South Med J 1980;73:1335–1338.
22. Wilson WR, Giuliani EF, Danielson GK, et al: General considerations in the diagnosis and treatment of infective endocarditis. Mayo Clin Proc 1982;57:81–85.
23. Hartman TL, Myers WK: Occurrence of bacterial endocarditis in older individuals. Geriatrics 1959;14:374–380.
24. King JW, Shehane RR, Lierl J: Infectious endocarditis at three hospitals in the same city: Two study periods a decade apart. South Med J 1986;79:151–158.
25. Cantrell M, Yoshikawa TT: Infective endocarditis in the aging patient. Gerontology 1984;30:316–326.
26. Watanakunakorn C: Streptococcus bovis endocarditis. Am J Med 1974;56:256–260.
27. Murray HW, Roberts RB: Streptococcus bovis bacteremia and underlying gastrointestinal diseases. Arch Intern Med 1978;138:1097–1099.
28. Klein RS, Recco RA, Catalan MT, et al: Association of Streptococcus bovis with carcinoma of the colon. N Engl J Med 1977;297:800–802.
29. Applefeld MM, Hornick RB: Infective endocarditis in patients over age 60. Am Heart J 1974;88:90–94.
30. Varma MP, McCluskey DR, Khan MM, et al: Heart failure associated with infective endocarditis. A review of 40 cases. Br Heart J 1986;55:191–197.
31. Cohen PS, Maguire JH, Weinstein L: Infective endocarditis caused by gram-negative bacteria: A review of the literature, 1945–1977. Prog Cardiovasc Dis 1980;22:205–242.
32. Watanakunakorn C: Prosthetic valve endocarditis. Prog Cardiovasc Dis 1979;22:181–192.
33. Cummings V, Furman S, Dunst M, et al: Subacute bacterial endocarditis in the older age group. JAMA 1960;172:137–141.
34. Lerner PI, Weinstein L: Infective endocarditis in the antibiotic era. N Engl J Med 1966;274:199–206, 259–266, 323–331, 388–393.
35. Jackson JF, Allison F: Bacterial endocarditis. South Med J 1961;54:1331–1339.
36. Tan JS, Watanakunakorn C, Terhune CA: Streptococcus viridans endocarditis: Favorable prognosis in geriatric patients. Geriatrics 1973;28:68–73.

37. Ziment I: Nervous system complications in bacterial endocarditis. *Am J Med* 1969;47:593–607.
38. Jones HR, Siekert RG, Geraci JE: Neurologic manifestations of bacterial endocarditis. *Ann Intern Med* 1969;71:21–28.
39. Pruitt AA, Rubin RH, Karchmer AW, et al: Neurologic complications of bacterial endocarditis. *Medicine* 1978;57:329–343.
40. Churchill MA, Geraci JE, Hunder GC: Musculoskeletal manifestations of bacterial endocarditis. *Ann Intern Med* 1977;87:754–759.
41. Levo Y, Nashif M: Musculoskeletal manifestations of bacterial endocarditis. *Clin Exp Rheumatol* 1983;1:49–52.
42. Werner AS, Cobb CG, Kaye D, et al: Studies on bacteremia of bacterial endocarditis. *JAMA* 1967;202:127–131.
43. Belli J, Waisbren BA: The number of blood cultures necessary to diagnose most cases of bacterial endocarditis. *Am J Med Sci* 1956;232:284–288.
44. Washington JA: Blood cultures. Principles and techniques. *Mayo Clin Proc* 1975;50:91–98.
45. Pazin GJ, Saul S, Thompson ME: Blood culture positivity. Suppression by outpatient antibiotic therapy in patients with bacterial endocarditis. *Arch Intern Med* 1982;142:263–268.
46. McGuire NM, Kauffman CA, Hertz CS, et al: Detection of bacteremia: Evaluation of the BACTEC antimicrobial re-moval system. *J Clin Microbiol* 1983;18:449–451.
47. Lutas EM, Robert RB, Devereux RB, et al: Relation between the presence of echocardiographic vegetations and the complication rate in infective endocarditis. *Am Heart J* 1986;112:107–113.
48. Mintz GS, Kotler MN, Segal BL, et al: Survival of patients with aortic valve endocarditis. The prognostic implications of the echocardiogram. *Arch Intern Med* 1979;139:862–866.
49. Mintz GS, Kotler MN: Clinical valve and limitations of echocardiography. **Evaluation of the BACTEC antimicrobial removal system.** *J Clin Microbiol* 1980;140:1022–1027.
50. Kaye D: Treatment of enterococcal endocarditis in experimental animals and in man, in Bisno AL (ed): *Treatment of Infective Endocarditis.* New York, Grune & Stratton, 1981, pp 97–112.
51. Dismukes WE: Prosthetic valve endocarditis: Factors influencing outcome and recommendations for therapy, in Bisno AL (ed): *Treatment of Infective Endocarditis.* New York, Grune & Stratton, 1981, pp 167–191.
52. Tuazon CU, Gill V, Gill F: Streptococcal endocarditis: single vs. combination antibiotic therapy and role of various species. *Rev Infect Dis* 1986;8:54–60.
53. Reller LB: Laboratory procedures in the management of infectious endocarditis, in Bisno AL (ed): *Treatment of Infective Endocarditis.* New York, Grune & Stratton, 1981, pp 252–256.
54. Schulman ST, Amren DF, Bisno AL et al: Prevention of bacterial endocarditis. *Circulation* 1984;70:1123a–1127a.

11
Infections of the Biliary Tract

Aksel G. Nordestgaard
Russell A. Williams

Biliary tract disease is the most common reason for abdominal surgery in the elderly.[1] This, coupled with the fact that there is a continuous increase in the mean age of the population in Western societies, underlines its importance as a source of morbidity and mortality, together with its economic cost, among the elderly.

Acute cholecystitis is associated with cholelithiasis in over 90% of cases.[2] The incidence of gallstones increases with age and differs with sex and race. Analysis of 26,895 consecutive autopsies showed that among white subjects older than 60 years, 30% of females and 15% of males had gallstones, whereas in those under 60 years old, the figures were 15% in females and 5% in males. The corresponding figures for blacks were about half.[3]

Little information is available on the likelihood of development of symptoms from cholelithiasis. However, in a recent study of partly unselected subjects the cumulative probability of developing biliary colic from gallstones was 18% at 20 years.[4] About 10% of subjects had acute cholecystitis.

In addition to the higher incidence of cholelithiasis and associated common bile duct stones among the elderly, there is also an increased frequency of bacteria in the bile (bactibilia).[5,6] Table 11-1 shows the bacteriologic findings in 102 of our patients undergoing elective cholecystectomy. Serious septic complications of acute cholecystitis develop more commonly in the older patients including empyema, gangrene, and perforation of the gallbladder.[7-10] This is explained in part by the delay that attends diagnosis of acute cholecystitis in this age group, as not atypically the elderly patient with abdominal sepsis has a deceptively

Table 11-1
Bacterial Findings in 102 Patients Undergoing Elective Cholecystectomy*

Gallbladder Bile Organism	No.	Gallbladder Wall Organism	No.
Escherichia coli	14	*Escherichia coli*	10
α-Hemolytic streptococcus, not group D	8	α-Hemolytic streptococcus, not group D	5
α-Hemolytic streptococcus, group D	4	γ-Hemolytic streptococcus, group D	5
Klebsiella pneumoniae	4	α-Hemolytic streptococcus, group D	4
γ-Hemolytic streptococcus, group D	3	*Klebsiella pneumoniae*	4
Group B *Streptococcus agalactiae*	2	*Propionibacterium* sp	3
α-Hemolytic streptococcus (microaerophilic)	2	γ-Hemolytic streptococcus, not group D	2
Staphylococcus epidermidis	2	*Klebsiella oxytoca*	2
Others†	9	*Peptostreptococcus* sp	2
		Others‡	7

* Twenty-six patients had positive cultures: Authors' unpublished data.
† *Staphylococcus aureus, Enterobacter cloacae, Bacillus* sp, *Citrobacter diversus, Citrobacter freundii, Klebsiella oxytoca, Bacteroides fragilis, Morganella morgani, Clostridium perfringens.*
‡ *S aureus, S epidermidis, E cloacae, C freundii, Aeromonas hydrophila, Aerococcus viridans, M morgani.*

benign clinical course until florid septic shock supervenes. Then there is need for additional caution that prolongs the resuscitation of these elderly patients because many have coexising cardiopulmonary disease. Thus the time is even further extended until the gallbladder, commonly in an advanced pathologic state, is removed at operation.

After cholecystectomy for acute cholecystitis in the older patient there is an increased morbidity that includes sepsis, heart and lung failure, and an increased mortality rate compared with younger patients. Glenn[11] found that patients older than 65 years operated on for acute cholecystitis had a mortality rate of 9.7% in contrast to 3.8% for all patients having the same treatment. This high mortality rate could in all likelihood be reduced if the older patient with acute cholecystitis were treated promptly rather than after the delay that now often occurs.[11,12]

PATHOPHYSIOLOGIC FEATURES

Bacterial infection is generally thought to be a secondary occurrence in acute calculous cholecystitis. Impaction of a gallstone in the cystic duct is the precipitating event and the resulting partial or complete obstruction to the egress of bile leads to biliary stasis and concentration, establishing a chemical inflammation of the mucosal lining of the gallbladder.

The mucosal layer once damaged, is likely to be followed by bacterial superinfection of the gallbladder. Bile is normally sterile, however bactibilia, extant with cystic duct obstruction, is believed to predispose to a more virulent pathologic course. Venous and lymphatic stasis together with local pressure from the impacted gallstone lead to tissue ischemia and necrosis that can become a major component of the acute inflammatory reaction. If it is extensive and involves the full thickness of the wall, gangrenous perforation of the gallbladder results.

Acute cholecystitis is often superimposed on chronic cholecystitis, known in the older patient to be associated with a high incidence of bactibilia.[7] This may account for the higher frequency of all the serious suppurative complications of acute cholecystitis recorded in the aged. Should the bile be sterile at the time of obstruction, it has been proposed that infection occurs via a hematogenous route, most likely the portal vein.[13]

Enteric organisms, particularly *Escherichia coli, Streptococcus faecalis, Klebsiella,* and *Pseudomonas aeruginosa* are recovered most often on culture from the gallbladder of patients with acute cholecystitis. The incidence of anaerobic bacteria cultured varies between 13% and 45% in different studies, in part explained by differences in anaerobic culture

Table 11-2
Bacterial Findings in Cultures from Bile in Acute Cholecystitis*

Aerobic Organisms	Total of 858 Isolates (%)	Anaerobic Organisms	Total of 858 Isolates (%)
Escherichia coli	20	*Bacteroides fragilis*	7
Streptococcus, group D	15	Other *Bacteroides* spp	1
Klebsiella	14	*Clostridium perfringens*	6
Pseudomonas aeruginosa	7	Other *Clostridium* spp	1
Viridans streptococci group	5	*Fusobacterium*	1
Enterobacter cloacae	3	Miscellaneous	2
Proteus mirabilis			
Staphylococcus epidermis	3		
Proteus morganii	2		
Citrobacter freundii	2		
Corynebacterium	1		
Pseudomonas	1		
Enterobacter aerogenes	1		
Staphylococcus aureus	1		
Miscellaneous	5		

*The findings are based on England and Rosenblatt's findings among 286 positive bile cultures.[15]

techniques.[14-18] *Bacteroides fragilis* and *Clostridium perfringens* are the most common anaerobes. The remaining microorganisms grown in acute cholecystitis from the gallbladder bile are listed, in decreasing frequency of isolation, in Table11-2. In more than 40% of positive bile cultures two or more different bacterial strains have been recovered.[15]

Experimental studies have shown that several of the anaerobic bacteria and the facultative anaerobe, *S faecalis*, deconjugate bile acids. Deconjugated bile acids are more toxic to the epithelial lining of the gallbladder than the usually present conjugated bile acids in bile.[19] The clinical significance of this is not known.

In 5% to 10% of patients with acute cholecystitis, no stones are found in the gallbladder. Acute acalculous cholecystitis develops in patients who are debilitated, particularly in the elderly during another illness or following an unrelated surgical procedure, major trauma, or while being treated for burns.[20,21]

No single etiologic agent is implicated in this type of cholecystitis. However, morphine or other opiate analgesics, anesthesia, prolonged fasting, and parenteral nutrition, any one or more of which may be a component of treatment for the foregoing conditions, impair that normal reflex emptying of the gallbladder that is stimulated by ingestion of food. The resulting bile stasis damages the mucosa, exciting a chemical inflammatory reaction. Another event that may underlie the origin of this disease is hypotension, particularly in those patients who have small vessel disease due to a connective tissue disorder, diabetes, atherosclerosis, or hypertensive arteriosclerosis. The hypotension may well be followed by thrombosis of the cystic artery or one of its more distal branches, especially the gallbladder fundus with consequent gallbladder necrosis.

CLINICAL FEATURES

Several authors[11,22,23] have pointed out that in the elderly there often is some delay in establishing the diagnosis of acute cholecystitis. Many of these patients with an intra-abdominal infective disorder have unimpressive symptoms, few physical findings, and laboratory tests that do not indicate underlying acute cholecystitis or other septic condition. Severe inflammation, gangrene, or even perforation may exist with few or none of the traditional clinical indicators. Localized pain and tenderness with or without a palpable right upper quadrant abdominal mass are the usual findings in a younger patient. However, these may not be found in the older patient who simply becomes disoriented or even delirious with the infection, making clarification of the clinical picture even more difficult.[11]

The clinical evolution of the inflammatory process in the typical patient with acute cholecystitis is somewhat analogous to acute appendicitis, although it usually evolves more slowly, probably because the bacterial population within the gallbladder is relatively sparse at the time of obstruction compared with the colon.

With initial obstruction of the cystic duct there may be only mild colicky epigastric pain known as biliary colic, followed by nausea and vomiting. If the obstruction is transient these symptoms subside within one to two hours, but if persistent the process may evolve into acute cholecystitis. The pain becomes increasingly severe and constant, shifting to the right upper quadrant and in many cases radiating to the right shoulder or interscapular region. The gallbladder is unlikely to be palpable if there is marked peritoneal irritation because the protecting reflex muscle obscures the mass. It is palpable in 30% to 40% of patients and about 20% of patients are slightly jaundiced. Fever is often moderate, reaching an average of 38°C in the absence of complications.

Laboratory abnormalities include leukocytosis ($>$ 10,000 WBC/μL), and a modest to moderately elevated total bilirubin, without a rise in alkaline phosphatase unless there is a gallstone in the common bile duct and some rise in the level of SGOT. At times there is a nonspecific elevation of the serum amylase.

The clinical and laboratory manifestations of acute cholecystitis are similar whether gallbladder calculi are present or not. But in the patient with acute acalculous cholecystitis, who typically may be undergoing treatment for another serious illness, the significance of these additional signs and symptoms is often misinterpreted, being attributed to the primary illness, until a late stage in the disease.

No specific clinical findings indicate that complications of acute cholecystitis such as empyema, gangrene, or perforation have developed. However, usually there is an unrelenting progressive deterioration of the patient's symptoms and signs with eventual decompensation into septic shock. These may be masked and follow a more protracted course if the patient is on antimicrobial therapy.

DIAGNOSIS

The clinical examination supplemented with laboratory chemistry makes the correct diagnosis of acute cholecystitis in up to 85% of patients.[24] Even higher diagnostic accuracy has been achieved in the past decade by the application of new bioimaging techniques, particularly ultrasonography and radionuclide scintigraphy. These have widely replaced the oral and intravenous (IV) cholangiogram in evaluating the patient suspected of having acute cholecystitis. However, the oral cholecystogram is still very useful in the patient with symptoms of chronic cholecystitis and cholelithiasis.

Although only 15% to 20% of gallstones are seen on a plain abdominal radiograph, it is nevertheless obtained as the initial diagnostic procedure; being simple and relatively inexpensive it gives information that excludes some of the conditions among the differential diagnoses, and it is highly specific for demonstrating emphysematous cholecystitis, in which gas is seen limited to the gallbladder wall and/or lumen (Fig.11-1).

The oral cholecystogram is of little use in evaluating suspected acute cholecystitis. It needs reasonable upper gastrointestinal (GI) function for uptake of the contrast material and at least 12 hours are required to allow hepatic conjugation of iopanoic acid. Furthermore, there is poor or no visualization of biliary structures in patients with bilirubin levels higher than 3 mg/dL.

An IV cholangiogram can provide useful diagnostic information in up to three quarters of patients,[25] but the dye used in this procedure produces hepatic, renal, and allergic toxicity and, similarly to the oral study, is not concentrated sufficiently to produce an image if there is a modest hyperbilirubinemia. Intravenous cholangiography has been replaced by radionuclide scintigraphy which is not associated with complications and does not have the practical limitations of the radiologic study. Visualization of the bile ducts and gallbladder excludes acute cholecystitis whereas visualization of the ducts but not the gallbladder, because the cystic duct is obstructed, makes the diagnosis of acute cholecystitis highly likely.

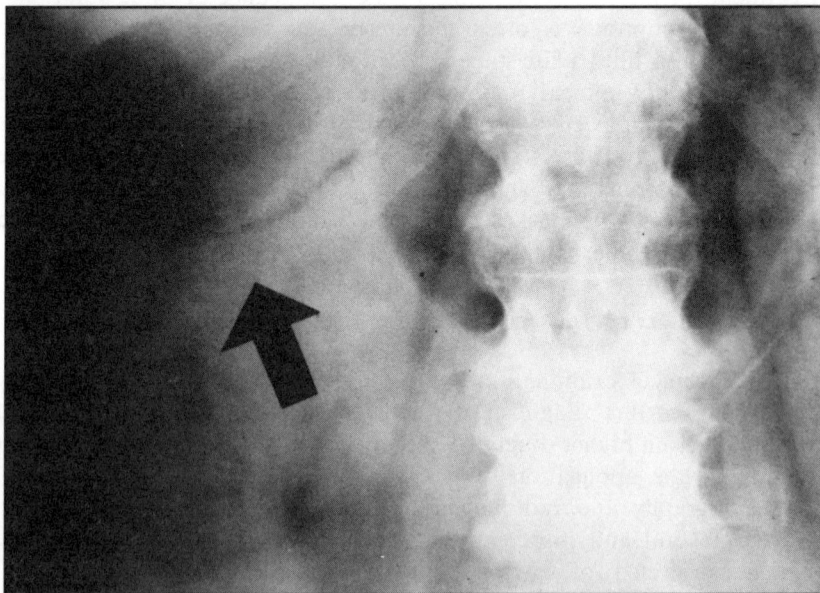

Figure 11-1 Abdominal radiograph showing emphysematous cholecystitis. Gas is seen filling the lumen of the gallbladder and extending intramurally (*arrow*).

Controversy still exists between ultrasonography and radionuclide scintigraphy as to which is the better method for evaluating the patient with suspected acute cholecystitis. Ultrasonography is a noninvasive, rapid, technique without exposure to radiation, has no side effects, and is relatively inexpensive. Its results are independent of liver function and it has a high sensitivity and diagnostic accuracy in patients with acute biliary tract disease. The ultrasonographic criteria for diagnosing acute cholecystitis are cholelithiasis together with secondary findings such as focal tenderness over the gallbladder (Murphy's sonographic sign), gallbladder enlargement and shape, the thickness of its wall, and the detection of sludge or intraluminal membranes[26] (Fig.11-2).

If the ultrasonographic study is equivocal or the patient has clinical signs of acute cholecystitis without calculi, an emergency radionuclide examination may be helpful. While ultrasonography provides detailed anatomical information, scintigraphy gives a dynamic representation of hepatobiliary function but with poor anatomical definition. Visualization of the gallbladder within one hour after administering the radiopharmaceutical agent virtually excludes the diagnosis of acute cholecystitis, including acalculous disease. Unfortunately, false-positive results (nonvisualization of the gallbladder in patients without cholecystitis) are not uncommon in alcoholic patients or those with severe liver disease,

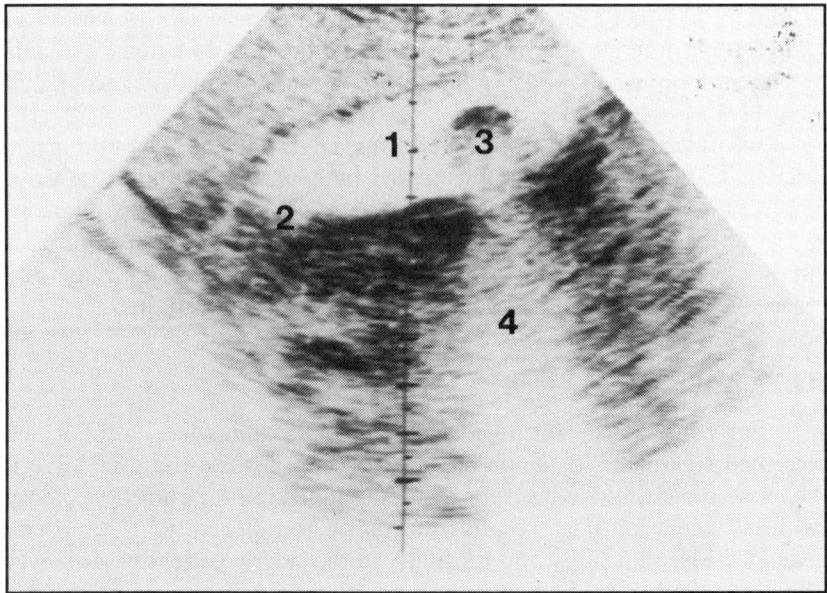

Figure 11-2 Ultrasonographic study in a patient who had acute calculous cholecystitis. The gallbladder (1) has a thickened wall (2) and contains one stone (3). The stone casts a sonic shadow (4).

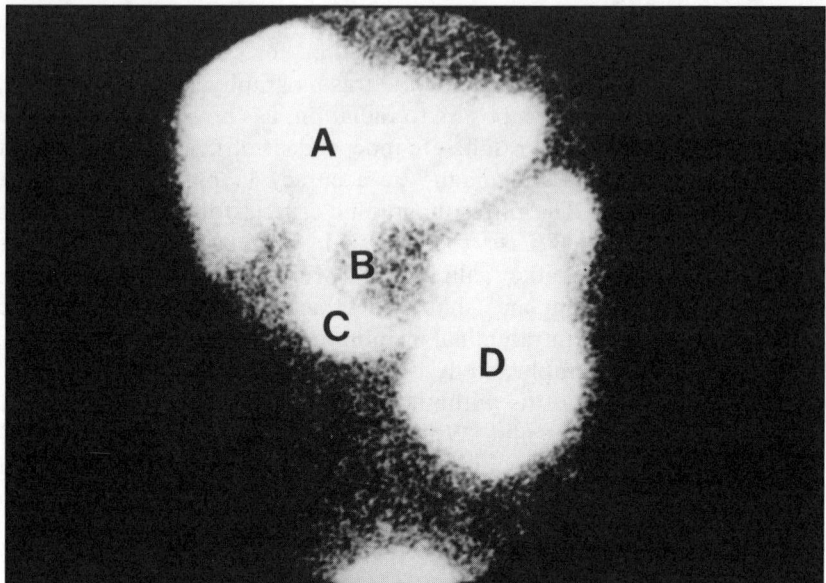

Figure 11-3 Scintigram (HIDA) showing no visualization of the gallbladder in a patient with acute cholecystitis. The liver (A), bile ducts (B), duodenum (C), and intestine (D) contain radionuclide.

common bile duct obstruction, patients on total parenteral nutrition, or with severe intercurrent illnesses.[26] Excluding the foregoing patients, cholescintigraphy too has high sensitivity and diagnostic accuracy[26] (Fig.11-3).

Information gained from both ultrasonography and the radionuclide excretory studies may be supplemented by concurrent administration of cholecystokinin (CCK). The obstructed gallbladder will be unaltered whereas the normal gallbladder is seen to contract and empty on each study. The algorithm shown in Figure 11-4 summarizes the diagnostic procedure in the patient suspected of having acute cholecystitis.

TREATMENT

Early operation, during the same hospital admission, is the widely accepted treatment for acute cholecystitis. It shortens the total time in hospital, obviating the need for a second admission for cholecystectomy, without increasing postoperative morbidity and mortality,[27,28] and may even decrease morbidity and mortality in the elderly patient.[12] Moreover, the nonoperative, medical management of acute cholecystitis in the elderly has an almost 100% failure rate, unlike the same disease in the younger patient, who typically recovers from the acute attack after several days.[11]

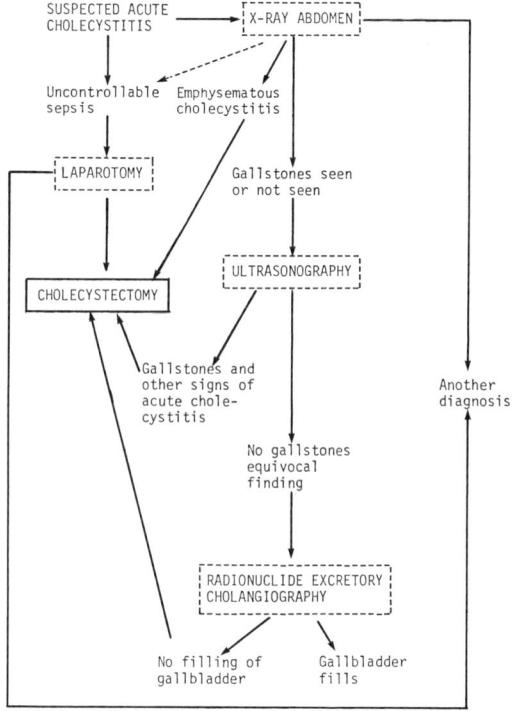

Figure 11-4 Algorithm for evaluation of patients with suspected acute cholecystitis.

It is recommended that the elderly patient suspected of having acute cholecystitis be admitted to a hospital for further expedient evaluation. On admission, if he or she is vomiting, nasogastric suction is started and maintenance, replacement fluids, and electrolyte requirements are given IV. Among the differential diagnoses are appendicitis, pancreatitis, perforated peptic ulcer, hepatitis, hepatic abscess, pyelonephritis and perinephrenic abscess, intestinal obstruction, myocardial infarction, and right lower lobe pneumonia.

Plain radiographs of the chest and abdomen are usually normal in patients with acute cholecystitis. Sometimes, however, atelectasis or even frank pneumonia is seen in the base of the right lung which has supervened because of splinting of the right diaphragm. This is not to be confused with a primary pulmonary infection. Gas in the lumen or within the gallbladder wall is specific for emphysematous cholecystitis (see Fig.11-1) whereas radioopaque gallstones are not, but have a sentinel function, focusing the physician's attention on the gallbladder. The ECG excludes acute myocardial disease and is required before any planned operation. Serum chemistry reflecting hepatic and pancreatic function and urine microscopy will be normal in many of the cases.

At times a moderate hyperbilirubinemia or hyperamylasemia is found. Bilirubin levels of 2–5 mg/dL without a rise in serum alkaline phosphatase may be found with simple acute cholecystitis. This has been called the "jaundice of sepsis" and in patients with severe infections may reflect the liver component of "multiple organ failure." In those patients, however, who are not so seriously ill, there is no good explanation for the hyperbilirubinemia.

Higher levels of bilirubin, with a rise in alkaline phosphatase, occur if there is concomitant obstruction of the common bile duct by a gallstone or compression of the duct by the enlarged gallbladder. Amylase levels may rise (200–1000 units; normal <200) with acute cholecystitis and many of the foregoing conditions included among the differential diagnoses.

Acute cholecystitis is confirmed by an ultrasound study, supplemented by a radionuclide liver excretory (HIDA) scan if necessary.

With the diagnosis made, plans are made for operation within the near future (24–48 hours) provided the patient does not have signs of advanced sepsis. Treatment with fluids and antimicrobial agents is continued. Signs that indicate serious sepsis include a high temperature, marked or even moderate leukocytosis, thrombocytopenia, tachycardia, and a low blood pressure, and blood cultures may grow one or more of the organisms previously described, found in the gallbladder or bile.

Antimicrobial agents are commonly given as part of the treatment for acute cholecystitis, usually controlling an accompanying bacteremia and preventing the progression of cellulitis adjacent to the gallbladder. The disease resolves if the stone disimpacts itself, re-establishing gallbladder drainage before severe tissue damage has occurred.

Elderly patients with their high frequency of bactibilia have an increased risk of developing wound and intra-abdominal infections after biliary surgery.[16] Perioperative ("prophylactic") antibiotics reduce this risk. The effectiveness of antibiotics in the treatment of biliary tract disease depends on achieving adequate serum and tissue levels rather than concentration in the bile as therapeutic bile levels cannot be achieved in the presence of biliary obstruction. Based on bacteriologic studies, antimicrobial regimens include agents such as an aminoglycoside (eg, gentamicin), which is effective against the gram-negative enteric organisms, particularly *Klebsiella* and *E coli*. Ampicillin, given in addition to the aminoglycoside, provides effective activity against enterococci and also against the most common anaerobe, *Clostridium* organisms, but not *B fragilis*.

Many surgeons use either an aminoglycoside alone or combined with ampicillin as either or both are effective against the overwhelming majority of organisms, largely gram-negative enteric flora, found in acute cholecystitis. If there is no resolution of the patient's condition within 24 to 36 hours after starting therapy, operation is done expeditiously; although thought could also be given to adding antimicrobials effective against the likely anaerobic organisms, it should not delay operation. The patient with florid sepsis not responding to these measures requires urgent operation to remove the focus of the sepsis — the gallbladder. This may preclude utilizing time to submit the patient to noninvasive studies before operation.

In many elderly patients, the acute biliary condition aggravates preexisting cardiac, renal, or diabetic disease. These organ systems are evaluated and treated beforehand to ensure that the patient is stable during anesthesia and operation.[11]

Cholecystectomy is the best treatment for acute cholecystitis. Cholecystostomy (drainage of the infected gallbladder) is reserved for patients judged too ill or in whom cholecystectomy is felt to be technically demanding, requiring extensive dissection, thus extending the anesthesia and operative time unnecessarily in a very sick, unstable patient.[29]

REFERENCES

1. Vartian CA, Septimus EJ: Intra-abdominal infections in the elderly: Diagnosis and management. *Geriatrics* 1986;41:51–56.
2. Arnold DJ, Zollinger RW, Bartlett RM, et al: 28,621 cholecystectomies in Ohio. *Am J Surg* 1970;119:714–717.
3. Lieber MM: The incidence of gallstones and their correlation with other diseases. *Ann Surg* 1952;135:394–405.
4. Gracie WA, Ransohoff DF: The natural history of silent gallstones. *N Engl J Med* 1982;307:798–800.
5. Farnell MB, van Heerden JA, Beart RW: Elective cholecystectomy. *Arch Surg* 1981;116:537–540.
6. Willis RG, Lawson WC, Hoare EM, et al: Are bile bacteria relevant to septic complications following biliary surgery? *Br J Surg* 1984;71:845–849.
7. Chetlin SH, Elliott DW: Biliary bacteremia. *Arch Surg* 1971;102:303–307.
8. Fry DE, Cox RA, Harbrecht PJ: Empyema of the gallbladder: a complication in the natural history of acute cholecystitis. *Am J Surg* 1981;141:366–369.
9. MacDonald JA: Perforation of the gallbladder associated with acute chloecystitis: 8-year review of 20 cases. *Ann Surg* 1966;164:849–852.
10. Fry DE, Cox RA, Harbrecht PJ: Gangrene of the gallbladder: a complication of acute cholecystitis. *South Med J* 1981;74:666–668.
11. Glenn F: Surgical management of acute cholecystitis in patients 65 years of age and older. *Ann Surg* 1981;193:56–59.
12. Morrow DJ, Thompson J, Wilson SE: Acute cholecystitis in the elderly. *Arch Surg* 1978;113:1149–1152.
13. Scott AJ, Khan GA: Origin of bacteria in bile duct bile. *Lancet* 1967;2:790–792.

14. Shimada K, Inamatsu T, Yamashiro M: Anaerobic bacteria in biliary disease in elderly patients. *J Infect Dis* 1977;135:850–854.
15. England DM, Rosenblatt JE: Anaerobes in human biliary tracts. *J Clin Microbiol* 1977;6:494–498.
16. Keighley MRB, Drysdale RB, Quoraishi AH, et al: Antibiotic treatment of biliary sepsis. *Surg Clin North Am* 1975;55:1379–1390.
17. Truedson H, Elmros T, Holm S: The incidence of bacteria in gallbladder bile at acute and elective cholecystectomy. *Acta Chir Scand* 1983;149:307–313.
18. Clasesson BE, Holmlund DE, Miatzsch TW: Microflora of the gallbladder related to duration of acute cholecystitis. *Surg Gynecol Obstet* 1986;162:531–535.
19. Shimada K, Urayama K, Noro T, et al: Biliary tract infection with anaerobes and the presence of free bile acids in bile. *Rev Infect Dis* 1984;6:S147–S151.
20. Howard RJ: Acute acalculous cholecystitis. *Am J Surg* 1981;141:194–198.
21. Glenn F: Acute acalculous cholecystitis. *Ann Surg* 1979;189:458–465.
22. Williams RA, Bennion RS, Wilson SE: Gallstone disease in the older patient: a call for early treatment. *Geriatr Med Today* 1983;2:66–70.
23. Glenn F, Hays DM: The age factor in the mortality rate of patients undergoing surgery of the biliary tract. *Surg Gynecol Obstet* 1955;100:11–18.
24. Essenhigh DM: Management of acute cholecystitis. *Br J Surg* 1966;53:1032–1038.
25. Cheung LY, Chang FC: Intravenous cholangiography in the diagnosis of acute cholecystitis. *Arch Surg* 1978;113:568–570.
26. Laing FC: Diagnostic evaluation of patients with suspected cholecystitis. *Surg Clin North Am* 1984;64:3–22.
27. McArthur P, Cuschieri A, Sells RA, et al: Controlled clinical trial comparing early with interval cholecystectomy for acute cholecystitis. *Br J Surg* 1975;62:850–852.
28. van der Linden W, Sunzel H: Early versus delayed operation for acute cholecystitis. *Am J Surg* 1970;120:7–13.
29. Joseph PK, Bizer LS, Sprayregen SS, et al: Percutaneous transhepatic biliary drainage. Results and complications in 81 patients. *JAMA* 1986;255:2763–2767.

12

Bacterial Infections of the Liver

Carlos E. Donayre
Samuel E. Wilson

The history of pyogenic hepatic abscess is a reassuring affirmation of the steadily improving prognosis for patients with serious intra-abdominal infection. Hepatic abscesses were recognized by Ochsner in the preantibiotic era as a surgical problem with considerable morbidity and mortality. The development of antibiotics and improvement in diagnostic microbiology made considerable impact on the treatment of this disease and the development of liver photoscanning in the 1960s made early diagnosis possible. The elderly population have the highest incidence of liver abscess and are at greatest risk. Early diagnosis decreased the mortality but was accompanied by an increase in morbidity due to complications of surgical drainage via a laparotomy in these older, and often poor-risk, operative candidates. The advent of needle aspiration and percutaneous closed drainage systems in the late 1970s allowed for treatment of this high-risk group with fewer complications and equivalent results. Soon the shift from surgical therapy to a medical form of treatment was complete. Thus this interaction between noninvasive technology and clinical ingenuity has resulted in a safer, more successful way of dealing with pyogenic liver abscesses in the 1980s.

The incidence of pyogenic hepatic abscesses is difficult to estimate accurately. The classic study of Ochsner et al, although now several decades old, clearly demonstrated a postmortem incidence of 0.29%, considerably higher than the reported incidence of 15 cases per 100,000 hospital admissions.[1] This discrepancy in clinical and postmortem incidence suggests that in Ochsner's time, at least, many patients had unrecognized liver abscesses. The true incidence of primary liver abscess in North America is unknown but is probably significantly lower than before widespread use of antibiotics. An estimate of the current incidence of pyogenic liver abscess is one per 7500 admissions. Review of the literature shows that the age of patients who have a hepatic abscess has changed over the last 40 years. In 1938 pyogenic liver abscesses were discovered most frequently in young adults, with the highest incidence in the third decade of life, but in the 1980s they occur predominantly in patients 50 years of age or older. The average age of 61 years for development of a liver abscess alerts the clinician to the importance of this entity in the differential diagnosis of intra-abdominal infection in the elderly patient. The amebic liver abscess, on the other hand, is a disease of the young male who is often an inhabitant of, or recent immigrant from an endemic area of amebiasis.[1-4]

PATHOPHYSIOLOGIC FEATURES

The causes of pyogenic liver abscesses may be derived from analysis of portal of entry of the bacteria: (1) bile duct, (2) portal vein, (3) hepatic artery, (4) direct extension, (5) blunt or penetrating trauma to the abdomen, and (6) cryptogenic, where no primary focus of infection is detected. Liver infections secondary to penetrating trauma are generally found in younger patients.[5]

The relative importance of each of the above routes of infection has also changed over the last 40 years. The majority of the patients in the preantibiotic era had an antecedent suppurative appendicitis or other intra-abdominal inflammation complicated by a pylephlebitis which was the source of blood-borne bacteria to the hepatic portal system. Aggressive early operation in patients with suspected appendicitis, accompanied by broad spectrum antibiotics, greatly reduced the incidence of peritoneal abscess and pylephlebitis and as a consequence shifted the incidence to an older group.[3]

Pyogenic liver abscess is often secondary to a distant primary focus. Consequently, abscess formation can result from within the abdomen or from any site drained by the portal vein, as with diverticulitis, infected hemorrhoids, perirectal abscess, and ulceration or perforation of the bowel. These types of abscesses are often multiple rather than single and are commonly found in the right lobe of the liver.

Liver abscesses can also result from direct extension of infection from an adjacent site, as can occur with empyema of the gallbladder, subphrenic abscess, pleural infection, or perinephric abscess.

Obstructive biliary tract disease, due either to calculus or tumor with subsequent development of suppurative cholecystitis and ascending cholangitis, has become the most common cause of pyogenic liver abscesses. These abscesses are again usually multiple but often are only confined to one lobe of the liver.

Blunt or penetrating injuries of the liver, which lead to laceration, hemorrhage, tissue necrosis, and bile extravasation, predispose devitalized liver to secondary infection. This type of abscess is usually single, well-localized, and typically presents some seven to ten days after the injury.

Generalized septicemia may also result in abscess formation.[6] Bacterial seeding occurs via the hepatic artery and may complicate bacterial endocarditis. In most reports of hepatic abscesses, no associated disease could be found in about 10% of cases. Buchman and Zuidema argue that cryptogenic hepatic abscesses arise by invasion of intestinal flora into hepatic microinfarcts of ischemic or thromboembolic origin.[7] They further propose that mechanisms of bacterial clearance such as opsonization and cellular lysosomal destruction become saturated because transit time through the portal system is fixed. Bacteria not opsonized proliferate within liver substance leading to abscess formation. The diagnosis of a cryptogenic hepatic abscess implies that the antecedent inflammation was undetectable or that the workup was insufficiently sensitive to identifying the underlying cause.

MICROBIOLOGY

Almost any organism may be implicated in a hepatic abscess, although gram-positive cocci were more common until 1960 (Table 12-1). Between 1952 and 1963 the incidences of staphylococcal and streptococcal pyogenic liver abscess were similar.[3] In 1964, however, Block et al[8] reported an increase in the percentage of gram-negative organisms. *Escherichia coli* became the most common pathogen isolated, accounting

Table 12-1
Organisms Isolated from Pyogenic Liver Abscesses

Aerobic	
Escherichia coli	*Alkaligenes fecalis*
Pseudomonas	Friedländer's bacillus
Aerobacter aerogenes	*Salmonella*
Klebsiella	ß-hemolytic streptococci s
Proteus	Hemolytic *Staphylococcus aureus*
Enterobacter organisms	*Staphylococcus epidermidis*
Nonhemolytic streptococci	*Mycobacterium tuberculosis*
Viridans streptococci	*Candida*
Anaerobic	
Peptostreptococcus	*Clostridium perfringenes*
Peptococcus	*Fusobacterium*
Bacteroides fragilis	*Actinomyces israelii*
Microaerophilic	
Streptococcis	

Adapted from Sabbaj et al.[9]

for 10% of all cases, followed by other Enterobacteriaceae, streptococci, staphylococci, enterococci, and occasionally clostridia. Gram-negative aerobic bacteria made up 67% to 72% of the isolates of all series and both aerobic and anaerobic organisms were found in 17% to 22% of patients.[8]

Bacteriologic data on liver abscess may be incomplete because of inadequate culture techniques, particularly for anaerobic or fastidious microaerophilic organisms. Also, prolonged use of antibiotics prior to obtaining the sample may have altered the flora. Recently the importance of anaerobes and *Streptococcus milleri* has been emphasized. In the study by Sabbaj et al, using proper technique anaerobes were found in 45% to 50% of all cases and they were the sole pathogens in 25% of the cases, with *Streptococcus milleri* group F being the most common isolate.[9] Bacteremia was seen in 30% of patients, with *Bacteroides fragilis* being the most common pathogen isolated from blood cultures. Organisms isolated from blood and from aspiration of abscesses were predominantly bowel flora and in no cases did culture of pus yield an organism not isolated from blood cultures. Thus the isolation of *Streptococcus milleri* or anaerobic organisms in an ill, febrile patient should alert one to the possible presence of an occult liver abscess.[10]

CLINICAL FEATURES

In the older patient the clinical presentation is usually one of sepsis with little or no localizing signs (Table 12-2). The onset of symptoms is insidious, making the presence of liver abscess obscure and its localization difficult. Most patients are seen with symptoms of less than 3 weeks' duration. Fever may be the only presenting complaint. The temperature varies from 101° to 106° F with intermittent spikes. Right upper quadrant

Table 12-2
Isolates Obtained on Direct Needle Aspiration of Liver Abscesses

Organism	No. of Patients	(%)
Streptococcus milleri	10	(62)
Streptococcus milleri +		
Fusobacterium necrophorum	3	(18)
Bacteroides fragilis		
Peptococcus spp		
Escherichia coli	2	(12)
Bacteroides fragilis		
Peptostreptococcus anaerobius		
Streptococcus pneumoniae (type 15)	1	(6)

Adapted from Sabbaj et al.[9]

Table 12-3
Clinical Manifestations of Pyogenic Hepatic Abscess

	No. of Patients	(%)
Symptoms		
Fever	29	(100)
Abdominal pain	18	(62)
Chills	16	(55)
nausea, vomiting	12	(41)
Physical findings		
Chest signs (rales, decreased breath sounds)	18	(62)
Hepatomegaly	8	(28)
Abdominal mass	8	(28)
Jaundice	4	(14)

Adapted from Hill and Laws.[12]

abdominal pain and tenderness is present in a significant number of patients.[11] If the abscess is secondary to biliary obstruction jaundice, right upper quadrant pain and chills will be the characteristic presentation. Occasionally patients with sepsis may be also mentally obtunded.

DIAGNOSIS

Laboratory Tests

Abnormal laboratory findings caused by pyogenic liver abscess are nonspecific and usually not helpful in establishing the diagnosis. Anemia is the most common finding with hematocrit usually less than 35%. Elevation of alkaline phosphatase occurs in 80% of cases and is seen in greater incidence in patients with underlying malignant conditions. The WBC count, although usually elevated, may be decreased in as many as 40% of patients, and hypoalbuminemia, hyperbilirubinemia, and elevation of SGOT was only demonstrated in a modest 60% of all patients. Hyperbilirubinemia is commonly seen only with abscesses secondary to biliary tract disease.[12] Tests of hepatic function do not deteriorate solely as a consequence of aging although decreased liver weight and reduced hepatic flow are seen as normal events in the older patient. Changes in function reflect the influence of illness or medications rather than the aging process.[13] Thus, in the management of a patient with a liver abscess, one can safely assume that an increase in SGOT or bilirubin is a direct consequence of the infective process.

Chest and *abdominal films* have been superseded by the more specific noninvasive technology but nevertheless are still abnormal in 50% of cases. A right-sided pleural effusion, elevation, and fixation of the diaphragm, changes in costophrenic angles, or basal pulmonary collapse should be looked for on upright, lateral, and decubitus views. Air-fluid levels in particularly large abscesses may be appreciated in upright abdominal films. Large abscesses can also contain gas produced by aerobic and anaerobic bacteria. Multiple pockets of gas may be seen in clostridial infection. Many of the above findings can be mistaken for pulmonary involvement.[11]

Radioisotope scanning. Liver scanning has been most useful in diagnosing and localizing liver abscesses. *The liver scan* depends on phagocytosis by the liver's reticuloendothelial system. Technetium-sulfur colloid is injected intravenously (IV) and selectively taken by the Kupffer cells where the technetium 99 undergoes isometric isolation to a lower energy state. The gamma radiation released is then measured by a photon crystal. Lesions are detected by differential phagocytotic activity between adjacent regions of liver. If liver is healthy, 2-cm lesions can be detected; if liver is diseased there will be decreased uptake and thus lesions need to be larger for detection.[7]

Ultrasonography. This noninvasive, safe, and well-tolerated diagnostic modality provides valuable information as to the presence and identification of hepatic lesions. Sonography can determine whether a lesion is cystic, complex, or solid. Thus a cystic or complex mass in the appropriate clinical setting is strongly suggestive of a hepatic abscess.

Limitations of ultrasonography include the presence of abscesses with high protein lipid content or many small bubbles of gas which can be confused for a solid mass or normal liver parenchyma. Fatty liver disease also produces a very echogenic liver that is difficult to evaluate. Abscesses present high in the dome of the liver are often missed. Ultrasonography should be used as a complementary diagnostic method to liver scanning, especially in those patients with equivocal studies. Recognizing the small false-negative rate, other tests should be pursued to confirm the diagnosis.[14]

Computed tomography (CT). The CT scan has revolutionized diagnosis of intra-abdominal infection and its impact is major in the diagnostic workup of hepatic abscesses. The CT image depends on the density of liver parenchyma and is not a physiologic scan but a physical one. By using composite imaging it is able to detect small lesions which may be lost in the shadow cast by a larger filling defect when using ultrasound or isotope modalities. Defects as small as 0.5 cm are readily displayed. Definition of the abscess and its relationship to adjacent structures provides landmarks for surgical or percutaneous drainage approaches. Studies have shown the CT scan to be ineffective in the diagnosis of liver abscesses when fatty infiltration of liver and alcoholic hepatitis was present. Its use is also limited by its expense, radiation exposure, and availability. Although highly sensitive in demonstrating liver abscesses, in many cases it fails to provide little more significant information than combined liver scan and ultrasound.[14]

Percutaneous transhepatic cholangiography (PTC). The benefits of this diagnostic modality are realized in patients with obstructive liver disease and complicating cholangitis since it can detect the presence and location of associated liver abscesses as well as initiate drainage in selected patients. PTC allows gram stain of infected bile obtained by aspiration for culture. Retrograde drainage of the obstructed infected bile can be obtained by indwelling catheter. Its use is limited by the morbidity of the procedure and highly specific use[15].

TREATMENT

Traditionally, surgical drainage and antibiotic coverage has been the accepted therapy of choice for all solitary and multiple liver abscesses. In patients with undrained abscesses the mortality approaches 100%. With the development of ultrasonography and the CT scan, exact localization of liver abscesses was possible and percutaneous drainage of hepatic abscesses was consistently successful. Percutaneous drainage is achieved by first entering the abscess with a Chiba needle guided by sonography or CT. Using guide wires, pigtail catheters can be introduced into the abscess and the contents of the cavity aspirated. The purulent material obtained is Gram-stained immediately and cultured for aerobic and anaerobic organisms and presumptive antibiotic therapy is instituted. The pigtail catheter draining pus to the outside is left securely in place until the abscess resolves. If the patient's condition does not improve and he remains febrile for 48 hours, it is recommended that a CT scan be repeated to rule out the presence of an undrained abscess and open drainage is considered. An adequately drained abscess shows a concomitant decrease in size on CT scan. The drainage catheter can be removed when clinical improvement of the patient is evident, the temperature is normal, resolution of the abscess is seen on CT ultrasound, and the character of the drainage changes to serous fluid.[16]

The advantages of percutaneous drainage are many: avoidance of a major operation, less patient discomfort, low cost when compared with surgical intervention, and lower risk of cross-contamination since it is a closed drainage system. It can be performed in elderly patients who are poor surgical risks, but should probably be avoided in patients with ascites because intraperitoneal contamination may lead to generalized peritonitis. A drainage catheter cannot be safely introduced if the proximity to vital structures such as lung and colon risks penetration. In addition, successful drainage by catheter requires that the contents of the abscess cavity not be too viscous to drain.

Surgical intervention is still necessary in selected patients with hepatic abscess but only in the following situations: rupture of the abscess into the peritoneum or pleura; when the abscess is secondary to biliary obstruction or other intra-abdominal problems that demand surgical correction; multiple small abscesses that are loculate or lack a safe drainage route; and in the case where percutaneous drainage has failed.

Patients with hepatic abscesses have been treated successfully with antibiotics alone.[17] Antibiotic coverage was determined by the antimicrobial susceptibilities of the organisms obtained from the blood and liver aspirate. Therapy consists of 3 to 4 weeks of broad spectrum IV antibiotics followed by 2 to 4 weeks of oral medications. If *Streptococcus milleri* is the dominant organism, penicillin is the agent of choice. Obligate anaerobes if present, may be susceptible only to metronidazole or clindamycin.

SUMMARY

The onset of pyogenic liver abscess is insidious, its presence obscure, and until recently its localization difficult. Early diagnosis is essential for the successful management of this disease. The elderly population is its main target.

Multiple imaging techniques are available but in most instances a liver scan and ultrasound will confirm the diagnosis in 90% of the cases if the lesion is greater than 2 cm. Computed tomography or ultrasound are also used to direct percutaneous drainage. After diagnosis adequate drainage of abscess is essential. Today, most cases can be managed successfully with percutaneous aspiration and catheter drainage. Morbidity is relatively low and the hospital stay shorter than when surgical drainage is undertaken. Surgery is indicated for multiple, small abscesses which cannot be adequately drained, a ruptured abscess, an abscess secondary to biliary obstruction, a coexistent intra-abdominal problem that demands surgical intervention, and of course, where percutaneous drainage has failed. Antibiotic coverage is determined by the antimicrobial susceptibilities of the organisms isolated from blood cultures or liver aspirates. If cultures are negative, anaerobic organisms, and Enterobacteriaceae must be covered. Clindamycin or metranidazole plus gentamicin or other aminoglycoside coverage is appropriate.

Prognosis of patients with pyogenic liver abscess is related less to the mode of therapy than to the patient's age, the presence of intercurrent disease, and the rapidity with which the diagnosis is made.

REFERENCES

1. Ochsner A, DeBakey M, Murray S: Pyogenic abscess of the liver. *Am J Surg* 1938;40:292.
2. Beaumont DM, Davis M: Clinical presentation of pyogenic liver abscess in the elderly. *Age Ageing* 1985;14:339–344.

3. Chattopadhyay B: Pyogenic liver abscess. *J Infect Dis* 1983;6:5–12.
4. Basile J, Klein SR, Worthen NJ, et al: Amebic liver abscess, the surgeon's role in management. *Am J Surg* 1983;146:67–71.
5. Rubin RH, Swartz MN, Malt R: Hepatic abscess: changes in clinical, bacteriologic and therapeutic aspects. *Am J Med* 1974;57:601–610.
6. Stenson WF, Eckert T, Avioli LA: Pyogenic liver abscess. *Arch Intern Med* 1983;143:126–128.
7. Buchman TG, Zuidema GD: The role of CT scan in the surgical management of pyogenic hepatic abscess. *Surg Gynecol Obstet* 1981;153:1–10.
8. Block MA, Schuman BM, Eyler WR, et al: Surgery of liver abscesses: use of newer techniques to reduce mortality. *Arch Surg* 1964;88:602–609.
9. Sabbaj J, Sutter VL, Finegold SM: Anaerobic pyogenic liver abscess. *Ann Intern Med* 1972;77:629–638.
10. Moore-Gillon JC, Eykyn SJ, Phillips I: Microbiology of pyogenic liver abscess. *Br Med J* 1981;283:819–821.
11. Conter RL, Pitt HA, Tompkins RK, et al: Differentiation of pyogenic from amebic hepatic abscesses. *Surg Gynecol Obstet* 1986;162:114–120.
12. Hill FS, Laws HL: Pyogenic hepatic abscess. *Am Surg* 1982;48:49–53.
13. Yoshikawa TT, Norman DC: Antimicrobial therapy of surgical infections in the elderly. *Infect Surg* 1984;8:805–812.
14. Rubison HA, Isikoff MB, Hill MC: Diagnostic imaging of hepatic abscesses: A retrospective analysis. *Am J Roentgenol* 1980;35:735–745.
15. Baumgarten F, Williams RA, Wilson SE: Patient selection and complications of transhepatic percutaneous cholangiography. *Surg Gynecol Obstet* 1987;165;199-203.
16. Attar B, Levendoglu H, Cursay NS: CT-guided percutaneous aspiration and catheter drainage of pyogenic liver abscesses. *Am J Gastroenterol* 1986;81:550–555.
17. Reynolds TB: Medical treatment of pyogenic liver abscess. *Ann Intern Med* 1982;96:373–374.

13

Viral Hepatitis

Inge Gurevich
Anne Sacks-Berg

Among the viruses that cause hepatitis in the elderly are those viruses whose main target is the liver itself — the hepatitis A, B, non-A, non-B viruses. There are others, such as the cytomegalovirus, whose main targets are various other organ systems, but which can coincidentally cause inflammatory hepatic disease. Because the hepatitis A and B viruses can now be readily identified, they are the focus of this discussion.

The prevalence of serologic markers denoting previous infection with the hepatitis virus increases with age. In those over 60 years old, it may be as high as 94% for hepatitis A and about 34% for hepatitis B.[1] Since past infection confers immunity, and because the risk factors for the acquisition of viral hepatitis in the elderly are generally fewer in number, new cases of hepatitis tend to be fairly infrequent. However, when hepatitis does occur in this population, it causes significantly greater morbidity. Mortality, which is less than 8% in the young, increases threefold above age 30, and even more so among the elderly, especially among women.[2] One reason for the increase in both severity and outcome of these infections is the normal decline in cell-mediated immunity with age and a concomitant increase in the formation of autoantibody. In contradistinction to the above findings, sex and race, but not age, were found to be statistically significant factors in predicting fatal outcome in a postmortem study of 60 subjects aged 7 to 79 years at Johns Hopkins in 1984.[3] Another reason for the increase in morbidity and mortality is the low index of suspicion for hepatitis in the elderly, some of whose symptoms are often ascribed to aging alone at first. Jaundice and weight loss often lead to an erroneous diagnosis of cancer. Surgery can be fatal in the presence of hepatitis.

CLINICAL FEATURES

In the young, viral hepatitis is an asymptomatic, subclinical, and self-limiting disease in 80% of cases. As with most viral diseases, severe clinical manifestations are more likely to occur with increasing age. In addition, manifestations such as fatigue and anorexia are present in 80% to 90% of affected patients and may be overlooked or ascribed to the normal fatigability and reduction of appetite suffered by many individuals with advancing age. Similarly, the constipation and arthralgias which may accompany hepatitis B may be thought of as "normally" occurring in older patients. If an early diagnosis is missed, and an elderly patient is on medications that are normally processed by the liver, hepatotoxicity may cause increasing problems. Often, the first signs may be nausea and vomiting, accompanied by hepatomegaly, increasing depression, dark urine, and light stools, which are usually followed by jaundice within about five days. Because an older individual is less likely to mount a febrile response, the low grade fever often present in the young adult may not occur. Additionally, in its early stages, hepatitis B often presents with flulike symptoms, such as cough and sore throat, as well as with musculoskeletal symptoms of arthralgia and myalgia. Dermatologic manifestations in the form of urticarial or maculopapular rashes are uncommon, as are glomerulonephritis and nephrosis (Table 13-1). With the appearance of jaundice, most symptoms diminish, with the exception of hepatomegaly and tenderness, and patients often complain of a feeling of fullness in the right upper quadrant. Cervical adenopathy may develop in up to 20% of patients.

Table 13-1
Common and Uncommon Manifestations of Viral Hepatitis

Common	Uncommon
Fatigue	Glomerulonephritis
Anorexia, weight loss	Pancreatitis
Nausea, vomiting	Transverse myelitis
Flulike syndrome (hepatitis B)	Myocarditis
Fever	Peripheral neuropathy
Hepatomegaly	Vasculitis
Constipation, diarrhea	Polyarteritis nodosa–like syndrome
Splenomegaly	Aplastic anemia
Dark urine, light stool	
Jaundice	
Pruritis	
Cervical adenopathy	
Mental confusion	
Rash (maculopapular, urticarial)	

Although most patients with hepatitis recover, among the elderly a progression to viral cholestatic disease may occur which mimics mechanical obstruction of the biliary system. Since extrahepatic obstruction is not uncommon in the elderly, it should be ruled out by the usual diagnostic visualization methods before a rising alkaline phosphatase and persistent jaundice in the face of rising transaminases can be ascribed to a viral epidemiology. Bile thrombi may be seen on histologic examination of biopsy material in conjunction with the dilatation of biliary canaliculi and ductules.

Fulminant hepatitis occurs in less than 0.5% of cases caused by hepatitis A, in about 1.5% of cases with hepatitis B, and in comparable number in non-A, non-B hepatitis. It is an outcome that is more likely to be seen in the elderly patient whose liver function may already be compromised by medications or other causes. Survival from fulminant hepatitis is rare above age 40.[2]

Asymptomatic carriage of the hepatitis B virus has been implicated in the high prevalence of primary liver cancer in Asian populations.[4] Although hepatoma is less common in the United States, its appearance during the later decades of life should raise the clinician's suspicion regarding possible carriage of the hepatitis B virus.

Chronic hepatitis may be due to either the hepatitis B or the non-A, non-B viruses. The chronic persistent form is a relatively benign condition which rarely progresses to liver failure or cirrhosis, and which in fact may resolve or "burn itself out" in the latter decades of life. In contrast, chronic active hepatitis brings with it the danger of portal hypertension and parenchymal liver failure, and few individuals survive much beyond their 60th year.[5]

DIAGNOSIS

Early diagnosis of hepatitis is helpful in all cases, especially so in an institutional setting, so that measures to prevent the spread to others can be instituted. Early diagnosis is especially important in the elderly if irreversible liver damage is to be avoided, since many of these patients are on medications that are hepatotoxic.

Although a definitive diagnosis can only be made by serologic testing for hepatitis A and B markers, a presumptive diagnosis can be entertained if certain parameters are present. Foremost of these is a history of exposure or other risk factors. For example, in a long-term institutional setting, hepatitis A is more likely to occur in an epidemic form, either from a common food source or from propagated spread. Hepatitis B or non-A, non-B hepatitis are more likely after surgery, and especially after administration of blood or blood products. The incubation period for hepatitis A is shorter (2–6 weeks) than that for hepatitis B (4 weeks–6 months) or non-A, non-B hepatitis (2 weeks – 6 months), and these temporal relationships may provide another clue.[6]

LABORATORY TESTS

Leukopenia and lymphocytosis with 10% to 20% atypical lymphocytes appear early in hepatitis as in most viral infections. Prolonged prothrombin times, urine bilirubin, and urobilinogen are also nonspecific. Liver function tests are required to narrow the focus toward the hepatobiliary systems. Elevations in bilirubin, serum glutamic-pyruvic transaminase (SGPT) or alanine aminotransferase (ALT), with a proportionally lesser elevation of alkaline phosphatase, are indicative of a hepatocyte-specific disease. When bilirubin levels exceed 2.5 mg/dL, jaundice is most likely to occur. Persistent levels above 20 mg/dL late in the course of hepatitis may be associated with more severe disease.[6] Extrahepatic obstruction should be ruled out if the more specific serologic tests are negative for hepatitis A or B viruses, and if posttransfusion hepatitis due to hepatitis non-A, non-B or cytomegalovirus is not a possibility.

Serologic Tests

Radioimmune assay (RIA) or enzyme-linked immunosorbant assay (ELISA) are sensitive tests and can indicate the type or stage of disease if a careful interpretation is made.[7] The presence of hepatitis A-specific antibody of the IgM class (anti-HA IgM) often appears about 4 weeks after exposure and usually persists for 8 to 10 weeks, although in some cases its presence can be detected at 3 months or more[8] (Fig. 13-1).

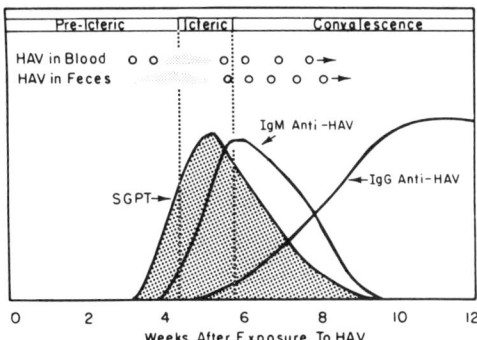

Figure 13-1 Relationship of liver enzyme elevation, stage of disease and antibody in hepatitis A. HAV = Hepatitis A virus. Reproduced with permission from Koff.[8]

Hepatitis A IgM thus indicates acute or convalescent hepatitis A virus infection. Hepatitis-specific antibody of the IgG class (anti-HA IgG) is usually detectable 6 to 8 weeks after exposure and persists for years, if not lifelong. It denotes past infection and presumptive immunity to the hepatitis A virus. False-positive tests are possible, unless carefully performed with a highly purified antigen preparation.[9]

The interpretation of tests for hepatitis B can be more complicated since both antigen and antibody detection is utilized and a variety of combinations can be found. Hepatitis B surface antigen (HBsAg), can be detected in 75% of patients in the late incubation period or early acute phase (Fig. 13-2). Antibody to the hepatitis B antigen (anti-HBc) is the second marker to appear in the serum, usually during the acute phase or very early during the recovery phase. Antibody to the hepatitis B surface antigen (anti-HBs) appears late in recovery and during convalescence, at which time the HBsAg is usually no longer detectable.[8] A complete interpretation of the tests is given in Table 13-2.

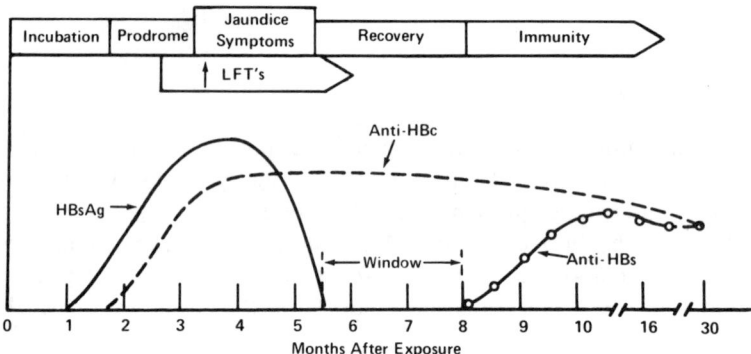

Figure 13-2 Relationships of serologic markers of hepatitis B infection with SGPT and course of disease. HBsAg = hepatitis B surface antigen; Anti-HBc = antibody to hepatitis B core antigen; Anti-HBs = antibody to hepatitis B surface antigen. (Reproduced with permission from Gurevich I, Cunha BA: *Viral Hepatitis.* Garden Grove, Calif, Medcom, Inc, 1985.)

When HBsAg is present alone or in combination with any other hepatitis B marker, the patient is considered infectious. Persistence of the surface antigen beyond 6 months should alert the clinician to the possibility of carriage or chronic disease. A combined finding of HBsAg and anti-HBc denotes the normal progression of disease unless the combination alone persists beyond 6 months. Anti-HBc alone may be found when HBsAg titers have declined beyond detection and before anti-HBs is detectable. This is called the window period and should be followed within about 3 months by the appearance of anti-HBs. If such progression is

Table 13-2
Interpretation of Hepatitis B Serologic Markers

HBsAg	Anti-HBc	Anti-HBs	Clinical Interpretation	Is Patient Infectious?
(−)	(−)	(−)	No infection — but in up to 25% of individuals, HBsAg titers are too low to be detected with present tests	No
(+)	(−)	(−)	Acute infection, carrier state, or chronic hepatitis	Yes
(+)	(+)	(−)	Late acute stage, carrier state, or chronic disease	Yes
(−)	(+)	(−)	Early convalescence — window period carrier state, or chronic hepatitis	If core antibody is of IgM class — yes; if IgG — probably not
(−)	(+)	(+)	Past infection (resolved)	No
(−)	(−)	(+)	Past infection—resolved, or response to hepatitis vaccine, or temporary passive antibody from hepatitis B immune globulin	No
(+)	(±)	(+)	Carrier state, or chronic hepatitis, or possible reinfection with different subtype (rare)	Yes

HBsAg = hepatitis B surface antigen; anti-HBc = antibody to hepatitis B antigen; anti-HBs = antibody to hepatitis B surface antigen. Reproduced with permission from Gurevich.[26]

absent, a diagnosis of carriage or chronicity should be entertained.[10] The presence of hepatitis B core antibody of the IgM class (anti-HBc IgM) in high titers denotes acute infection, although it may remain detectable for 1 to 2 years in chronic cases, whereas anti-HBc IgG denotes that the patient is less likely to be infectious and that infection has probably resolved.[11] However, liver biopsy is required to establish this type of differential diagnosis.

A combination of anti-HBc and anti-HBs shows resolution of the infection; the patient is not infectious and is usually considered immune to further hepatitis B infection. One or both of these markers usually persists for life, but titers may decline with age. Additional combinations and their interpretations are featured in Table 13-2.

In cases where persistent infectivity must be ruled out (especially in young, pregnant women), the third antigen-antibody system, consisting of the hepatitis B e component, can provide some insight. The hepatitis B e antigen (HBeAg) is detectable only in patients who are also HBsAg-positive, whether it be during the acute stage or in persistent carriage or disease. Its presence denotes a high degree of infectivity, but there is some controversy about its prognostic value.[12] Hepatitis B e antigen when absent, or the presence of antibody to the hepatitis B e antigen (anti-HBe), makes infectivity much less likely, but does not rule it out completely.[13]

In recent years, an increasing number of infections with an additional hepatitis agent, the delta virus, have been identified. This occurs mainly via shared drug paraphernalia. The delta hepatitis virus (HDV) is an incomplete RNA virus which cannot express itself without the presence of the hepatitis B viral DNA. Therefore delta hepatitis poses a risk only to those already infected and carrying the HB virus, or to those acquiring both hepatitis B and delta hepatitis concomitantly.[14,15] When **intravenous (IV) drug abuse is not a factor,** as in the elderly population, acquisition of HDV would occur mainly via contaminated units of blood or blood products.[16]

NON-A, NON-B HEPATITIS

There are at least two, and probably three or more viruses that differ antigenically from both hepatitis A and hepatitis B, and that have not as yet been fully identified. These non-A, non-B (NANB) viruses are reportedly part of a group of viruses demonstrating particle-associated reverse transcriptase activity, and they are thus tentatively classified as retroviruses or retroviruslike agents.[17] One of these viruses, with a short (2-week) incubation period, has been implicated in outbreaks of hepatitis A-like disease in India, one of which affected 2752 persons and caused 12 deaths. Others in the group cause manifestations similar to hepatitis B. This NANB group is the most likely of all the hepatitis viruses to have an impact on the geriatric age group, because it is the cause of 80% of posttransfusion hepatitis, (the other 20% of cases are due to cytomegalovirus [15%] and hepatitis B [5%]).[18] Since medical conditions, such as chronic renal failure with hemodialysis, and surgical conditions, such as cholecystectomy, and open-heart surgery, occur comparatively frequently in the older age group, posttransfusion hepatitis NANB is a considerable risk factor among that subgroup of elderly patients. The outcome of posttransfusion NANB hepatitis is similar to that of hepatitis B, as are its clinical manifestations, laboratory findings, and management. The diagnosis of hepatitis NANB, however, is one of exclusion. A patient, especially one who has undergone surgery during a preceding 4-week to 6-month period and who develops manifestation of hepatitis, whose serologic tests for acute hepatitis A and B are negative, and in whom hepatitis due to CMV can be ruled out, the most likely etiologic agent will be one of the NANB hepatitis viruses.

MANAGEMENT OF HEPATITIS

There is no specific treatment for hepatitis, and therapy is mainly supportive and directed to relief of symptoms. In younger patients, judgment of the patient's tolerance for activities and diet have replaced rigidly enforced bed rest, with the exception of alcohol and dietary restrictions. Fat intake may have to be curtailed in the presence of steatorrhea. In older persons, activities should also be geared to the patient's tolerance, taking into account the pre-existing level of fatigability. Of much greater concern is the possibility that the patient's nutritional status may already be suboptimal. Hepatitis-related CNS involvement may result in behavioral changes and depression which, when coupled with the additional anorexia that accompanies hepatitis, may present a real crisis. Hospitalization for parenteral hydration and maintenance of fluid, electrolyte, and caloric balance, may be required for such patients. Hospitalization is also recommended for anyone with excessive vomiting. Changes in carbohydrate metabolism have been described, and very close monitoring of the elderly who may be suffering from diabetes is most important. Cholestyramine may be helpful in relief of pruritus, and vitamin K should be given to those whose prothrombin time is prolonged. Corticosteroids should not be used for treatment of acute viral hepatitis, and their use is contraindicated in fulminant disease.

The use of immunosuppressive or anti-inflammatory agents in chronic active hepatitis is still controversial. Prolonged immunosuppressive treatment has been reported to have deleterious effects on the course of the disease.[19,20] However, a postmortem study from Johns Hopkins found significantly lower frequency of chronic active hepatitis, cirrhosis, and fulminant hepatic necrosis in those patients who had received immunosuppressive therapy and chemotherapeutic agents for conditions other than their hepatitis.[3]

Clinical trials with interferon and vidarabine (ara-A) seem to hold out some hope for achieving clinical improvement and reversal of histopathologic damage, and may lead to firm recommendations in the near future.[21,22]

Of importance is the prevention of further hepatotoxicity in the elderly by a careful review of a patient's existing medical regimen. Drugs that are metabolized by the liver should be avoided if at all possible.

PREVENTION AND PROPHYLAXIS

Although a safe, effective vaccine against hepatitis B is available, its widespread use in a low-incidence population such as the elderly is not generally recommended.[23,24] For individuals at high risk, such as spouses or sexual partners of a newly diagnosed case of acute or chronic hepatitis, use of the vaccine should be considered, along with hepatitis B immune globulin. Vaccine may also be indicated for patients newly enrolled in a chronic hemodialysis program if the patient demonstrates no serologic markers of previous exposure to the virus. Three doses of the vaccine are required over 7 months.

Postexposure prophylaxis for exposed individuals who are not immune to the type of hepatitis in question is also available.[25] Immune globulin may prevent or ameliorate hepatitis A if given within 2 weeks of exposure. Hepatitis B immune globulin is recommended for high-risk exposure, and a second dose must be given 28 days after the first unless a concomitant vaccination is undertaken. There are no firm recommendations for prophylaxis after exposure to NANB hepatitis, although immune globulin can be administered

Both endemic and epidemic occurrences of hepatitis should be reported to the local health department, so that potential outbreaks can be recognized and averted, and contacts eligible for prophylaxis can be notified. Any patient who is in the infectious stages of hepatitis, be it acute or chronic, should be handled with certain precautions according to the mode of transmission of the particular type of disease.[26]

Hepatitis A virus is transmitted through food, or person to person, and "enteric precautions" should be maintained for 2 weeks. Although two cases of hepatitis A due to blood transfusion have been reported, blood is not usually implicated in its transmission. Hepatitis B and NANB are transmitted parenterally or per mucosa, both directly person to person, and indirectly from contaminated equipment and the environment. Virus is present in all body fluids, but saliva, urine, semen, and blood are especially infectious. These patients, therefore, require "body fluid precautions." Although outbreaks in nursing homes are uncommon, one such outbreak which occurred in one of the Scandinavian countries involved six of 59 residents, and was probably related to the shared use of bath brushes. If an infectious patient is to be hospitalized or admitted to a nursing home, it is the physician's responsibility to bring the patient's status to the attention of the admissions clerk and/or the charge nurse of the unit to which the patient is admitted. Patients who are asymptomatic carriers of hepatitis B or NANB, or who have chronic disease, must be reminded to so inform their dentists, surgeons, or podiatrists, to prevent transmission of their infection to those individuals.

SUMMARY

The geriatric age group, although at cumulatively lesser risk of endemic viral hepatitis, is nevertheless at risk of serious disease when hepatitis does occur. This is especially true if the index of suspicion is low and the disease is compounded by continuous administration of the many drugs commonly required with advanced age, many of which may be hepatotoxic. Early detection can decrease the mortality faced by this population, and in an institutional setting, can substantially reduce transmission of disease to patients and personnel.

REFERENCES

1. Finkelstein MS, Freedman ML, Shenkman L, et al: Evidence of prior hepatitis B and hepatitis A infections in an ambulatory geriatric population. *J Gerontol* 1981;32:202–205.
2. Gross PA: Gastrointestinal infections: Viral hepatitis, in: Gurevich I, Tafuro P, Cunha BA (eds): *The Theory and Practice of Infection Control*. New York, Praeger Publishing, 1984; pp 324–350.
3. de la Monte SM, Hutchins GM, Moore GW: Risk factors for development of lethal sequelae after hepatitis B infection in humans. *Am J Med* 1984;77:482–488.
4. Beasly RP: The risk of hepatocellular carcinoma in hepatitis B virus infections: A prospective study in Taipan. Presented at the International Symposium on Viral Hepatitis. New York, March–April, 1981.
5. Gamen D: Persistent infection of humans with hepatitis B virus: mechanisms and consequences. *Rev Infect Dis* 1982;4: 1026–1047.
6. Dienstag JJ, Wards JR, Koff RS: Acute hepatitis A and chronic hepatitis, in Isselbacher KJ, et al (eds): *Harrison's Principles of Internal Medicine*, ed 10. New York, McGraw-Hill Book Co, 1983, pp 1789–1804.
7. Hollinger FB, Dienstag JL: Hepatitis viruses, in *Manual of Clinical Microbiology*. Washington, American Society for Microbiology, 1980, pp 899–921.
8. Koff RS: *Viral Hepatitis*. New York, John Wiley & Sons, 1978.
9. Snydman DR, Dienstag JL, Stedt B, et al: Use of IgM hepatitis A antibody testing: investigating a common-source food-borne outbreak. *JAMA* 1981;245:827–830.
10. McMahon BJ, Bender TR, Berquist KR, et al: Delayed development of

antibody to hepatitis B surface antigen after symptomatic infection with hepatitis B virus. *J Clin Microbiol* 1981;14:130 – 134.
11. Lemon SM, Gates NL, Simms TE, et al: IgM antibody to hepatitis B core antigen as a diagnostic parameter of acute infection with hepatitis B virus. *J Infect Dis* 1981;143:803-809.
12. Overby LR: The new serology of liver disease, in Gitnick GL (ed): *Current Gastroenterology and Hepatology.* Boston, Houghton Mifflin Co, pp 276 – 309.
13. Francis DP, Maynard JF: The transmission and outcome of hepatitis A, B, and NANB. A review. *Epidemiol Rev* 1979;1:17 – 31.
14. De Cook KM, Govindarajan S, Chin KP, et al: Delta hepatitis in the Los Angeles area. A report of 126 cases. *Ann Intern Med* 1986;105:108 – 114.
15. Govindarajan S, Valinluck B, Peters L: Relapse of acute B viral hepatitis-role of delta agent. *Gut* 1986;27:19 – 22.
16. Rosina F, Saraggo G, Rizzetto M: Risk of post-transfusion infection with the hepatitis delta virus. *N Engl J Med* 1985;312:1488 – 1491.
17. Seto B, Iwarson S, Coleman WG, et al: Detection of reverse transcriptase activity in association with the non-A, non-B hepatitis agent(s). *Lancet* 1984;1:941 – 943.
18. Robinson WS: The enigma of non-A, non-B hepatitis. *J Infect Dis* 1982;145:387 – 395.
19. Scullard GH, Robinson WS, Merigan TC, et al: The effect of immunosuppressive therapy on hepatitis B viral infection in patients with chronic hepatitis, abstracted. *Gastroenterology* 1979;77:A40.
20. Scullard GH, Smith LI, Merigan TC, et al: Effects of immunosuppressive therapy on viral markers in chronic active hepatitis B. *Gastroenterology* 1981;81:987 – 991.
21. Scullard GH, Andres LL, Greenberg HB, et al: Antiviral treatment of chronic hepatitis B virus infection: improvement in liver disease with interferon and adenine arabinoside. *Hepatology* 1981;1:228 – 232.
22. Weller IVD, Bassendino MF, Craxi A, et al: Successful treatment of HBs and HBeAg positive chronic liver disease: prolonged inhibition of viral replication by highly soluble adenine arabinoside-5-monophosphate (ARA-AMP). *Gut* 1982;23:717 – 713.
23. Immunization Practices Advisory Committee: Update on hepatitis B prevention. *MMWR* 1987;36(23):353 – 365.
24. Centers for Disease Control: Hepatitis B vaccine: evidence confirming lack of AIDS transmission. *MMWR* 1984;33:685 – 686.
25. Immunization Practices Advisory Committee: Postexposure prophylaxis of hepatitis B. *MMWR* 1985;34:313 – 337.
26. Gurevich I: Editorial commentary: Practical infection control aspects, in Gurevich I, Tafuro P, Cunha BA (eds): *The Theory and Practice of Infection Control.* New York, Praeger Publishers, 1984, pp 345 – 350.

14
Intra-Abdominal Infections

John G. Bartlett

Intra-abdominal infections refer to infectious processes within the abdominal cavity that are external to the gastrointestinal (GI) tract. These infections are usually due to bacteria, and most frequently involve components of the resident flora of the lumen that actually represent the "milieu exterieur" of Claude Bernard. Exogenous pathogens are rarely implicated so that these patients seldom pose a problem in terms of transmissible disease. The clinical features are variable depending to a large extent on the nature of the pathogenic process. Nevertheless, the anticipated findings are fever, leukocytosis, and abdominal pain with or without nausea, vomiting, diarrhea, or constipation. These infections are particularly important in the elderly, since the incidence of intra-abdominal sepsis in this patient population is relatively high and the frequency of atypical presentation seems to correlate almost directly with age.[1]

APPENDICITIS

Studies from three decades ago indicated that only about 1% to 3% of all cases of acute appendicitis occurred in patients over the age of 60 years, but more recent studies indicate that this age group now accounts for 7% to 9% of cases. The diagnosis of appendicitis in this age category may be particularly elusive since it is usually viewed as a disease of younger persons and the elderly are more likely to show atypical presentation. Further, a consistent clinical experience has been that elderly patients have a high incidence of advanced disease at the time the diagnosis is established.[2-4] The incidence of perforation is 3 to 5 times higher in persons over the age of 60 years. Other complications that occur more frequently include gangrene, which has been found in as many as 60% of elderly patients, periappendiceal abscess in up to 50%, and generalized peritonitis in 15%. It is not certain if this advanced stage of disease reflects a delay in presentation or more rapid progression due to degenerative changes within the appendix associated with the aging process. In any event, there is a notable increase in the mortality rates and the incidence of postoperative complications which presumably reflects both host factors and advanced pathology. Mortality rates are generally reported at 3% to 10% in the elderly compared with less than 1% in younger patients.[3] Furthermore, a skeptical note has been passed on the incidental appendectomy for patients over 65 years who undergo laparotomy since it is estimated that a thousand appendectomies would be necessary to prevent a single case.[5]

DIVERTICULITIS

Diverticular disease is largely a phenomenon of twentieth-century, Western civilization, reduced crude fiber in the diet, and the aging process. The incidence of diverticulosis is less than 10% in persons aged under 40 years, 30% in those over 60 years, and about 50% in persons over 80 years.[6] The most common location is the sigmoid colon and the most frequent form is the pulsion type with a mucosal pouch projecting through circular layers of muscle. Long-term studies show that most patients remain asymptomatic throughout life and, in fact, a major portion show no progression in terms of the total number or size of diverticuli.[6,7] The incidence of inflammatory complications is a function of age and duration. Diverticulitis occurs in approximately 10% of patients followed 5 years or less, in 25% followed 6 to 10 years, and in about one third of patients followed for up to 20 years.[7]

Management guidelines vary according to the severity of the attack and the presence of complications. Upright films of the abdomen and chest or a cross-table lateral view may show free air indicating perforation. This is rare, but obviously represents a serious complication that requires emergent surgery. Barium enema examinations are almost always abnormal, but the changes are usually nonspecific. The only diagnostic findings of particular merit are the detection of a fistula or a luminal compression as a result of a pericolonic abscess. The preferred studies for the detection of a peridiverticular abscess, which represents the most common complication, are computed tomography (CT) or ultrasound studies to be described below. Endoscopy is rarely indicated except to rule out other diagnostic considerations such as colonic carcinoma, inflammatory bowel disease, or enteric infections.

Most patients with diverticulitis respond to medical management. Patients with mild disease may often be treated successfully with dietary modification, and "a little antibiotic" treatment using ampicillin or tetracycline on an ambulatory care basis. Patients with more severe disease require hospitalization for more aggressive treatment and observation to exclude complications that might necessitate surgical intervention. This would apply to most patients with fever, leukocytosis, and moderately severe abdominal pain or tenderness; it would also apply to patients who have roentgenographic evidence of a complication, progression of symptoms during observation as an outpatient, and patients who have other diagnostic considerations such as ischemic colitis, inflammatory bowel disease, or inflammation or perforation as a complication of colonic carcinoma.

Complications requiring surgical intervention occur in approximately 25% of patients hospitalized with diverticulitis.[8] The most frequent indication is a diverticular abscess; less frequent indications include free perforation with generalized peritonitis, GI tract obstruction, or fistula formation. About 7% of those requiring surgery have a "malignant" form characterized by extensive inflammation, fistulization, and obstruction.[9] Occasional patients have giant diverticula with gas trapping by a ball-valve mechanism and require segmental resection.[10] Patients with small abscesses may be treated with a primary resection and anastomosis. Patients with larger abscesses or free perforation usually undergo a two-stage procedure with a diverting or proximal colostomy and primary resection as the initial procedure followed by colostomy closure and reanastomosis at the second stage.

INTRA-ABDOMINAL ABSCESSES

Intra-abdominal abscesses usually represent complications of GI trauma, surgery, and perforations. Regardless of location, there are two sequential stages in the evolution of the infection which usually involve the intestinal flora.[11] The initial phase is inflammation, which may be widespread, as with generalized peritonitis following free perforation, or localized, such as a "phlegmon," diverticulitis, or appendicitis. The second stage is the abscess phase in which there is the characteristic collagen wall containing leukocytes, necrotic debris, and bacteria.

Intra-abdominal abscesses are classified as intraperitoneal, retroperitoneal, and visceral.[12] These collections may appear adjacent to the portal of entry as with a periappendiceal abscess, a peridiverticular abscess, or an abscess at a site of an anastomotic leak. Alternatively, there may be extension to distant sites due to a failure to localize the infection at the portal of entry. The most common sites when there is distant spread is a subphrenic location due to cephalad movement reflecting negative pressure created by diaphragmatic movements, or a lower quadrant abscess reflecting gravitational flow. Intraperitoneal abscesses usually occur in association with diseases or operations involving the intestinal lumen, although some cases occur with no apparent explanation. Posterior retroperitoneal abscesses generally reflect a contiguous renal infection, but anterior retroperitoneal abscesses occur in association with diverse conditions including appendicitis, diverticulitis, colonic carcinoma, pancreatitis, gastric or duodenal peptic ulcer disease, biliary tract infections, and inflammatory bowel disease. Visceral abscesses are most common in the liver, pancreas, and biliary tract. Subphrenic and subhepatic infections are both common and especially elusive in the diagnostic evaluation. These infections may result from diverse causes including diseases or surgery of the stomach, colon, appendix, pancreas, spleen, and biliary tract, often as a result of the cephalad flow, noted previously, via the paracolic gutters.

Table 14-1
Source of Intra-Abdominal Abscess: Analysis of 501 Cases

Primary Disease	No. of Cases (%)	Average Age (yr)	Mean Temperature (°F)	Mean WBC (1000/mL)	Mortality
Appendicitis	97 (19%)	32	102	19	2%
Pancreatitis or pancreatic tumor	60 (12%)	58	102	18	44%
Genitourinary tract	91 (18%)	44	101.7	22	9%
Diverticulitis	37 (7%)	60	103	16.4	21%
Biliary tract	41 (8%)	62	103	18.7	4%

Adapted from Altemeier et al.[12]

The conclusion from the above is that intra-abdominal abscesses represent loculated collections that are usually located either at the portal of entry or at widely distant sites reflecting diverse traffic patterns within the abdominal cavity. Regardless of the location, these infections are particularly common in the elderly due in part to the high incidence of the most common associated conditions in this age group. These abscesses have traditionally presented a formidable diagnostic challenge since the abdominal cavity is especially difficult to evaluate for loculated abscesses compared with other anatomical sites using physical examination and the usual laboratory tests. Most patients have fever, although this may be deceptively low or absent in elderly patients, patients receiving corticosteroids or antipyretics, and patients with gram-negative bacteremia.

Patients with a recent laparotomy often have fever, but elevated temperatures that persist beyond four days suggest intra-abdominal sepsis as a complication.[13] Most patients have leukocytosis and, again, prolonged leukocytosis following laparotomy specifically suggests this diagnosis.[13] The physical examination may be deceptive or unimpressive and is especially difficult to evaluate in postoperative patients. Abdominal plain films and contrast studies are often either negative or show only nonspecific findings. The most frequent observation regarded as specific is extraluminal gas, but this is found in a relatively small portion of cases. The availability of new scanning techniques has revolutionized the diagnostic evaluation for intra-abdominal sepsis, although there continues to be considerable controversy regarding the relative merits and indications of various tests.[14]

Radioactive gallium 67 scans show a sensitivity of up to 80% for detecting intra-abdominal abscesses. One advantage is that images of the entire body are readily obtained. Limitations with the technique include an unacceptably high rate of false-positive tests, the prolonged interval of 48 to 72 hours required to complete the study, and the lack of specificity since gallium uptake occurs with tumors and at postoperative sites as well as with active infectious processes. Furthermore, the tracer is excreted in the gut making interpretation of intra-abdominal collections especially difficult. An alternative is the use of indium 111–labeled white cells, which provides an earlier answer and appears to be more specific.

Ultrasonography shows a sensitivity of 90% or more for detecting intra-abdominal abscesses and has the advantage that it can be performed at the bedside for patients who may be too seriously ill for transport. One potential problem is that fluid collections in the gallbladder or bowel may cause occasional false-positive tests, intestinal gas may preclude adequate examination of some areas, and it may be difficult to distinguish purulent collections, hematomas, and serous collections.

Computed tomography is probably the most useful examination in terms of specificity and sensitivity. Purulent collections show attenuation values which are different for soft tissue, blood, and serous fluid. Additionally, the surrounding wall of an abscess may be enhanced with intravenous (IV) contrast material, and orally administered contrast substances are useful for distinguishing fluid collections within the bowel. False-negative CT scans are extremely uncommon, the major causes being very small abscesses or misinterpretation. Nevertheless, the choice of a particular study should be influenced by the availability of local expertise, resources, scheduling availability, and the severity of the illness. It should also be noted that these scans may be complementary. An example is the use of the gallium scan or ultrasound to identify the particular area of interest so that subsequent CT scans may be performed with more frequent imaging in the area of suspicion.

TREATMENT

Surgical

The treatment of intra-abdominal abscesses consists of drainage combined with antibiotic administration. The traditional method of choice for drainage is with surgery. The extraserous approach is obviously attractive since it is associated with the best prognosis. However, the transperitoneal approach is often preferred since this permits detection of multiple abscesses as well as associated conditions that account for the abscess when the cause is unclear. At the present time, most drainage operations are performed using a transperitoneal approach. The extraserous approach is generally restricted to large unilocular abscesses that are likely to be single, such as a subphrenic abscess following left colectomy and splenectomy, a right subphrenic abscess following a Bilroth II resection, or a pelvic abscess after low anterior resection, or abscesses contiguous with the abdominal wall.

An alternative to surgical drainage is percutaneous drainage using ultasonic or CT guidance.[15,16] The advantage with this method is that it avoids general anesthesia and some postoperative complications. This may be particularly attractive in some elderly, debilitated patients who are not considered good surgical candidates. The initial published experience with percutaneous drainage shows an overall success rate of about 80% to 85%, a record that is at least as good as that noted with traditional surgical drainage. Nevertheless, this must be recognized as a relatively new procedure which should be reserved for clinical situations that satisfy stringent criteria: (1) Technical expertise is mandatory; (2) percutaneous drainage should be restricted to single, well-defined, unilocular abscesses; (3) there needs to be a safe percutaneous drainage route; and (4) there needs to be immediate operative capability in the event of a complication, the major complication being hemorrhage.

Antibiotic Therapy

Most cases of intra-abdominal sepsis involve a polymicrobial flora with bacteria that normally colonize the GI tract. With infections following a colonic portal of entry, the dominant isolates are coliforms, especially *Escherichia coli*, and anaerobic bacteria, especially *Bacteroides fragilis*. Infections associated with a gastric or small bowel portal of entry tend to involve streptococci, gram-positive bacilli, and only occasionally coliforms or *Candida*. Coliform bacteria, such as *E coli*, *Klebsiella*, *Enterobacter*, and *Proteus* spp, tend to be the dominant isolates in biliary tract infections, pancreatic infections, and spontaneous peritonitis. These idiosyncrasies in the distribution of bacteria account for some of the vagaries in antibiotic recommendations for both treatment and prophylaxis in various settings under the category of "intra-abdominal sepsis." In addition, there are some situations where the clinician has the benefit of defined bacteriology, either as a result of positive blood cultures or the results of cultures of exudate from the infected site that will obviously influence the therapeutic decisions. Nevertheless, there is a significant portion of patients who have no defined bacteriologic findings, in whom the site of infection is not entirely clear, and empiric decisions are necessary.

Most authorities now advocate regimens for intra-abdominal sepsis that include antibiotics active against both coliforms and anaerobes based on the prevalence of these organisms at the infected site. Commonly advocated regimens include an aminoglycoside for activity against coliforms such as gentamicin, tobramycin, or amikacin. A second drug, utilized for activity against anaerobes, may be clindamycin, cefoxitin, metronidazole, chloramphenicol, or ticarcillin (or other antipseudomonad penicillins). Comparative clinical trials indicate that the regimens noted are equally meritorious according to criteria used to judge outcome (Table 14-2).

Table 14-2
Comparative Clinical Trials of Antibiotic Regimens
in the Treatment of Intra-Abdominal Sepsis and
Pelvic Infections

Source	Regimens	No. of Treatment Failures/ No. treated (%)
Klastersky et al, 1979[17]	Clindamycin ± gentamicin	4/24 (17)
	Cefoxitin ± gentamicin	4/22 (18)
Smith et al, 1980[18]	Clindamycin + tobramycin	3/23 (13)
	Metronidazole + tobramycin	5/34 (15)
Harding et al, 1980[19]	Clindamycin + gentamicin	4/42 (10)
	Chloramphenicol + gentamicin	10/53 (19)
	Ticarcillin + gentamicin	4/39 (10)
Tally et al, 1981[20]	Cefoxitin ± amikacin	3/37 (8)
	Clindamycin + amikacin	8/37 (22)
Collier et al, 1981[21]	Clindamycin ± other agent	5/87 (6)
	Metronidazole + other agent	1/83 (1)
Drusano et al, 1982[22]	Cefoxitin ± aminoglycoside	10/46 (22)
	Clindamycin + aminoglycoside	11/44 (25)
Canadian Study Group, 1983[23]	Clindamycin + gentamicin	3/69 (4)
	Metronidazole + gentamicin	4/72 (6)
Van Scoy et al, 1984[24]	Clindamycin ± aminoglycoside penicillin	3/34 (9)
	Chloramphenicol ± aminoglycoside-penicillin	5/36 (14)
Nichols et al, 1984[25]	Clindamycin + gentamicin	7/75 (9)
	Cefoxitin	6/70 (9)

However, most of the trials cited have been criticized for the common failure to include seriously ill patients, inclusion of heterogeneous patient populations, the common failure to account for causes of failure, and the use of inadequate numbers to permit meaningful stratification based on severity or type of infection.[26] The implication is that the demonstration of differences will require a multi-institutional study. Until that time, most clinicans will utilize regimens selected empirically based on personal experience and justified by clinical trials which, despite notable deficiencies, still represent the "best show in town." There are a few factors that may influence the specific regimen selected.

The aminoglycosides are considered equally effective against susceptible coliforms, although sensitivity profiles within a given institution may vary and this should influence the choice, especially for patients with hospital-acquired infections. In general, tobramycin is somewhat more active than gentamicin versus *Pseudomonas aeruginosa*, gentamicin is somewhat more active against *Serratia marcescens*, and amikacin is active against many isolates resistant to the other two aminoglycosides. Tobramycin is probably the least nephrotoxic, although the data are somewhat controversial, and the prevalent impression that tobramycin is preferred in patients with pre-existing renal dysfunction is probably erroneous.[27] The major problem with aminoglycosides in most cases is usually not the selection of a specific drug from the group, but the use of an inadequate dose to achieve therapeutic levels in patients who are seriously ill. This point is emphasized in the study by Moore et al[28] of 89 patients with gram-negative bacteremia treated with aminoglycosides. The mortality rate was only 2% (one) among 41 patients with therapeutic levels compared to 21% (nine) among 43 patients with subtherapeutic levels.

Cefoxitin may be used as a single agent due to activity against both coliforms and anaerobes.[20] An attractive feature of this "monotherapy" is that it avoids aminoglycosides with the attendant risks of nephrotoxicity and the necessity of therapeutic monitoring. However, this approach can be advocated only in patients who acquire their infection prior to hospitalization and have not received other forms of antibiotic treatment during the preceding 2 weeks. It should be noted that cefoxitin appears to be the betalactam antibiotic of choice for intra-abdominal sepsis due to its enhanced activity versus *B fragilis* compared with other cephalosporins.[28] Alternative strategies to permit avoidance of aminoglycosides include the use of third-generation cephalosporins with anti-*B fragilis* activity, but most authorities do not currently advocate this approach due to reduced activity of these drugs versus penicillin-resistant anaerobes.

The regimens recommended above generally lack activity versus the enterococcus. Many authorities feel this organism is not especially important in mixed infections, although there are certain notable exceptions. Treatment versus the enterococcus is recommended when this organism is recovered in blood cultures, when it is found in exudate in pure culture, and for patients who fail to respond with no apparent alternative explanation. Some authorities advocate the routine use of drugs active against this organism for intra-abdominal sepsis using either ampicillin or penicillin G combined with an aminoglycoside.

Drugs utilized for the anaerobic component of the infection are controversial, particularly for the "*B fragilis* group." In vitro sensitivity studies of over 1000 strains isolated from multiple centers[29] showed that virtually all were susceptible to chloramphenicol and metronidazole, 5% to 10% were resistant to clindamycin and cefoxitin, and 10% were resistant to antipseudomonad penicillins; third-generation cephalosporins other than moxalactam were notably inferior. One particularly important observation is that resistant profiles for some drugs appeared to reflect utilization rates. Thus over 25% of strains were resistant to cefoxitin at Tufts-New England Medical Center where this drug had been used as the preferred agent for intra-abdominal sepsis for several years. The apparent message is that the same painful lesson learned with the evolution of resistance by coliforms in response to antibiotic pressure may apply to at least some drugs with anaerobic bacteria as well.

Patients with intra-abdominal sepsis often have persistent signs of infection or recurrence of these findings despite what appears to be the necessary surgery combined with rational antibiotic regimens. In many instances, these patients either require simply more time to respond, or they are inadequate hosts and cannot respond to any regimen, or there is a need for further drainage procedures. Changes in the antibiotic regimen are only occasionally effective. Factors to consider in such cases are the in vitro sensitivity profiles of gram-negative bacilli, the presence or absence of enterococci, and the detection of other organisms that may have unusual sensitivity profiles such as *Candida* sp. Metronidazole is the most active of all available drugs against *B fragilis* and most other anaerobes; this would be an appropriate choice for the patient with persistent sepsis involving anaerobes in which the original regimen included an alternative drug. This approach would especially apply to patients with persistent or recurrent *Bacteroides* bacteremia.

REFERENCES

1. Vartian CA, Septimus EJ: Intra-abdominal infections in the elderly: Diagnosis and management. *Geriatrics* 1986;41:51 – 56.
2. Peltokallio P, Tykka H: Evolution of the age distribution and mortality of acute appendicitis. *Arch Surg* 1970;100:140.
3. Coran AG, Wheeler HB: Early perforation in appendicitis after age 60. *JAMA* 1966;197: 745.
4. Williams JS, Hale HW Jr: Acute appendicitis in the elderly: review of 83 cases. *Ann Surg* 1965;162:208.

5. Nockerts SR, Detmer DI, Fryback DG: Incidental appendectomy in the elderly? No. *Surgery* 1980;88:301−306
6. Parks TG: Natural history of diverticular disease of the colon. *Clin Gastroenterol* 1975;4:53.
7. Horner JL: Natural history of diverticulosis of the colon. *Am J Dig Dis* 1958;3:343.
8. Mitty WF, Befeler D, Gross C, et al: Surgical management of complications of diverticulitis in patients over seventy years of age. *Am J Surg* 1969;117:270.
9. Morgenstern L, Weiner R, Michael SL: "Malignant" diverticulitis: a clinical entity. *Arch Surg* 1979;114:1112−1116.
10. Gallagher JJ, Welch JP: Giant diverticula of the colon. *Arch Surg* 1979;114:1079−1183.
11. Bartlett JG, Onderdonk AB, Louie T, et al: A review. Lessons from an animal model of intra-abdominal sepsis. *Arch Surg* 1978;113:853−857.
12. Altemeier WA, Culbertson WR, Fullen WD, et al: Intraabdominal abscess. *Am J Surg* 1973;125:70−79.
13. Lennard ES, Dellinger EP, Wertz MJ, et al: Implications of leukocytosis and fever at conclusion of antibiotic therapy for intra-abdominal sepsis. *Ann Surg* 1982;195:19−24.
14. Ferrucci JT Jr, vanSonnenberg E: Intra-abdominal abscess. *JAMA* 1981;246:2728−2733.
15. Percutaneous drainage of the abdominal abscess, editorial. *Lancet* 1982;1:889−890.
16. Gerzof SG, Robbins AH, Johnson WC, et al: Percutaneous catheter drainage of abdominal abscesses. *N Engl J Med* 1981;305:653−657.
17. Klastersky J, Coppens L, Mombelli G: Anaerobic infection in cancer patients: comparative evaluation of clindamycin and cefoxitin. *Antimicrob Agents Chemother* 1979;16:366−371.
18. Smith JA, Skidmore AG, Forward AD, et al: Prospective randomized, double-blind comparison of metronidazole and tobramycin with clindamycin and tobramycin in the treatment of intra-abdominal sepsis. *Ann Surg* 1980;192:213−220.
19. Harding GKM, Buckwold FJ, Ronald AR, et al: Prospective randomized comparative study of clindamycin, chloramphenicol and ticarcilin, each in combination with gentamicin, in therapy for intra-abdominal and female genital tract sepsis. *J Infect Dis* 1980;142:384−393.
20. Tally FP, McGowan K, Kellun JM, et al: A randomized comparison of cefoxitin with or without amikacin and clindamycin plus amikacin in surgical sepsis. *Ann Surg* 1981;193: 318−323.
21. Coller J, Colhoun EM, Hill PL: A multicentre comparison of clindamycin and metronidazole in the treatment of anaerobic infections. *Scand J Infect Dis* 1981;26 (suppl): 96−100.
22. Drusano GL, Warren JW, Saah AJ, et al: A prospective randomized controlled trial of cefoxitin versus clindamycin-aminoglycoside in mixed anaerobic-aerobic infections. *Surg Gynecol Obstet* 1982;154:715−720.
23. Canadian Study Group: Prospective randomized comparison of metronidazole and clindamycin, each with gentamicin, for the treatment of serious intra-abdominal infection. *Surgery* 1983;93:221−229.
24. Van Scoy RE, Wilkowske CJ, O'Fallon WM, et al: Clindamycin versus chloramphenicol in treatment of anaerobic infections: a prospective randomized, double-blind study. *Mayo Clin Proc* 1984;59: 842−846.
25. Nichols RL, Smith JW, Klein DB, et al: Risk of infection after penetrating

abdominal trauma. *N Engl J Med* 1984; 311:1065 – 1070.
26. Solomkin JS, Meakins JL, Allo MD, et al: Antibiotic trials in intra-abdominal infections. A critical evaluation of study design and outcome reporting. *Ann Surg* 1984;200:29 – 39.
27. Moore RD, Smith CR, Lipsky JL, et al: Risk factors for nephrotoxicity in patients treated with aminoglycosides. *Ann Intern Med* 1984;100:352 – 357.
28. Moore RD, Smith CR, Lietman PS: The association of aminoglycoside plasma levels with mortality in patients with gram-negative bacteremia. *J Infect Dis* 1984;149:443 – 448.
29. Cuchural GJ Jr, Talley FP, Jacobus NV, et al: Antimicrobial susceptibilities of 1,292 isolates of the *Bacteroides fragilis* group in the United States: comparison of 1981 with 1982. *Antimicrob Agents Chemother* 1984;26:145 – 148.

15

Urinary Tract Infections

Jerome A. Boscia
Donald Kaye

Urinary tract infection is very common in the elderly and presents a series of problems of major concern to the practitioner of geriatrics. The epidemiology, pathogenesis, etiology, clinical manifestations (especially their absence), and management of urinary tract infection in the geriatric population differs significantly from urinary tract infection in the general population. This chapter reviews urinary tract infection in the elderly with particular emphasis on the differences from urinary tract infection in the younger population. Also, catheter-associated urinary tract infection, which is a serious problem in elderly patients residing in nursing homes, extended care facilities, and hospitals, is reviewed.

Bacteriuria literally means bacteria in the urine. The presence or absence of infection in the bladder can be determined by quantitating numbers of bacteria by culture techniques in voided urine and/or in urine obtained via urethral catheterization. The term "significant bacteriuria" describes the numbers of bacteria in midstream clean-catch–voided urine that exceed the numbers usually due to the contamination of urine by bacteria present in the urethra (ie, $\geq 10^5$ bacteria/mL). The possibility of urinary tract infection should be considered when the presence of more than 10^5 bacteria/mL of urine is detected by culture.

Asymptomatic bacteriuria is a frequently used term in the elderly and refers to significant bacteriuria in a subject without symptoms. Urinary tract infection may involve the lower urinary tract alone or both the upper and lower urinary tracts. The term *cystitis* describes the symptom complex involving dysuria, urgency, and frequency, and refers to lower urinary tract infection. These symptoms may be caused by urethritis due to sexually transmissible infections (eg, gonorrhea or chlamydia) but these appear to be rare diagnoses in the geriatric population. The presence of symptoms of lower urinary tract infection without upper urinary tract symptomatology by no means excludes upper urinary tract involvement. The term *acute pyelonephritis* describes the syndrome characterized by fever and flank pain and/or tenderness, often accompanied by dysuria, urgency, and frequency.

Urinary tract infection may be a recurrent problem. Recurrences may be either relapses or reinfections. The term *relapse* refers to recurrence of bacteriuria with the same organism that was present before antimicrobial treatment. This is due to persistence of the organism in the urinary tract despite therapy. The term *reinfection* refers to a new episode of bacteriuria, often with a different organism than was present before antimicrobial treatment. Occasionally reinfection may occur with the same organism which may have persisted in the vagina or perineal area.

PATHOGENESIS

There are two known routes by which bacteria can invade the urinary tract. These are the ascending and hematogenous routes. The urethra, in particular the anterior portion, is usually colonized by bacteria. The presence of small numbers of organisms in the bladders of uninfected subjects has occasionally been found via suprapubic puncture.[1] Apparently, both urethral massage and sexual intercourse can force bacteria into the bladder in women.[2-4] Urinary tract infection has been shown to develop following one bladder catheterization in about 1% of ambulatory subjects and within three or four days in almost all patients with indwelling bladder catheters with open drainage systems.[5,6]

Urinary tract infection is much more common in women than in men, supporting the importance of the ascending route of infection. The female urethra is short and is close to the bacterially colonized vagina and perineum, making contamination of the urethra likely. Organisms that cause urinary tract infection in women colonize the periurethral area before urinary tract infection results.[7] Once bacteria gain access to the bladder via the urethra they may multiply and pass up the ureters to the kidneys, especially if vesicoureteral reflux is present.

Infection of the kidneys by the hematogenous route clearly occurs but is much less frequent than kidney infection caused by the ascending route. For example, the kidney is frequently the site of abscess formation in patients with staphylococcal bacteremia.[8] However, infection of the kidney with gram-negative bacilli rarely occurs by the hematogenous route.

The end result of bacterial colonization and invasion of the urinary tract depends on the inoculum size and the virulence of the organism involved and the status of the host defense mechanisms. In the elderly, inoculum size would appear to be increased by soiling of the perineum from fecal incontinence in demented women[9] and increased urethral catheterization or instrumentation in both sexes. The most important virulence factor of organisms capable of causing urinary tract infection has been reported to be their capacity to adhere to uroepithelial cells.[10] Sobel and Kaye studied adherence of *Escherichia coli* to uroepithelial cells in young uninfected women and men as well as elderly uninfected and infected women and men.[11] This study showed no evidence to support the hypothesis that increased adherence is a factor in the high prevalence of urinary tract infection in the elderly (Fig. 15-1).

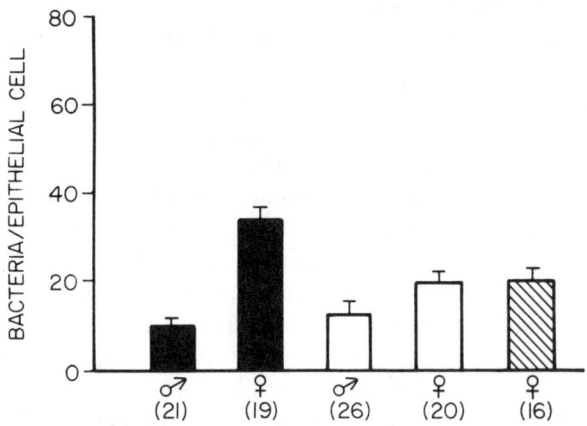

Figure 15-1 Comparison of in vitro adherence of a mannose-sensitive strain of *Escherichia coli* to uroepithelial cells obtained from healthy uninfected young control subjects (*black bars*), uninfected elderly subjects (*white bars*), and infected elderly women (*stippled bars*). Number of subjects is in parentheses.

Host defense mechanisms against bacterial colonization and invasion of the urinary tract appear to begin with antiadherence mechanisms such as vaginal and periurethral antibodies.[12] It is unknown whether or not these antibodies are underproduced in the elderly. It has also been reported that a low vaginal pH is the most important factor related to lack of colonization of uropathogens.[13] It is unclear if the vaginal pH changes in the elderly. Urine is generally considered to be a good culture medium for bacteria but it does possess some antibacterial activity. Urine defenses that inhibit bacterial growth include a low pH, extremes of osmolality, a high urea, a high organic acid concentration, and prostatic secretions.[14,15] It is likely that with the decline of renal function that occurs with aging, the ability of the kidney to acidify the urine, achieve extremes of osmolality, and excrete a high urea load would be diminished.

Glucose in the urine of diabetic patients provides a better culture medium for the growth of bacteria.[16]

Bladder defense mechanisms include micturition with complete emptying of the bladder and a possible intrinsic antiadherence mechanism.[17,18] Complete emptying of the bladder is less likely to occur in the elderly with obstructive uropathy from the prostate in men, bladder prolapse in women, and neurogenic bladders in both sexes.[11,19] With the occurrence of bladder infection, secondary defense mechanisms such as mobilization of neutrophils followed by phagocytosis with subsequent bacterial destruction are called on to remove bacteria.[20]

Renal defense mechanisms include the flow of urine, which is undoubtedly important in washing bacteria down the ureters.[11] During pyelonephritis, neutrophils are mobilized to limit bacterial spread and persistence within the kidney. Also renal infection induces a systemic antibody response.[21] The latter does not usually occur with bladder infection.[22]

EPIDEMIOLOGY

Bacteriuria is much more common in elderly than in young subjects. In young to middle-aged women and men the prevalence of bacteriuria is less than 5% and less than 0.1% respectively.[23] At least 20% of women and 10% of men over 65 years of age have bacteriuria.[24] In contrast to young adults where bacteriuria is approximately 30 times more frequent in women than men over 65 years of age the ratio of women to men with bacteriuria decreases progressively to approximately 2–3:1. In the elderly in both sexes the prevalence of bacteriuria rises substantially with advancing age. Epidemiologic studies have shown that about 20% of women and 2% to 3% of men 65 to 70 years of age have bacteriuria on a single survey as compared with approximately 23% to 50% of women and 20% of men over 80 years of age.[25,26] Elderly subjects living at home are less likely to have bacteriuria than those living in nursing homes, who in turn are less likely to have bacteriuria than those in hospitals.

Table 15-1 lists ranges of prevalence of bacteriuria in subjects over 65 years of age compiled from various series.[25–29] These single-survey studies have shown that about 20% of elderly women and 10% of elderly men living at home have bacteriuria. These figures increase to about 25% and 20% respectively in nursing homes and extended care facilities and to 30% for both sexes in hospitals. The longer the stay in the hospital, the greater the chance of developing bacteriuria. The higher rates of bacteriuria associated with institutions are probably related to the more debilitated state of the residents, with more perineal soiling from fecal incontinence, less complete bladder emptying, and more bladder catheterization.

Table 15-1
Prevalence of Bacteriuria in Subjects over 65 Years of Age

	Percent with Bacteriuria	
	Women	Men
Living at home	17–33	6–13
Nursing home or extended care facility	23–27	17–26
Acute hospital	32–34	30–33
Long-term hospital	34–50	34

Data compiled from Sourander,[25] Brocklehurst et al,[26] Akhtar et al,[27] Gladstone and Recco,[28] and Lye.[29]

We conducted an epidemiologic study that investigated the dynamic aspects of asymptomatic bacteriuria in a large ambulatory geriatric population (184 women and 76 men over age 68), including and differentiating subjects who resided in apartments or a nursing home. We examined the patterns of bacteriuria on three surveys performed at 6-month intervals. Although only 16% of women and 5% of men had bacteriuria on the first survey, the cumulative percentage infected on at least one survey was 30% of women and 11% of men by the third survey (Fig. 15-2).[30] In a study of 101 women and 87 men over age 65 in Finland, 24% of women and 8% of men had bacteriuria on one survey; an additional survey was performed 5 years later and the cumulative percentage infected on at least one of the two surveys was 38% of women and 15% of men.[31] In a study of 231 women and 121 men over age 70 in Greece, 27% of women and 19% of men had bacteriuria on an initial survey; a second survey was performed 1 year later and the cumulative percentage with bacteriuria on one of the two surveys was 44% of women and 28% of men.[32]

In our study and the studies from Finland and Greece additional surveys would have undoubtedly increased the percentage of the population that had asymptomatic bacteriuria at least once. Thus it should be clear that asymptomatic bacteriuria in the elderly is much more common than is apparent from performing one survey. The lines in Figure 15-2 may continue to ascend at the same rate with subsequent surveys and it is possible, and in fact likely, that the majority of the geriatric female population experiences episodes of asymptomatic bacteriuria.

The geriatric population with asymptomatic bacteriuria is not a stable one. In our study, 17% of women and 6% of men with negative cultures initially developed bacteriuria by the second and/or third survey.[30] In this same study 40% of women and 75% of men with positive cultures initially had lost their bacteriuria by the second and/or third survey. In the study from Finland, of the women and men with negative

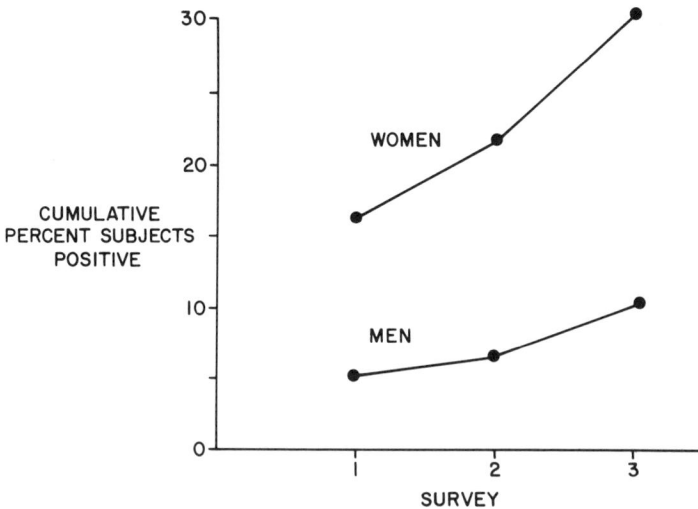

Figure 15-2 Cumulative percentage of subjects with at least one positive urine culture survey after three surveys performed at 6-month intervals.

cultures intially, 18% and 8% respectively developed bacteriuria when recultured 5 years later.[31] In this same study, of the women and men with positive cultures initially, 58% and 86% respectively had lost their bacteriuria when recultured 5 years later. In the study from Greece, 23% of women and 11% of men with negative cultures initially developed bacteriuria when recultured 1 year later.[32] In this same study, 27% of women and 22% of men with positive cultures initially had lost their bacteriuria when recultured 1 year later. All three of these studies reveal a considerable acquisition rate of asymptomatic bacteriuria among previously uninfected elderly women and men and an impressive rate of loss of bacteriuria in previously infected women and men.

In our study persistence of bacteriuria with the same organism on all three surveys was found in only 6% of women and 1% of men.[30] In the study from Greece persistence of bacteriuria with the same organism on three surveys also performed at 6-month intervals was found in 11% of women and 7% of men.[32] In our study the bacteriuric nursing home subjects were significantly more likely to have persistence of bacteriuria than the bacteriuric subjects who resided in apartments.[30]

MICROBIOLOGY

Young adults with urinary tract infection have *E coli* as the etiologic pathogen in 80% to 90% of cases.[33,34] Although *E coli* is the most common infecting organism in the geriatric population, elderly subjects are less likely than younger subjects to be infected with *E coli* and more likely to have bacteriuria with *Proteus, Klebsiella-Enterobacter, Serratia,* and *Pseudomonas* spp, and enterococci.[35-37] In our epidemiologic study of asymptomatic bacteriuria in a geriatric population, the organisms isolated from 77 positive urine cultures in a single survey of 523 subjects (373 women and 150 men, mean age 85) were predominantly Enterobacteriaceae in women, but predominantly gram-positive bacteria in men.[30] Ninety-three percent of isolates from women and only 44% of isolates from men were Enterobacteriaceae whereas 7% of isolates from women and 56% of isolates from men were gram-positive bacteria. This increase in gram-positive organism infections in men has not been reported in previous studies of bacteriuria in the elderly.[35-37] The explanation for the high percentage of gram-positive isolates observed in men with bacteriuria in our study is not known.

Part of the explanation for the increased prevalence of non–*E coli* isolates in the elderly with bacteriuria is the greater likelihood of hospitalization in this population. The hospital environment is an important determinant of the nature of the bacterial flora in urinary tract infection. *Proteus, Klebsiella-Enterobacter, Serratia,* and *Pseudomonas* spp, and enterococci are more often isolated from in-hospital patients with bacteriuria as compared with a greater preponderance of *E coli* in out-of-hospital urinary tract infections.[38] Other possible reasons for the increased prevalence of non–*E coli* isolates in the elderly with bacteriuria include an increased frequency of structural abnormalities of the urinary tract (obstructive uropathy from the prostate in men, bladder prolapse in women, and neurogenic bladders in both sexes) and increased urethral catheterization or instrumentation in both sexes. Repeated courses of antimicrobial therapy for recurrent bacteriuria or for other infections in the elderly might select for multiple antimicrobial-resistant bacterial isolates.

CLINICAL FEATURES

The clinical manifestations of symptomatic urinary tract infection are relatively easy to recognize. Lower urinary tract symptoms result from inflammation of urethral and bladder mucosa causing dysuria, urgency, and frequency. Micturition produces small amounts of turbid and sometimes bloody urine. Occasionally patients complain of suprapubic pain. Fever is usually absent with infection limited to the lower urinary tract. Classic upper urinary tract symptoms include fever and flank pain often accompanied by dysuria, urgency, and frequency. Flank pain and tenderness are more intense when obstructive disease of the urinary tract is present. Patients with urinary tract infection in the presence of an indwelling bladder catheter usually have no lower tract symptoms, but fever and flank pain are common with upper tract infection.

The vast majority of elderly subjects with bacteriuria do not have urinary symptoms.[36,39] Pyuria has been reported to be present in only 36% to 79% of elderly subjects with bacteriuria.[25,27,40] Even when symptoms are present, they are often difficult to interpret since uninfected elderly subjects commonly experience dysuria, urgency, frequency, and incontinence[26,29] We recently conducted a study to determine if asymptomatic bacteriuria in a geriatric population is really asymptomatic.[41] Seventy-two elderly subjects (59 women and 13 men, mean age 85) were questioned about urinary symptoms (dysuria, urgency, frequency, incontinence, suprapubic pain, flank pain, fever) and symptoms indicating lack of well-being (malaise, fatigue, weakness, anorexia, insomnia) both when they were with and without bacteriuria. In 22 subjects bacteriuria had resolved spontaneously; 24 nonbacteriuric subjects had developed bacteriuria; and in 26 subjects bacteriuria resolved with antimicrobial therapy. Symptoms indicating lack of well-being were commonly present, and urinary symptoms (especially stress incontinence) were occasionally reported. However, no differences were found in either the frequency or severity of symptoms whether subjects were with or without bacteriuria. Thus asymptomatic bacteriuria in the elderly really appears to be asymptomatic.

Acute pyelonephritis in elderly uncatheterized patients was recently reviewed.[42] The diagnosis was initially missed in 21% of cases because of attention given to pulmonary or gastrointestinal symptoms. Bacteremia and shock were present in a much higher percentage of patients (61% and 26% respectively) than would be true in a younger population. Another study has shown that acute pyelonephritis is the most common cause of bacteremic sepsis in the elderly.[43]

SIGNIFICANCE OF BACTERIURIA

While symptomatic urinary tract infections should be treated in patients of any age, the significance of asymptomatic bacteriuria for the well-being of elderly patients is unknown. One group of investigators found decreased renal function in elderly subjects with bacteriuria.[44-46] However, others have not been able to confirm this observation[27,29] Hypertension has been associated with bacteriuria in the elderly in some studies[40] but not in others.[27,29,46] At present, no cause-and-effect relationship between uncomplicated urinary tract infection in the elderly and renal insufficiency has been demonstrated. Therefore it is not warranted to use prevention of renal insufficiency as an indication for antimicrobial treatment of asymptomatic bacteriuria in the elderly. Also, because of the high prevalence and recurrence rates, it is not feasible to attempt to eradicate all bacteriuria in the elderly. In addition, the adverse reaction rate to antimicrobials is sufficiently high in the elderly to warrant caution in adopting too vigorous an approach to the treatment of asymptomatic bacteriuria.

On the other hand, urinary tract infection in the elderly can lead to progressive renal damage in the presence of urinary tract obstruction.[47] In fact, urinary tract infection in elderly men suggests the possibility of obstructive uropathy from an enlarged prostate gland. An effort should be made in any man with urinary tract infection to determine whether or not prostatic obstruction exists. A good history and physical examination is of primary importance. Determination of postvoiding residual urine in the bladder by urethral catheterization, an intravenous pyelogram with a postvoiding film of the bladder, or preferably ultrasonography of the bladder, should document the presence or absence of obstruction.

Two studies in the elderly have demonstrated decreased survival in bacteriuric subjects compared with nonbacteriuric subjects.[31,46] Whether the decreased survival and the bacteriuria are causally related is not clear. Increased susceptibility to bacteriuria may be due to immobility, dementia, cerebrovascular disease, or other disease resulting in soiling of the perineum from fecal incontinence in women and incomplete bladder emptying in both sexes.[9] These underlying diseases, rather than the bacteriuria, may result in the decreased survival. On the other hand, bacteriuria may be a cause of silent bacteremia and subsequent death or may in some other unknown way predispose to decreased survival.

In both of the studies in the elderly demonstrating an association between asymptomatic bacteriuria and decreased survival, subjects were categorized as bacteriuric or nonbacteriuric according to the results of an initial urine culture.[31,46] The problem with this design is that despite subsequent loss or acquisition of bacteriuria, which are common in the elderly, the subject's category was not changed. Our recent epidemiologic study of asymptomatic bacteriuria in a geriatric population, alluded to earlier, revealed different patterns of bacteriuria on three surveys performed at 6-month intervals.[30] These different patterns of bacteriuria may correlate with decreased survival differently. It is possible and even likely that occasional episodes of bacteriuria, persistent bacteriuria, and frequent reinfections have different relationships to decreased survival. It is conceivable that persistent bacteriuria may correlate more with decreased survival than occasional episodes of bacteriuria. It is also possible that frequent reinfections may have the worst prognosis. Subjects who have serious underlying disease may be more prone to frequent reinfections than to persistent bacteriuria and thus there can be an apparent association between reinfections and decreased survival. Also, frequent reinfections may be more prone to cause bacteremia than persistent bacteriuria where protective antibody is more likely to be present. A more recent study in the elderly did not demonstrate decreased survival in bacteriuric subjects compared with nonbacteriuric subjects.[39]

It is apparent that much more information is needed on the association between asymptomatic bacteriuria in the elderly and decreased survival, particularly with regard to the different patterns of bacteriuria that the elderly experience. Even if it is established that asymptomatic bacteriuria in the elderly somehow results in decreased survival, before antimicrobial therapy for bacteriuria can be advocated it will be necessary to demonstrate that eliminating bacteriuria lengthens survival. In a study on bacteriuria in elderly institutionalized men, attempts to eradicate bacteriuria with antimicrobial therapy was ineffective and did not alter mortality compared with bacteriuric subjects who received no therapy.[37]

DIAGNOSIS

Microscopic examination of the urine is one of the most useful tests for presumptive diagnosis of urinary tract infection. Smaller numbers of bacteria can be detected microscopically in centrifuged rather than in uncentrifuged urine and in gram-stained rather than in unstained urine.[48] The presence of at least one bacterium per high dry field in centrifuged, unstained urine or per oil immersion field in uncentrifuged, gram-stained urine correlated with the presence of more than 10^5 bacteria/mL.[24] The absence of bacteria in several oil immersion fields in centrifuged, gram-stained urine indicates the probability of less than 10^4 bacteria/mL.[24]

The diagnosis of urinary tract infection is usually determined by quantitative cultures of midstream, clean-catch urine specimens. In patients unable to cooperate, due to such illnesses as dementia and neuromuscular disease in both sexes, or obstructive uropathy from the prostate in men, bladder catheterization may be necessary to obtain a urine specimen. Since the urethra and periurethral areas are difficult or impossible to sterilize, even carefully collected urine specimens (including those obtained by bladder catheterization) are frequently contaminated. By quantitating bacteria in midstream, clean-catch urine, or in urine obtained by bladder catheterization, it is possible to separate contamination ($< 10^4$ bacteria/mL) from significant bacteriuria ($\geqslant 10^5$ bacteria/mL) which is indicative of infection.[6,24,49]

In patients with symptoms of urinary tract infection, one midstream, clean-catch urine culture with more than 10^5 bacteria/mL of urine has a 95% probability of representing true infection.[24] One midstream, clean-catch urine culture with more than 10^5 bacteria/mL of urine from an asymptomatic woman has an 80% chance of indicating true bacteriuria.[24] Two urine cultures with more than 10^5 of the same bacteria per milliliter of urine from an asymptomatic woman increases the probability to 95% that true infection is present.[24] Thus two midstream, clean-catch urine specimens should be collected in an asymptomatic woman to confirm urinary tract infection. In men where contamination of midstream, clean-catch urine specimens is less likely, more than 10^4 bacteria/mL of urine is suggestive of urinary tract infection.[50]

One study has challenged the validity of midstream, clean-catch urine cultures in elderly women.[51] This study compared cultures of midstream, clean-catch, and suprapubic bladder aspirate urine from elderly hospitalized women and found 30% of midstream cultures to be positive but only 13% of suprapubic aspirate cultures to be positive. This yields a 57% false-positive rate for midstream cultures or only a 43% probability of a positive culture representing infection. Other studies have reported much lower false-positive midstream, clean-catch urine culture results (eg, 17%) in elderly women.[9,39] The accuracy of such cultures is undoubtedly related to the effort given to obtain true midstream urine after proper cleansing.

Further confusion has arisen from the observation that at least 25% of young sexually active women with acute symptomatic coliform infection of the lower urinary tract have less than 10^5 bacteria/mL isolated from midstream, clean-catch urine specimens (documented by cultures of suprapubic bladder aspirates or bladder-catheterized urine specimens).[52,53] It is likely that symptomatic men of any age, symptomatic elderly women, and possibly asymptomatic women and men also have lower urinary tract infection with less than 10^5 bacteria/mL in midstream, clean-catch urine specimens. However, this needs to be documented by cultures of suprapubic aspirates or bladder-catheterized urine specimens.

Detection of antibody-coated bacteria (ACB) in urine has been used to differentiate lower urinary tract infection from upper urinary tract infection.[54,55] A positive test result for ACB in urine has been associated with infection of the kidney and/or prostate while a negative test result for ACB in urine has been associated with bladder bacteriuria.[56] The main use for ACB testing of urine is in the study of the pathogenesis, epidemiology, and/or treatment of urinary tract infection. It has not played a major role clinically in the routine management of patients with urinary tract infections.

In our epidemiologic study of asymptomatic bacteriuria in a geriatric population, three urine culture surveys were performed at 6-month intervals.[30] Urine specimens from bacteriuric subjects were examined using the ACB technique and correlated with persistent and nonpersistent bacteriuria. Table 15-2 shows that a positive test result for ACB in urine was significantly more common (60%) in subjects with persistent bacteriuria (at least two consecutive surveys positive for the same

Table 15-2
Results of Antibody-Coated Bacteria Test (ACB) on Urine Specimens of 64 Elderly Subjects with Bacteriuria

	Subjects (N = 260)	
	Total	One or More Positive ACB (%)
Subjects with persistent bacteriuria	25	15* (60.0)
Subjects with nonpersistent bacteriuria	39	11* (28.2)

* $P < .05$.

organism) compared with that (28%) in subjects with nonpersistent bacteriuria.[30] A positive test result for ACB in the urine of subjects with persistent bacteriuria appears to indicate a correlation between persistent bacteriuria and a focus of infection in the kidney and/or prostate. A negative test result for ACB in the urine of subjects with nonpersistent bacteriuria indicates a correlation between nonpersistent bacteriuria and bladder bacteriuria.

Radiologic procedures play an important role in the evaluation of patients with urinary tract infection.[57] The most important contribution provided by radiologic evaluation is the detection of surgically correctable abnormalities of the urinary tract. Elderly subjects with urinary tract infection in whom evaluation should be considered include all men (see Significance of Bacteriuria above) and women who have bacteremia or pyelonephritis that does not respond well to antimicrobial therapy. In these groups urinary tract obstruction or intrarenal or perinephric abscess formation should be considered. Radiologic evaluation should consist of ultrasonography and/or an intravenous pyelogram.[57] Computed tomography (CT) is of particular value in the diagnosis of intrarenal or perinephric abscess.[58] It is not necessary to obtain radiologic evaluation in the vast majority of elderly women with urinary tract infection. However, after multiple episodes, radiologic evaluation may be indicated.

TREATMENT

Symptomatic urinary tract infection should always be treated. Elderly patients with acute pyelonephritis should usually be hospitalized to receive parenteral antimicrobial therapy, especially if bacteremia is suspected (high fever, shaking chills, hypotension). Empiric antimicrobial therapy will depend on microscopic examination of urine including a gram stain. When gram-positive cocci resembling streptococci are observed, parenteral ampicillin 6−12 g/day is usually the agent of choice. When gram-negative bacilli are seen and the infection is community acquired, appropriate initial therapy can be a parenteral first-generation cephalosporin (eg, cefazolin sodium 3−4 g/day) plus a parenteral aminoglycoside (eg, gentamicin sulfate 5 mg/kg/day), a parenteral aminoglycoside alone, a parenteral third-generation cephalosporin (eg, cefotaxime sodium 6−12 g/day), or parenteral trimethoprim-sulfamethoxazole (320−480 mg trimethoprim plus 1600−2400 mg sulfamethoxazole/day). All of these antimicrobial regimens will be adequate for the most common gram-negative bacilli seen in community-acquired infection.

For hospital- or nursing home−acquired acute pyelonephritis due to gram-negative bacilli, empiric antimicrobial therapy should be with cefpatazidine 3−6 g/day or a parenteral antipseudomonas penicillin (eg, piperacillin sodium 12−18 g/day) with or without a parenteral aminoglycoside to cover most gram-negative bacilli including *P aeruginosa*. Elderly subjects have fewer vestibular and cochlear end organ sensory hair cells and nephrons than younger subjects, and therefore aminoglycosides with their potential for ototoxicity and nephrotoxicity should be used with caution. Doses of antimicrobial agents (especially aminoglycosides and trimethoprim-sulfamethoxazole) must be adjusted to compensate for the diminished renal function and therefore slower excretion of these drugs in the elderly.

Once the infecting organism has been identified by urine culture and the antimicrobial susceptibilities are known, therapy can be altered to the most innocuous, least expensive antimicrobial agent to which the infecting organism is sensitive. In general the penicillins and cephalosporins are the agents least likely to result in serious adverse reactions in the elderly. Oral therapy can be substituted for parenteral therapy once a good clinical response has occurred. Therapy should be continued to a total of 14 days.

Acute pyelonephritis complicated by urinary tract obstruction will usually require bladder catheterization in men with obstruction due to prostatic enlargement. Pyelonephritis behind a ureter obstructed by a calculus requires a percutaneous nephrostomy in either sex followed by removal of the stone. Perinephric abscesses usually require percutaneous[58] or open surgical drainage. Intrarenal abscesses can usually be successfully treated with about 4 weeks of appropriate antimicrobial therapy,[59,60] with percutaneous or surgical drainage only occasionally being necessary.

In the past, seven to 14 days of two to four doses per day of oral antimicrobial therapy was routinely recommended for patients with symptomatic lower urinary tract infection. Many different antimicrobial agents have been successfully used including sulfisoxazole, ampicillin, amoxicillin, cephalexin, cephradine, naladixic acid, nitrofurantoin, trimethoprim, and trimethoprim-sulfamethoxazole.[61]

There is now substantial evidence that several days of oral antimicrobial therapy or even a single oral dose of certain agents gives results comparable to the conventional seven- to 14-day course of therapy in women (but not men) with lower urinary tract infection (negative ACB test).[62,63] Single oral dose therapy has been successful with amoxicillin (3 g), trimethoprim (400 mg), trimethoprim-sulfamethoxazole (320 mg and 1600 mg), and various sulfonamides.[63,64] The advantages of single-oral dose antimicrobial therapy include a high compliance rate, low cost, and fewer adverse reactions to the antimicrobial agents. In the absence of an ACB test of urine (which has not become a major clinical tool), women with symptoms of lower urinary tract infection can be treated with single-oral dose therapy and if relapse of symptoms occurs (indicating probable upper urinary tract infection), antimicrobial therapy should then be administered for 14 days. An alternative to single-oral dose therapy is three days of conventional oral therapy[65,66] (eg, amoxicillin 500 mg every eight hours or trimethoprim-sulfamethoxazole 160 mg/800 mg every 12 hours).

Eradication of urinary tract infections, including asymptomatic bacteriuria, among the elderly is usually no more difficult than among younger patients. However, reinfection rates are high.[9,37] In one study, elderly hospitalized patients (mainly women) with urinary tract infections were treated with conventional courses of antimicrobial therapy and the urine was sterilized in all.[9] However, reinfection was noted in 43% of these patients within 1 year. Another study reported the results of single-dose antimicrobial therapy in a group of uncatheterized, hospitalized elderly men with asymptomatic bacteriuria.[37] Persistence or relapse of bacteriuria occurred in 67% of the treatment courses, with reinfection following another 30% of the treatment courses within 18 months.

At present, many authorities believe that asymptomatic bacteriuria in the elderly is a benign disease in the absence of obstructive uropathy and should not be treated, especially considering the high reinfection rate and the high adverse reaction rate to antimicrobial agents in this population. Furthermore, the cost of screening elderly subjects repeatedly for asymptomatic bacteriuria and treating those infected would be difficult to justify with the current state of knowledge.

The most likely reasons for patients to relapse after appropriate antimicrobial therapy for urinary tract infections are (1) renal involvement, (2) a structural abnormality of the urinary tract, or (3) chronic bacterial prostatitis. Relapses may require a longer duration of antimicrobial therapy. One study has demonstrated that a 6-week course of therapy resulted in a higher cure rate than a 2-week course in patients who relapsed after 2 weeks of therapy.[67] If relapse occurs after a 6-week course of antimicrobial therapy, courses lasting 6 months or even longer may be considered. In the elderly long courses of antimicrobial therapy should not be used for relapses unless symptoms are present. Long-term suppressive therapy with low doses of antimicrobial agents (eg, amoxicillin 250 mg every 12 hours or trimethoprim-sulfamethoxazole 80 mg and 400 mg every 24 hours) may be indicated in patients who cannot be cured and who promptly relapse with symptoms when therapy is discontinued.

Patients with reinfection of the urinary tract following cure of an infection can generally be divided into two groups: (1) those who have relatively infrequent reinfections (eg, several reinfections a year) and (2) those who develop frequent reinfections (eg, patients who become reinfected shortly after each course of antimicrobial therapy). With infrequent reinfections, each new episode of symptomatic infection should be treated separately with antimicrobial agents. Asymptomatic infection should not be treated in the absence of obstructive uropathy. Occasionally elderly patients (particularly women) develop symptomatic reinfections so frequently that they can be incapacitated. In these patients long-term antimicrobial prophylaxis may be indicated to decrease the number of reinfections. However, long-term antimicrobial prophylaxis is not indicated for asymptomatic reinfections unless obstructive uropathy is present. Low-dose, once-daily trimethoprim-sulfamethoxazole (40 mg and 200 mg) or trimethoprim (100 mg) alone are particularly useful for long-term prophylaxis for frequent symptomatic reinfections.[68] Although nitrofurantoin in a once-daily dose of 100 mg is also effective,[68] the pulmonary and neurologic adverse reactions of this agent make its long-term use inappropriate.

CATHETER-ASSOCIATED URINARY TRACT INFECTION

The urinary tract is one of the most common sites of hospital- and nursing home—acquired infection and most of these infections occur in elderly patients who have undergone bladder catheterization.[38]
Intermittent straight catheteriyation is less likely to result in infection than an indwelling bladder catheter and should be used if possible when catheterization is necessary.[69] When a bladder catheter is to remain in place for long periods of time, infection is unavoidable. With open drainage systems, 50% of patients with sterile urine prior to catheterization develop significant bacteriuria within 24 hours and virtually all are infected within three or four days.[6] Antimicrobial bladder rinses (neomycin plus polymyxin) with an open drainage system using a triple-lumen catheter have been shown to delay bacteriuria for up to ten days in 50% of patients. Closed drainage systems are equally effective.[70] However, antimicrobial bladder rinses add little to the protective effect of

the closed drainage system.[71] We prefer the closed drainage system to the open drainage system plus antimicrobial bladder rinses because the former is less expensive, easier to maintain, and if infection occurs, the organism is less likely to be resistant to multiple antimicrobial agents.

One study using a closed drainage system showed that with systemic antimicrobial therapy the initial infecting organism could usually be eradicated even though the bladder catheter remained in place.[72] However, when the bladder catheter remained in place, subsequent reinfection was common, usually with organisms resistant to multiple antimicrobial agents. When bacteriuria occurs in the presence of an indwelling bladder catheter, antimicrobial therapy should be withheld unless fever, flank pain, or other symptoms or signs of urinary tract infection occur.

Long-term antimicrobial prophylaxis in patients with indwelling bladder catheters is contraindicated. Such an approach does not prevent the development of bacteriuria but rather predisposes to infection with organisms resistant to multiple antimicrobial agents. It also risks adverse reactions to the antimicrobial agent, which are more common in the elderly.[73]

SUMMARY

Bacteriuria in the elderly is common and usually asymptomatic. In the absence of symptoms and/or obstructive uropathy (which is rare in women), asymptomatic bacteriuria in the elderly appears to be a benign disease and therefore antimicrobial therapy is probably not warranted. When symptomatic lower urinary tract infection occurs, single—oral dose or short-course (three days) antimicrobial therapy appears to be indicated initially. Fourteen days of therapy is indicated in patients with upper urinary tract infection.[74]

REFERENCES

1. Monzon OT, Ory EM, Dobson HL, et al: A comparison of bacterial counts of the urine obtained by needle aspiration of the bladder, catheterization and midstream-voided methods. *N Engl J Med* 1958;259:764–767.
2. Bran JL, Levison ME, Kaye D: Entrance of bacteria into the female urinary bladder. *N Engl J Med* 1972;286:626–629.
3. Buckley RM, McGuckin M, MacGregor RR: Urine bacterial counts following sexual intercourse. *N Engl J Med* 1978;298:321–324.
4. Nicolle LE, Harding GKM, Preiksaitis J, et al: The association of urinary tract infection with sexual intercourse. *J Infect Dis* 1982;146:579–583.
5. Turck M, Goffe B, Petersdorf RG: The urethral catheter and urinary tract infection. *J Urol* 1962;88:834–837.
6. Kass EH: Asymptomatic infections of the urinary tract. *Trans Assoc Am Physicians* 1956;69:56–64.

7. Stamey TA, Timothy M, Millar M, et al: Recurrent urinary infections in adult women. The role of introital enterobacteria. *Calif Med* 1971;155:1 – 19.
8. Cluff LE, Reynolds RC, Page DL, et al: Staphylococcal bacteremia and altered host resistance. *Ann Intern Med* 1968;69:859 – 873.
9. Brocklehurst JC, Bee P, Jones D, et al: Bacteriuria in geriatric hospital patients, its correlates and management. *Age Ageing* 1977;6:240 – 245.
10. Svanborg-Eden C, Hagberg L, Hanson LA, et al: Adhesion of *Escherichia coli* in urinary tract infection. *Ciba Found Symp* 1981;80:161 – 187.
11. Sobel JD, Kaye D: Host factors in the pathogenesis of urinary tract infections. *Am J Med* 1984;76 (suppl 5A):122 – 130.
12. Stamey TA, Wehner N, Mihara G, et al: The immunologic basis of recurrent bacteriuria: role of cervicovaginal antibody in enterobacterial colonization of the introital mucosa. *Medicine* 1978;57:47 – 56.
13. Stamey TA, Timothy MM: Studies of introital colonization in women with recurrent urinary infections. I. The role of vaginal pH. *J Urol* 1975;114:261 – 270.
14. Kaye D: Antibacterial activity of human urine. *J Clin Invest* 1968;47:2374 – 2390.
15. Stamey TA, Fair WR, Timothy MM, et al: Antibacterial nature of prostatic fluid. *Nature* 1968;218:444 – 447.
16. Ascher AW, Sussman M, Weiser R: Bacterial growth in human urine, in O'Grady F, Brumfitt W (eds): *Urinary Tract Infection*. London, Oxford University, 1968, pp 3 – 13.
17. Cox CE, Hinman F Jr: Experiments with induced bacteriuria, vesical emptying and bacterial growth on the mechanism of bladder defense to infection. *J Urol* 1961;86:739 – 748.
18. Parsons CL, Greenspan C, Mulholland SG: The primary antibacterial defense mechanism of the bladder. *Invest Urol* 1975;13:72 – 76.
19. Sourander LB, Ruikka I, Gronroos M: Correlation between urinary tract infection, prolapse conditions and function of the bladder in aged female hospital patients. *Geront Clin* 1965;7:179 – 184.
20. Cobbs CG, Kaye D: Antibacterial mechanisms in the urinary bladder. *Yale J Biol Med* 1967;40:93 – 108.
21. Hanson LA, Fasth A, Jodal U, et al: Biology and pathology of urinary tract infection. *J Clin Pathol* 1981;34:695 – 700.
22. Rene P, Dinolfo M, Silverblatt FJ: Serum and urogenital antibody response to *Escherichia coli* pili in cystitis. *Infect Immun* 1982;38:542 – 547.
23. Kaye D: Urinary tract infections in the elderly. *Bull NY Acad Med* 1980;56:209 – 220.
24. Sobel JD, Kaye D: Urinary tract infections, in Mandell GL, Douglas RG Jr, Bennett JE (eds): *Principles and Practice of Infectious Diseases*. New York, John Wiley & Sons, Inc, 1985, pp 426 – 452.
25. Sourander LB: Urinary tract infection in the aged — an epidemiological study. *Ann Med Intern Fenn* 1966;55 (suppl 45):7 – 55.
26. Brocklehurst JC, Dillane JB, Griffiths L, et al: The prevalence and symptomatology of urinary infection in an aged population. *Geront Clin* 1968;10:242 – 253.
27. Akhtar AJ, Andrews GR, Caird FI, et al: Urinary tract infection in the elderly: a population study. *Age Ageing* 1972; 1:48 – 54.
28. Gladstone JL, Recco R: Host factors and infectious diseases in the elderly. *Med Clin North Am* 1976;60:1225 – 1240.
29. Lye M: Defining and treating urinary infections. *Geriatrics* 1978;33:71 – 77.

30. Boscia JA, Kobasa WD, Knight RA, et al: Epidemiology of bacteriuria in an elderly ambulatory population. *Am J Med* 1986;80:208–214.
31. Sourander LB, Kasanen A: A 5-year follow-up of bacteriuria in the aged. *Geront Clin* 1972;14:274–281.
32. Kasviki-Charvati P, Drolette-Kefakis B, Papanayiotou PC, et al: Turnover of bacteriuria in old age. *Age Ageing* 1982;11: 169–174.
33. Braude AI: Current concepts of pyelonephritis. *Medicine* 1973;52:257–264.
34. Winickoff RN, Wilner SI, Gall G, et al: Urine culture after treatment of uncomplicated cystitis in women. *South Med J* 1981;74:165–169.
35. Walkey FA, Judge TG, Thompson J, et al: Incidence of urinary infection in the elderly. *Scott Med J* 1967;12:411–414.
36. Wolfson SA, Kalmanson GM, Rubini ME, et al: Epidemiology of bacteriuria in a predominantly geriatric male population. *Am J Med Sci* 1965;250:168–173.
37. Nicolle LE, Bjornson J, Harding GKM, et al: Bacteriuria in elderly institutionalized men. *N Engl J Med* 1983;309:1420–1425.
38. Turck M, Stamm WE: Nosocomial infection of the urinary tract. *Am J Med* 1981;70:651–654.
39. Nordenstam GR, Brandberg C, Oden AS, et al: Bacteriuria and mortality in an elderly population. *N Engl J Med* 1986;314: 1152–1156.
40. Freedman LR, Phair JP, Seki M, et al: The epidemiology of urinary tract infections in Hiroshima. *Yale J Biol Med* 1963; 37:262–282.
41. Boscia JA, Kobasa WD, Abrutyn E, et al: Lack of association between bacteriuria and symptoms in the elderly. *Am J Med* 1986;81:979–982.
42. Gleckman R, Blagg N, Hibert D, et al: Acute pyelonephritis in the elderly. *South Med J* 1982;75:551–554.
43. Esposito AL, Gleckman RA, Cram S, et al: Community-acquired bacteremia in the elderly: analysis of one hundred consecutive episodes. *J Am Geriatr Soc* 1980;28:315–319.
44. Dontas AS, Papanayiotou P, Marketos S, et al: Bacteriuria in old age. *Lancet* 1966;2:305–306.
45. Marketos SG, Papanayiotou PC, Dontas AS: Bacteriuria and nonobstructive renovascular disease in old age. *J Gerontol* 1969;24:33–35.
46. Dontas AS, Kasviki-Charvati P, Papanayiotou PC, et al: Bacteriuria and survival in old age. *N Engl J Med* 1981;304:939–943.
47. Freedman LR: Natural history of urinary tract infection in adults. *Kidney Int* 1975;8(suppl):S96–S100.
48. Cobbs CG: Presumptive tests for urinary tract infection, in Kaye D (ed): *Urinary Tract Infection and Its Management.* St Louis, CV Mosby Co, 1972, pp 43–51.
49. Sanford JP, Favour CB, Mao FH, et al: Evaluation of the "positive" urine culture: an approach to positive differentiation of significant bacteria from contaminants. *Am J Med* 1956;20:88–93.
50. Stamey TA, Govan DE, Palmer JM: The localization and treatment of urinary tract infections: the role of bactericidal urine levels as opposed to serum levels. *Medicine* 1965;44:1–36.
51. Moore-Smith B: Bacteriuria in elderly women. *Lancet* 1972;2:827.
52. Stamm WE, Wagner KF, Amsel R, et al: Causes of the acute urethral syndrome in women. *N Engl J Med* 1980;303:409–415.
53. Stamm WE, Counts GW, Running KR, et al: Diagnosis of coliform infection in acutely dysuric women. *N Engl J Med* 1982;301:463–468.
54. Thomas V, Shelokov A, Forland M: Antibody-coated bac-teria in the urine and the site of urinary tract infection. *N Engl J Med* 1974;290:588–590.

55. Jones SR, Smith JW, Sanford JP: Localization of urinary tract infections by detection of antibody-coated bacteria in urine sediment. *N Engl J Med* 1974;290:591–593.
56. Thomas VL, Forland M: Antibody-coated bacteria in urinary tract infections. *Kidney Int* 1982;21:1–7.
57. Filly R: Ultrasonography, in Friedland GW, Filly R, Goris ML, et al (eds): *Uroradiology, An Integrated Approach.* New York, Churchill Livingstone, 1983, vol 1, pp 311–312.
58. Gerzof SG, Gale ME: Computed tomography and ultrasonography for diagnosis and treatment of renal and retroperitoneal abscesses. *Urol Clin North Am* 1982;9:185–193.
59. Schiff M Jr, Glickman M, Weiss RM, et al: Antibiotic treatment of renal carbuncle. *Ann Intern Med* 1977;87:305–308.
60. Hoverman IV, Gentry LO, Jones DW, et al: Intrarenal abscess — report of 14 cases. *Arch Intern Med* 1980;140:914–916.
61. Levison ME, Kaye D: Management of urinary tract infection, in Kaye D (ed): *Urinary Tract Infections and Its Management.* St Louis, CV Mosby Co, 1972, pp 188–226.
62. Kunin CM: Duration of treatment of urinary tract infections. *Am J Med* 1981;71:849–854.
63. Souney P, Polk BF: Single-dose antimicrobial therapy for urinary tract infections in women. *Rev Infect Dis* 1982;4:29–32.
64. Tolfoff-Rubin NE, Wilson ME, Zuromskis P, et al: Single-dose amoxicillin therapy of acute uncomplicated urinary tract infections in women. *Antimicrob Agents Chemother* 1984;25:626–629.
65. Charlton CAC, Crowther A, Davies JG, et al: Three-day and ten-day chemotherapy for urinary tract infections in general practice. *Br Med J* 1976;1:124–126.
66. Fair WR, Crane DB, Peterson LJ, et al: Three-day treatment of urinary tract infections. *J Urol* 1980;123:717–721.
67. Turck M, Ronald AR, Petersdorf RG: Relapse and reinfection in chronic bacteriuria. II. The correlation between site of infection and pattern of recurrence in chronic bacteriuria. *N Engl J Med* 1968;278:422–427.
68. Stamm WE, Counts GW, Wagner KF, et al: Antimicrobial prophylaxis of recurrent urinary tract infection. Double-blind placebo control trial. *Ann Intern Med* 1980;92:770–775.
69. Kunin CM: New developments in the diagnosis and treatment of urinary tract infections. *J Urol* 1975;113:585–594.
70. Grahm D, Norman DC, White ML, et al: Validity of urinary catheter specimens for diagnosis of urinary tract infection in the elderly. *Arch Intern Med* 1985;145:1858–1860.
71. Warren JH, Platt R, Thomas RJ, et al: Antibiotic irrigation and catheter-associated urinary tract infection. *N Engl J Med* 1978;299:570–573.
72. Butler HK, Kunin CM: Evaluation of specific antimicrobial therapy in patients while on closed catheter drainage. *J Urol* 1968;100:567–572.
73. Sanford JP: Hospital-acquired urinary tract infections. *Ann Intern Med* 1964;60:903–914.
74. Roberts JA: Urinary tract infections: In-depth review. *Am J Kidney Dis* 1984;4:103–117.

16
Prostatitis

William J. Holloway

Infections of the prostate gland usually occur in association with infection elsewhere in the lower genitourinary (GU) tract. The gonococcus was the most common cause of prostatitis prior to the availability of effective antibiotic therapy. This began as severe acute prostatitis followed by chronic recurrent infection. Now prostatic infection accompanies bladder infection and the common pathogens are the coliforms and enterococci which most often cause urinary infection.

The exact incidence of bacterial prostatitis is not known, probably because the clinical picture is variable and the diagnosis is difficult. Recent authoritative monographs have outlined the proper steps in the clinical and laboratory diagnosis of this disease.[1-3]

Infecting organisms can gain access to the prostate gland by several possible avenues. These include the ascending route by way of the urethra; reflux of urine from the posterior urethra into the prostate gland; direct extension from the rectum via lymphatics and bacterial seeding from the bloodstream. While any of these four mechanisms can be important in individual cases, it would appear that reflux of urine from the urethra into the prostate gland represents the most common route of infection. This hypothesis is strengthened by the fact that bacterial prostatitis is usually associated with bacterial urinary infection and by the recent observations that prostatic calculi often contain chemicals of urinary origin which are not found in the prostatic gland. This suggests that reflux of urine from the urethra into the prostate is much more common than once suspected.[3,4]

The data on age relationship to prostatic infections are confusing. Some authorities report an increase in infection in older men and a linear increase in incidence associated with age. Since bacterial infection of the urinary tract is more likely to occur in men with obstructive uropathy, acute and chronic bacterial prostatitis should be more common in men past the age of 60 years. However, this assumption is based on the finding of infection in prostatic tissue obtained by transurethral resection and at autopsy. This evidence could be misleading since infection acquired at an early age might still be detectable in later years when prostatic resection is more likely to be carried out. Since prostatitis is often a sexually transmitted disease, it should be common under the age of 50. In fact, the most common prostatic infection, nonbacterial prostatitis, occurs most often in men aged 30 to 45.[2-5]

CLINICAL FEATURES

Acute Bacterial Prostatitis

Acute bacterial prostatitis is a fulminant disease characterized by chills, fever, and other signs of systemic infection including, on occasion, septic shock. Urinary symptoms such as urgency, hesitancy, frequency, and dysuria can be present as well as severe pain in the perineal area or inner surface of the thighs. Rectal examination reveals an exquisitely tender, hard, swollen prostate gland and prostatic massage or frequent prostatic examination is not recommended because of the potential for producing bacteremia and worsening of the sepsis.

Acute bacterial prostatitis can occur as a complication of acute infection of the urinary tract or it can be a result of seeding from the hematogenous route. When this infection complicates infection elsewhere in the urinary tract, the coliform organisms are most often the pathogen. When the infection occurs by way of the hematogenous route, the most common pathogen is *Staphylococcus aureus* though a variety of organisms may be responsible. This type of infection usually occurs in critically ill compromised patients in a hospital setting.

Acute bacterial prostatitis also occurs in patients with indwelling bladder catheters, particularly in a situation where there have been frequent catheter changes or manipulation such as occurs in patients moved frequently for diagnostic procedures in the hospital. Any hospital patient with an indwelling catheter who develops unexplained sepsis should be examined immediately for the possibility of acute prostatitis.

The first step in the treatment of acute bacterial prostatitis is to assure adequate urinary drainage. Acute bacterial prostatitis is frequently associated with urethral obstruction, and bladder drainage by way of a suprapubic tube is frequently preferred to attempting to force an indwelling catheter through the prostatic portion of the urethra.[3]

If the offending organism is not identified from a current urine culture, empiric antibiotic therapy should be instituted immediately. An aminoglycoside combined with ampicillin would cover the gram-negative rods and enterococci, the most likely pathogens in greater than 95% of the patients. In patients with hospital-acquired urinary tract infection and prostatitis, a knowledge of the most common urinary pathogens in that institution might aid further in selecting specific antibiotic therapy. If *S aureus* is a possible pathogen, a penicillinase-resistant penicillin should be added to the therapeutic regimen. The identification of unusual causes of acute bacterial prostatitis such as *Haemophilus influenzae* and *Staphylococcus saprophyticus* would prompt refinements in antibiotic selection.[6,7]

The risk of acute bacterial prostatitis in the hospital patient can be reduced by appropriate catheter care, appropriate antibiotic therapy for urinary tract infection and the removal of indwelling bladder catheters as promptly as possible.

Chronic Bacterial Prostatitis

Chronic infection of the prostate gland is more common than acute infection and is almost always associated with chronic infection in the lower urinary tract. In fact, the diagnosis of chronic bacterial prostatitis should be suspected in patients who have recurrent lower urinary infection with the same infecting organism. Chronic bacterial prostatitis can also occur in association with chronic bacterial urethritis without bladder involvement but this is probably uncommon. Chronic bacterial prostatitis from hematogenous spread can occur due to *Mycobacterium tuberculosis, Cryptococcus neoformans*, or other indolent pathogens. In this situation, it is difficult to determine whether the organism reaches the prostate by the hematogenous route or by excretion in the urine and reflux into the prostatic ducts.

The clinical picture of chronic bacterial prostatitis is variable and never diagnostic. Since it is most often associated with recurrent lower urinary infection it is more common in older males who have some degree of prostatic obstruction. The most common symptoms of chronic bacterial prostatitis are those of the associated recurrent urinary infection with the customary urgency, hesitancy, frequency, and dysuria. Some patients may report perineal, lower abdominal, or thigh discomfort as well as systemic symptoms of infection. Rectal spasms have been associated with chronic infection of the prostate.

The diagnosis of chronic bacterial prostatitis is suspected when patients with lower urinary infection tend to have recurrences after adequate antibacterial therapy. The precise diagnosis is made by the demonstration of infection in the expressed prostatic secretion as well as the localization of bacteria to the prostate gland. Following prostatic massage, the prostatic secretion is examined microscopically under the high power field and the presence of 12 to 15 leukocytes or more in association with fat-laden macrophages suggests the presence of an inflammatory process. In bacterial prostatitis (in contradistinction to nonbacterial prostatitis) the leukocyte counts are quite high, more than 50 leukocytes per high power field.

The subsequent step in diagnosing bacterial prostatitis is localization of infection to the prostate using the technique described by Stamey.[2] Patients report with a full bladder and urine specimens are collected in the following manner; The initial voided urine is collected (VB1) and then a midstream specimen is obtained after 50 to 100 mL of urine has been passed (VB2). Then the prostate is massaged and the expressed prostatic secretion is collected in a sterile container. Following the prostatic massage, a third urine specimen is collected (VB3) and the three urine specimens and prostatic secretion are examined microscopically and by culture. Bacteria found in a larger quantity in the bladder urine following prostatic massage are thought to represent bacteria residing in the prostate gland. As a cost-saving procedure, the first and third voided specimens only are cultured and if the colony count is significantly higher in VB3, prostatic infection is confirmed. In questionable situations the expressed prostatic secretions should be cultured. A heavy growth of bacteria in the prostatic secretion confirms the diagnosis of chronic bacterial prostatitis.

The organisms most often implicated in chronic bacterial prostatitis are the Enterobacteriaceae and other gram-negative organisms including *Proteus* organisms and *Pseudomonas aeruginosa*. Enterococci are also frequently the cause of chronic bacterial infection, particularly in older males. Some controversy exists as to whether commensal, urethral organisms such as coagulase-negative staphylococci and corynebacteria can cause chronic bacterial prostatitis. While some reports suggest that these organisms can be pathogenic,[8] the consensus of opinion at the present time is that they are rarely, if ever, the cause of chronic infection.[3]

The bacteria isolated from the urine or prostatic secretions in patients with chronic bacterial prostatitis are antibody-coated so it is not surprising that increased levels of immunoglobulins and bacterial antibody have been detected in the blood and prostatic fluid of patients with prostatitis. Measuring antibody or immunoglobulins has been suggested as an ancillary means of making the diagnosis of chronic bacterial prostatitis in difficult cases.[9,10] However, these techniques are only available in research facilities so are of no value to the practicing physician.

One of the consistent findings in patients with chronic bacterial prostatitis is a decrease in the level of zinc in the prostatic fluid. Whether this is a cause or effect of the chronic infection is not clear at the present time. There is no decrease in the serum zinc levels in these patients and despite recent reports there is no scientific basis for oral zinc administration.[11]

The role of prostatic calculi in the pathogenesis of chronic bacterial prostatitis is not clear at present. A large percentage of older men are found to have prostatic calculi even though they cannot always be detected by x-ray or digital examination of the prostate gland. It has been suggested that prostatic calculi may be a nidus for the infecting organism preventing sterilization of the prostate by antibiotic agents.[12]

The history and physical examination of the patient with chronic bacterial prostatitis are usually unrewarding since there is no typical clinical picture and the prostate gland is most often normal.

The treatment of chronic bacterial prostatitis is limited to antibiotic therapy and, on rare occasions, transurethral resection of the prostate. There is no evidence that prostatic massage, increased or decreased sexual activity, or abstinence from certain foods or drink have any influence on the course of chronic infection of the prostate.

There is considerable confusion in the medical literature concerning antibacterial agents of choice in the treatment of chronic prostatitis. Some of this confusion arises from the fact that the human model does not lend itself to clinical investigation and the pH of prostatic secretion in dogs is significantly different from that in the infected human. The prostatic secretion in the patient with chronic bacterial prostatitis tends to be slightly alkaline while the prostatic secretion in the dog and in the noninfected young male tends to be slightly acid. The pH tends to increase with age so that the older male patient with chronic bacterial prostatitis tends to have a higher alkaline pH than the younger patient. The literature on antibiotic selection in patients with chronic bacterial prostatitis has emphasized three factors that are important in the antibiotic gaining access to the prostatic tissue in a form that retains significant antibacterial activity. The pH lipid solubility and serum protein binding are important. Another factor is the pH partition or ion trapping by prostatic secretions since antibiotics that are less highly ionized in the prostatic fluid are thought to be less active in the treatment of infections of the prostate gland. The degree of inflammation present in the prostate also is an important factor in antibiotic efficacy since a significant degree of inflammation tends to override all of the other factors and allow good concentration of most antibiotic agents in the prostate gland.[2,3,13,14]

While reports of the efficacy of antibacterial agents used in the treatment of prostatic infections vary greatly, it would appear that most, if not all, of the agents used in the treatment of recurrent urinary tract infection are also efficacious in the treatment of chronic bacterial prostatitis. Trimethoprim alone or in combination with sulfamethoxazole has been the most widely used agent in the treatment of chronic bacterial prostatitis with varying degrees of success. Most authorities suggest that this agent be used first and treatment continued for a period of 4 to 6 weeks in patients with chronic bacterial prostatis. At the end of therapy, repeat studies should be done to demonstrate a cure. If chronic infection persists, other agents can be tried or the patient can be placed on long-term suppressive therapy. Other oral agents that have been used successfully in the treatment of chronic bacterial prostatitis include the tetracyclines (particularly doxycycline and minocycline), the oral inandyl ester of carbenicillin, other penicillins, and the cephalosporins. Prolongation of the course of therapy is probably as important as the antibiotic selected.

In refractory cases of chronic bacterial prostatitis, particularly those associated with prostatic calculi, extensive transurethral resection of the prostate has been reported to be effective. Before undertaking such a radical step, the side effects of extensive transurethral resection should be weighed against the inconvenience of long-term therapy for suppression of symptoms of recurrent bacterial prostatitis.

Nonbacterial Prostatitis

The diagnosis of nonbacterial prostatitis is made when the expressed prostatic secretion shows an inflammatory response ($>12-15$ pus cells with fat-laden macrophages) in the absence of bacterial infection. The symptoms of this type of infection are similar to but less specific than those present in patients with chronic bacterial prostatitis; probably because patients with chronic nonbacterial prostatitis are less likely to have associated urinary tract infection. Nonbacterial prostatitis is most common in the age group 30 to 45 years, and since it is a sexually transmitted disease is less likely to occur in the older patients. Agents implicated as possible pathogens in nonbacterial prostatitis include trichomonads, anaerobic bacteria, fungi, and a variety of viruses as well as *Chlamydia trachomatis* and *Ureaplasma urealyticum*. The latter two organisms are now the prime suspects but the pathogenicity of these organisms has not been conclusively confirmed. Improved techniques for isolation of chlamydia and mycoplasma should make it possible to culture them from the expressed prostatic secretion or postprostatic massage bladder urine in the future. Until that time, it is appropriate to treat patients suspected of having nonbacterial prostatitis with a course of tetracycline since both of these microorganisms respond to therapy with that agent. If there is no clinical response, repeated courses of antibiotic therapy are not justified.[15,16] Suggested alternative therapy for nonbacterial prostatitis include the anti-inflammatory drugs, hot sitz baths, and prostatic massage. Controlled studies are not available to support any of these modalities of therapy and the efficacy of prostatic massage is frequently questioned.[1-3]

Prostatodynia

The term *prostatodynia* is used to describe a clinical syndrome with symptoms suggestive of prostatitis such as perineal discomfort and vague distress related to voiding. There is no history of recurrent urinary infection. Urine and prostatic expressate cultures are negative and the prostatic expressate does not show an inflammatory response. These patients frequently suffer from psychosexual dysfunction or problems with sexual identity. Fortunately, this problem is seldom seen in patients over the age of 50 years.

Prostatic Infections Associated with Genitourinary Surgery

A significant percentage of men over age 50 will undergo transurethral resection of the prostate. There is a typical infectious morbidity associated with this surgical procedure, most often manifested as urinary sepsis at times complicated by septic shock. Patients should be screened for bacteriuria prior to transurethral resection and those with positive cultures given appropriate antibiotic therapy before and during the operative procedure. Less clear-cut is what should be done with patients who have negative urine cultures prior to GU surgery. Is prophylaxis indicated in such patients? Reports in the literature indicate that a high percentage of patients undergoing transurethral resection have bacteria present in the prostatic chips obtained at the time of the surgical procedure. The problem is determining whether the presence of bacteria in these prostatic chips represent a threat to the patient undergoing transurethral resection. The evidence is inconclusive. In some reports the organisms present in the prostatic chips were never implicated in subsequent clinical infection while in other instances the reverse is true. Obviously, further studies are needed to assess the significance of organisms present in the prostate gland during transurethral resection. In the meantime, it would not be unreasonable to administer prophylactic antibiotic therapy preoperatively in patients undergoing transurethral resection of the prostate. Such therapy might not eradicate the organism from the prostate gland but would at least prevent the sequelae of bacteremia. An aminoglycoside in combination with ampicillin or a broad spectrum penicillin would seem to be the most appropriate antibiotic regimen for such prophylaxis. Cephalosporin antibiotics have been touted in this situation but their uniform lack of activity against the enterococcus, a common infecting organism in older men, make use of these agents inappropriate.[17-20]

REFERENCES

1. Meares EM: Prostatitis syndromes, in Remington JS, Swartz MN (eds): *Current Clinical Topics in Infectious Diseases.* New York, McGraw-Hill Book Co, 1980, pp 1–24.
2. Stamey TA: Prostatitis. *JR Soc Med* 1981;74:22–40.
3. Meares EM: Prostatitis syndromes: New perspectives about old woes. *J Urol* 1980;123:141–147.
4. Blacklock NJ: Prostatitis. *Practitioner* 1979;223:318–322.
5. Ireton RC, Berger RE: Prostatitis and epididymitis. *Urol Clin North Am* 1984;11:83–94.
6. Goetz MB, Craig WA: Haemophilus influenzae prostatitis. *JAMA* 1982;247:3118.
7. Carson CC, McGraw VD, Zwadyk P: Bacterial prostatitis caused by *Staphylococcus saprophyticus. Urology* 1982;19:576–578.
8. Drach GW: Prostatitis: Man's hidden infection. *Urol Clin North Am* 1975;2:499–520.
9. Wishnow KI, Wehner N, Stamey TA: The diagnostic value of the immunologic response in bacterial and nonbacterial prostatitis. *J Urol* 1982;127:689–694.
10. Madsen PO, Jensen KM, Iversen P: Chronic bacterial prostatitis: Theoretical and experimental considerations. *Urol Res* 1983;11:1–5.
11. Marmar J, Katz S, Praiss D, et al: A protocol for evaluation of prostatitis. *Urology* 1980;16:261–265.
12. Chronic bacterial prostatitis, editorial. *Lancet* 1983;1:393–397.
13. Ristuccia AM, Cunha BA: Current concepts in antimicrobial therapy of prostatitis. *Urology* 1982;20:338–345.
14. Barza M, Cuchural G: The penetration of antibiotics into the prostate in chronic bacterial prostatitis. *Eur J Clin Microbiol* 1984;3:503–505.
15. Weidner W, Schiefer AG: Re: Isolation of *Chlamydia trachomatis* from the prostatic cells in patients affected by nonacute abacterial prostatitis, letter. *J Urol* 1986;136:690.
16. Ridgway JL: Chlamydial infections in man. *Postgrad Med J* 1986;62:249–253.
17. Gibbons RP, Stark RA, Correa RJ, et al: The prophylactic use — or misuse — of antibiotics in transurethral prostatectomy. Chicago, American Urological Association, 1977, pp 381–383.
18. Morris MJ, Golovsky D, Guinness MD, et al: The value of prophylactic antibiotics in transurethral prostatic resection: a controlled trial, with observations on the origin of postoperative infection. *Br J Urol* 1976;48:479–484.
19. Nielsen OS, Maigaard S, Frimodt-Moller N, et al: Prophylactic antibiotics in transurethral prostatectomy. *J Urol* 1981;126:60–62.
20. Neu HC: Chemotherapy of infections, in Braunwald E, Isselbacher K, Petersdorf RG, et al (eds): *Harrison's Principles of Internal Medicine,* ed 11. New York, McGraw-Hill Book Co, 1987, pp 485–501.

17

Skin and Soft Tissue Infections

Leon G. Smith
John W. Sensakovic

The integument is not only the largest organ system in the human body, it is also the system most directly exposed to the chemical and mechanical effects of the environment. These "wear-and-tear" effects are compounded by the natural aging process, which at least partly involves decreases in turgor, elasticity, and resistance to infections. Combining these deleterious factors with other processes commonly seen in the elderly such as the small vessel disease of diabetes, or the presence of peripheral vascular disease, it is no wonder skin and soft tissue infections are so frequent in the elderly. Indeed, skin and soft tissue infections are exceedingly common in the elderly. Unfortunately, these infections are often not benign. The skin and soft tissue as a recognizable focus for sepsis in the elderly are the third most common site of infections, preceded only by urinary tract and respiratory tract infections.

In addition to their common occurrence in elderly patients, some skin and soft tissue infections are unique to the elderly, either by their distinct manifestations or by their occurrence. Thus the elderly patient may present with a toxic form of erysipelas, or a toxic necrotizing fasciitis, or a chronic *Pseudomonas* folliculitis, all rather unique to this patient population. Likewise, the all too frequent diabetic foot infection, or infected decubitus ulcer with recurrent sepsis are often monumental problems in the elderly.

Because of the frequency of skin and soft tissue infections, as well as their often unusual presentation in the elderly, and occasionally their severity, a thorough understanding of these entities is absolutely necessary in dealing with the medical problems of geriatric patients.[1]

STAPHYLOCCCOCAL AND STREPTOCOCCAL INFECTIONS

Typically, the primary skin infections are due to *Staphylococcus aureus* and group A streptococcus. The streptococcus can colonize all of the skin and its growth is enhanced by increased humidity during the summer months. Colonization is enhanced by contact with certain serotype strains, some of which are nephrogenic, especially in children. *Staphylococcus aureus* on the other hand colonizes the anterior nares in a very high percentage of hospital-associated and nursing home people. Such carrier rates not only put the carrier at risk, but also those with whom the carrier is in contact. Persons with small boils are at high risk of spreading staphylococcus via contact of hands all around them. These two organisms can be extremely lethal for the elderly for several reasons: Elderly people have more portals of entry from skin lesions like decubiti; traumatized skin in the elderly repairs itself more slowly; and older people tend to cluster together, such as in nursing homes and retirement villages. *Staphylococcus aureus* and streptococcal infections can manifest in many different ways, including both cellulitis, deep and superficial (erysipelas), ecthyma, toxic shock syndromes, bullous impetigo, pustules, folliculitis, abscesses, and gangrene.

Usually the *S aureus* is methicillin-sensitive, although methicillin-resistant organisms have occurred in nursing home outbreaks. The group A streptococcus remains penicillin-sensitive. Group B streptococcus, which affects primarily the diabetic, may require the addition of an aminoglycoside for eradication.

There is no absolute clinical way of differentiating *S aureus* from group A streptococcal lesions. Erysipelas is usually streptococcal, but not always, as *S aureus* has hyaluronidase as well. Toxic shock syndromes are usually due to *S aureus*, but a few strains of group A streptococcus are toxin-producing. Lymphangitis is more common with the streptococcus. Myositis is most often due to *S aureus*.

Erysipelas is a rapidly moving erythematous, raised lesion usually on the face or an edematous leg that can produce marked toxicity. The organisms are occasionally demonstrable at the moving edge of the lesion. Immediate anti–streptococcal and staphlyococcal therapy is needed. The response may be slow at first with resultant scaling of the skin developing later.

Ecthyma is often not appreciated and its deep scar looks like excoriations, Bazin's disease, fever acne, or foreign body reactions. After uncovering the lesion, swarms of *S aureus* are demonstratable. Long-term oral dicloxacillin is curative.

Toxic shock syndrome (TSS) in the elderly is associated with minor wounds and postoperative infections. A rapidly falling blood pressure, rapid pulse, generalized erythema, and toxicity characterize this entity. There is no pus associated with TSS, even though the organism can be found occasionally.

Scalded skin syndrome can also develop in the very old, with nearly a 100% mortality. The skin is completely denuded like a burn from the toxins of *S aureus*, usually phage type II. Often there is an underlying malignancy in these patients.

The major therapy for *S aureus* is still the methicillin family of penicillins, with nafcillin or oxacillin the safest of this group, giving less neutropenia, hepatitis, and renal problems. Oral dicloxacillin provides higher blood levels per gram than other oral members of this family. Vancomycin is the best alternate drug in penicillin-sensitive individuals, as well as those with methicillin-resistant *S aureus* infections. Such infections are being recognized with increasing frequency.

Tolerance of *S aureus* to penicillins has been described in the laboratory. In tolerant strains the minimal inhibitory concentrate (MIC) differs enormously from the maximum bactericidal concentration (MBC). Tolerance is of no significance in skin and soft tissue infection unless bacteremia is present. The group A streptococcus is sensitive to penicillin, and also responds to erythromycin, vancomycin, clindamycin, and first-generation cephalosporins. Immunologic complications such as nephritis are extremely rare in the elderly. Streptococcal purpura fulminans can occur if the infection is not treated rapidly.[1]

PSEUDOMONAS SKIN INFECTIONS

In the elderly, pseudomonas infections of the skin manifest themselves in various ways. They range from a simple chronic folliculitis to a fulminant cellulitis. With the increase in use of water therapy in the elderly, whether swimming for exercise or hot tub baths for therapy, the skin is subject to develop pruritic, pustular eruptions. Often, these lesions are erythematous macules, papules, and follicular pustules that are usually concentrated around the buttocks. The trunk, face, and neck are less common sites of involvement. In older women involvement of the areolar surfaces of the breasts is a unique manifestation of *Pseudomonas*. Patients remain afebrile. Earache and sore throat are common symptoms associated with negative objective findings. Regional lymphadenopathy is a rare consequence of this form of chronic folliculitis.

The pathogenesis of *Pseudomonas* folliculitis is quite distinctive from other bacteria in that *Pseudomonas aeruginosa* is a rare component of normal flora because of its sensitivity to dryness. *Pseudomonas* produces proteolytic enzymes that impart an alkaline pH to the skin. Acetic acid and other acid compresses neutralize this action and reduce the virulence of the *Pseudomonas* organism. On the other hand, occlusive dressings, incontinence of urine, contaminated pools, hot tubs, and whirlpools foster growth of these bacteria to as high a level as 10^8/sq cm. The severity of the illness and the rash correlates with the colony count. Only free chlorine inhibits the growth of *Pseudomonas*. The usual test kit for pools uses orthotoludine, which does not always reflect the free chlorine content. The US Department of Health suggests keeping the free chlorine at levels from 1.0 through 1.5 ppm with a pH of 7.2 through 7.8. The bacterial colony count for all water products is of less value, because it is usually not precise. Serotyping the *Pseudomonas* organisms is of epidemiologic importance, with types 0:11 and 0:9 predominating. Swimming pools are not as common a source of folliculitis as they are of otitis externa.

Other cutaneous *P aeruginosa* lesions are green nail syndrome, severe toe web infections, ecthyma gangrenosum, and blastomycosis-like pyoderma. One of the most virulent forms is found in diabetics. Diabetics can develop otitis externa with a swollen external auditory canal and swollen and macerated cartilage. Movement of the ear produces pain in varying degrees. If not treated vigorously, the lesion can extend to the brain and cranial nerves, producing death in 50% of the cases. This is called malignant otitis externa.

The green nail syndrome is a rare infection. The nail is nontender and contains a pyocyanin pigment of various shades of green. This colors the nail thumb plate. Usually, there is heavy use of water and detergent with the hands. Too often, the lesion can be mistaken for a malignant melanoma. Biting and poor manicuring of nails predispose to this syndrome. Topical anti-*Pseudomonas* therapy over a period from 1 to 4 months are usually corrective.

The toe web infection can develop in individuals who have poor hygiene or a poor vascular supply to the area. Wet feet are secondarily infected with pyocyanin-producing *Pseudomonas* bacteria. This entity was first described in military personnel in the swamplands. Associated dermatophytosis is also common in these circumstances. Topical and systemic therapy with anti-*Pseudomonas* drugs is often needed.

Ecthyma gangrenosum is a life-threatening complication of debilitated individuals, especially older patients with malnutrition. Diabetes mellitus, cancer, chemotherapy, acquired immunodeficiency syndrome (AIDS), and burns are also predisposing factors. The initial lesion is a benign-looking erythematous macule that progresses rapidly from a vesicular, pustular lesion to a black, gangrenous ulcer with a central eschar. The lesion is deep with *P aeruginosa* collected within the necrotic blood vessel walls. Early aggressive anti-*Pseudomonas*, systemic antibiotics are necessary.

Pseudomonas pyoderma is a superficial lesion, with a bluish discharge and grapelike odor. The border is eroded. The lesion develops after decubitus and ischemic ulcers of the leg. Hair transplants also face the rash of *Pseudomonas* pyoderma. Blastomycosis-like pyoderma (botryomycosis) is a rare *Pseudomonas* infection. It is characterized by verrucous plaques with overlying pustules. There is an elevated border similar to blastomycosis. It can be seen with some squamous cell carcinomas. Other organisms, such as *S aureus*, can also be present in the lesion.

Systemic therapy of *Pseudomonas* infections in general requires the combined use of an anti-*Pseudomonas* penicillin or new cephalosporin, along with an aminoglycoside.[1-3]

NECROTIZING FASCIITIS

Necrotizing fasciitis is the most often missed diagnosis of the skin and soft tissue diseases. The major reason for this is the lack of experience with this entity. Clinically, necrotizing fasciitis is characterized by acute pain at the site of involvement. The sites are primarily the leg, abdominal wall, and inguinal area. On examination the skin is surprisingly near normal in appearance with varying degrees of edema and redness. It is this lack of local skin changes and a negative aspiration of the area that can mislead the examining physician. Severe pain and toxicity out of proportion to the clinical findings is the hallmark of necrotizing fasciitis. It is at this stage that exploration with wide excision of the necrotic fascia must be done. The excision must be extensive beyond the normal adjacent areas, and the surgery should be designed to allow later plastic repair. Antibiotics alone will not affect the outcome. Local skin changes of tenseness with shiny and smooth texture progress to purplish discoloration and necrosis. Bullae develop on occasion. Lymphadenitis and lymphangiitis are very rare. Marked gangrene develops in the terminal stages.

Associated with the toxicity and toxic encephalopathy are consumption of platelets and fibrinogen and marked elevation of the white cells with toxic granulation. Dehydration and electrolyte abnormalities develop rapidly, similar to those seen in burns. Occasionally the calcium drops to produce carpopedal spasm and a positive Chvostek's sign. Toxic hepatitis with jaundice can develop along with shock lung and cardiovascular collapse. Gas in the tissue as an x-ray finding occurred in 19 (73%) of 26 cases in one series. The causative organisms can be found best at the center of the lesion. In older persons the flora is mixed with anaerobes and *Escherichia coli, Pseudomonas* sp, and streptococci are commonly present.

Except for narcotic addicts, diabetics, and posttrauma cases, the predisposing factors are rarely known. The differential diagnosis includes erysipelas, gas gangrene, both clostridial and nonclostridial, and Fournier's perineal gangrene. The mortality has been reduced only to 39% with aggressive early surgery — the key to success. Concomitant diabetes mellitus and atherosclerosis increase the mortality. Venous thrombosis is a common complication. Early nutritional support is helpful.

Fournier's disease may be an anaerobic variant of necrotizing fasciitis involving the scrotum. It is characterized by a profound foul odor associated with testicular and adjacent wall necrosis. *Bacteroides* organisms are associated with 50% of the cases. Once again early aggressive surgery is the key to survival, with antibiotics playing a lesser role. Antibiotic coverage must be that for anaerobic organisms such as *Bacteroides fragilis* as well as a drug effective against gram-negative bacilli.[4-7]

GAS GANGRENE

Gas gangrene can be classified by causation as clostridial or nonclostridial. Clostridial gas gangrene is less common in the aged than nonclostridial. The classic clostridial syndromes do develop with fever, toxicity, crepitation, rotten-apple odor, and progressive necrosis, which necessitates radical surgery and penicillin therapy. This type of gangrene generally follows a puncture wound and a closed anaerobic environment which enhances clostridial growth. *Clostridium perfringens* is the primary pathogen in this group and may have an incubation period of a few hours to many weeks. *Clostridium tetani* can coinfect the host on occasion.

Nonclostridial gangrene can be caused by numerous organisms, generally including *Klebsiella, Enterobacter, Proteus, E coli,* and anaerobes. The portal of entry is from an ischemic area, decubitus, or a skin ulcer. More often the condition is chronic and slowly progressive. Gas is demonstrable on soft tissue x-ray films. Diabetes mellitus is the most common underlying disease. Extensive surgery and antibiotics effective against the appropriate pathogen is the state-of-the-art treatment. Plastic repair of the area later may be necessary because of the extensive filleting procedures. Hyperbaric oxygen therapy has been disappointing. Many patients have an associated osteomyelitis. Long-term suppressive therapy makes sense since the relapse rate is very high because of the persistence of the ischemic baseline conditions.

A variant of nonclostridial gangrene is synergistic gangrene, which describes the relationship of the aerobic pathogen enhancing the anaerobic bacteria to exert its full potential as a pathogen. Synergistic gangrene can be quite virulent. The therapy is identical with other nonclostridial gangrenes with extensive surgery and sometimes amputation as the main ingredient. The foul odor is quite characteristic.[1]

FOOT INFECTIONS ASSOCIATED WITH DIABETES MELLITUS AND PERIPHERAL VASCULAR DISEASE

The frequent occurrence of diabetes mellitus and the often associated peripheral vascular disease in the elderly patient make foot infections an all too common geriatric problem. The factors leading directly to the development of foot infections in the elderly diabetic include peripheral sensory neuropathy; trauma, which is usually unnoticed due to the neuropathy; small vessel disease, which contributes to delayed healing of injured tissue; the often associated peripheral vascular disease; and the well-described leukocyte defects, which contribute to lowered resistance of tissue to infection. All of these factors contribute directly and significantly to the frequent occurrence of serious foot infections in the elderly diabetic patient. The management of such infections depends on prevention wherever possible, and prompt diagnosis and treatment should prevention fail.

Tissue breakdown occurs in the foot of the elderly diabetic mainly because of weight shifts on the neuropathic joints of the diabetic foot. These shifts place unusual pressure upon the plantar skin below the metatarsophalangeal joints, leading to necrosis and uloceration. The sensory neuropathy allows significant trauma and, all too often, advanced infection to go unnoticed.

Education of the elderly diabetic patient concerning awareness of foot care, along with frequent inspection, early treatment of minor trauma, proper nail care, and use of properly fitting or even molded shoes, can alleviate many of these problems. When infection does occur in the foot of the elderly diabetic, it must be recognized promptly and treated aggressively and appropriately.

Diabetic foot infections occur in two distinct forms, which differ in their causative bacterial agents, their clinical presentation, and their respective appropriate therapies. Diabetic foot infections can occur as a cellulitis due to gram-positive organisms such as *Staphylococcus aureus*, *Streptococcus pyogenes*, or group B streptococcus, or as the more characteristic synergistic gangrene with mixed anaerobes and gram-negative organisms. Cellulitis is recognized by the presence of notable erythema and edema, whereas synergistic gangrene is associated with pathognomonic tissue necrosis and a pungent, fetid odor. Proper anaerobic cultures in this infection will invariably reveal the presence of *Bacteroides* organisms in addition to facultative gram-negative rods.

The therapies appropriate for these two entities are as distinctly different as their respective presentations and causes. Cellulitis in the foot of an elderly diabetic is best treated with anti-gram-positive agents such as nafcillin or vancomycin, whereas synergistic gangrene requires an antibiotic regimen active against both anaerobes as well as facultative gram-negative organisms (clindamycin, gentamicin, metronidazole, extended spectrum cephalosporins). In addition, this type of infection requires frequent and meticulous local care and debridement, all of which, when done properly and patiently, can result in the cure of infections which may have initially looked unsalvageable. In those instances where significant peripheral vascular disease is amenable to bypass surgery, such surgical revascularization procedures can be critical for effective control and healing of infection.[8-11]

INFECTION OF DECUBITUS ULCERS

Infections of decubitus ulcers are frequent and serious causes of morbidity and mortality in the elderly. Because of the normal aging process, the lowered nutritional status, the decreased fat pads, and increased recumbency of this population, decubitus ulcers are very common. Because of the rapidity with which such ulcers become colonized and infected, progressive infection and resultant sepsis are also common. In fact, sepsis in a geriatric patient mandates an immediate search for pneumonia, urinary tract infection, or an infected decubitus ulcer.

There are three primary factors responsible for the development of decubitus ulcers: (1) external pressure, (2) ischemic necrosis, and (3) bacterial infection. External pressure is the primary factor leading to decubitus formation. Such pressure in the immobile or bedridden patient is greatest over the bony prominences of the sacrum, ischium, greater trochanter, and heel. These are the most common sites for development. The ill effects of this pressure in the elderly debilitated patient are complicated by the absence of subcutaneous fat pads, poor nutritional status, decreased skin temperature and blood flow in these areas, and abnormal sheer forces. These factors contribute to occlusion of blood flow to the skin, causing the associated ischemic necrosis. Because the skin is supplied with blood by so-called "candelabra" vessels perforating from the subcutaneous tissue, each supplying a significant overlying area, point pressure can lead to ischemic necrosis of a relatively large area of skin.

The necrotic tissue that develops is rapidly colonized by the multitude of organisms found on the lower trunk. Colonization rapidly results in infection with anaerobes as well as facultative gram-negative organisms (*Bacteroides, Ecoli, Proteus, Pseudomonas*), to levels greater than 10^5 organisims per gram of tissue. At these levels, healing is prevented, and the risk of subsequent sepsis is high. Progresion of the ulcer is now the rule, frequently to an extent leading to an underlying osteomyelitis. Once bony involvement occurs, persistence and progression of the lesions become more certain.

The treatment of decubitus ulcers is directed at preventing and reversing the causative factors. External pressure over bony prominences must be alleviated by proper positioning and frequent turning of the patient. Special apparatus may or may not be a useful adjunct. Sheepskins and egg crates are routinely used, but probably do little. Special mattresses, which distribute pressure evenly, such as water mattresses (Rolo Mattresses) can be extremely useful and are available at a moderate cost. Special self-cleaning "air beds" can be very effective, but such devices are extremely costly and tend to be greatly overused.

Nutrition is critical in the treatment of any bed sore. A positive nitrogen balance must be achieved, and if the serum albumin is less than 3.0 g, it is unlikely that any regimen will be successful. Vitamin and trace element supplementation, especially zinc, is mandatory.

Ischemic necrosis must be reversed by frequent and adequate debridement, both surgical and chemical. Removal of dead tissue is necessary to reduce bacterial growth and to promote good granulation tissue and healing.

Bacterial growth must be reduced. Healing will not occur with bacterial counts greater than 10^5 organisms per gram of tissue. Debridement is the first step in this process. Frequent cleansing is mandatory. Topical antimicrobial agents, such as iodine solutions (povidone-iodine) or silver sulfadiazine cream have a definite role, provided local irritation or an allergic reaction does not occur. The role of systemic antibiotics in reducing local growth is limited. They should be reserved for those instances in which significant cellulitis or abscess, osteomyelitis, or septicemia occur. When used, they must be directed at both anaerobic as well as facultative gram-negative bacteria. In the case of large, deep decubitus ulcers, once the bacterial growth has been reduced, surgical imposition of a myocutaneous flap can be dramatically helpful.[9-11]

VIRAL SKIN INFECTIONS

Just as the normal aging process of the skin and soft tissues make them susceptible to various bacterial skin infections, the elderly frequently suffer from various viral infections involving the skin. These viral infections, however, are related to the diminished cellular immune system in the elderly rather than to the aging processes in the skin itself. They are occasionally associated with secondary bacterial infection. The commonly seen viral infections in the geriatric patient include herpes zoster (shingles), herpes simplex, and papilloma virus (warts).

Herpes zoster is clearly an infection of the elderly, the peak incidence being between 50 and 70 years of age. The infection is caused by the spontaneous reactivation of a latent virus contained in the dorsal root ganglion of the patient from a prior infection which was manifest as chickenpox. Many precipitating factors have been suggested including stress, trauma, radiotherapy, immunosuppressive drugs, and underlying malignancy. None have truly been proved. Certainly a depressed cell-mediated immune system is involved, to some often unclear degree. In most instances this must be temporary, as in the majority of cases no underlying predisposing illness or condition becomes manifest.

Clinical shingles or herpes zoster often is heralded by a burning sensation in a dermatomal distribution of the skin several days before the development of viral skin lesions. Occasionally malaise, headache, and low-grade fever may occur. The viral lesions then appear as erythematous papules confined usually to a single dermatome. They progress through edematous, vesicular, pustular, erosive, and crusting stages. Rarely the lesions are hemorrhagic. Although on occasion, the lesions can involve more than one dermatome, and a few lesions may appear outside the typical distributions, more than ten to 12 lesions outside the area of involvement suggests dissemination. The thorax is the most frequently involved area, followed by the trigeminal, cervical, lumbar, and lumbosacral areas.

Although these infections are usually self-limited, serious problems can result from complications due to dissemination, secondary bacterial infection, ocular involvement, and prolonged severe pain due to postherpetic neuralgia.

The clinical presentation is usually characteristic. A Tzanck smear made from cells at the base of a vesicle shows characteristic multinucleated giant cells with intranuclear inclusions, diagnostic of *Herpes-virus* infection. The herpes zoster virus can be isolated from cell culture, though not as quickly or as easily as with herpes simplex.

The use of the antiviral drug acyclovir, by intravenous (and possibly also by oral) route can dramatically alter herpes zoster infections. Disseminated herpes zoster can respond dramatically to acyclovir therapy, and there are many experts who feel that such therapy is also effective in modifying the course of any severe attack. More importantly, some studies suggest acyclovir therapy may prevent the development of postherpetic neuralgia. Supportive care is also essential, including adequate analgesia and open wet dressings. Proper isolation techniques are important to prevent the spread of the virus to other individuals who have either never had chickenpox, or, more importantly, are immunocompromised and prone to develop disseminated infection if exposed.

Herpes simplex is not specifically a geriatric problem; it is common to all ages. It is important as a viral skin infection to be differentiated from herpes zoster. It is estimated that 20% to 30% of the population have recurrent herpes simplex. These lesions appear as grouped vesicles on an erythematous base. Although most frequently located around the mouth, lesions can appear anywhere on the skin or mucous membranes. Recurrent herpes simplex of the buttocks is not uncommon in elderly women. In contrast, herpes genitalis due to herpes type II is rarely seen in the elderly. Serious complications of herpes simplex infection include ocular infection, encephalitis, dissemination in immunocompromised patients, secondary bacterial infection, and the development of erythema multiforme. Tzanck smear preparations and virus culture are useful in the diagnosis of herpes infections.

Therapy of herpes simplex infection is generally symptomatic for local disease, with all of the commercial as well as antidotal therapies probably being equally (in)effective. Topical acyclovir probably adds no advantage beyond the initial infection.

For ocular infection, topical adenine arabinoside is very effective. Systemic acyclovir therapy is effective for disseminated infection, and encephalitis can be treated effectively with both systemic adenine arabinoside and, more recently, high-dose acyclovir.

Human warts are benign virus-induced tumors. Although warts are common to all ages, they do seem to resolve spontaneously at a less frequent rate in the elderly. This may be related to the aging immune system. Filiform and pedunculated warts of the face and neck, especially the eyelids, are especially common in the elderly. In addition to the cosmetic difficulty, the lesions are often important for differentiation from actinic keratosis and squamous cell carcinomas. Removal for biopsy is warranted in these situations. Generally, however, cryosurgery with liquid nitrogen or electrodesiccation are effective therapies.[1,12]

REFERENCES

1. Hirschmann JV: Localized infections and abscesses, in Braunwald E, Isselbacher K, Petersdorf RG, et al (eds): *Harrison's Principles of Internal Medicine*, ed 11. New York, McGraw-Hill Book Co, 1987, pp 478–484.
2. Meislin HW: Pathogen identification of abscesses and cellu-litis. *Ann Emerg Med* 1986;15:329–332.
3. Hook EW III, Hooton TM, Horton CA, et al: Microbiologic evaluation of cutaneous cellulitis in adults. *Arch Intern Med* 1986;146:295–297.
4. Miller JD: The importance of early diagnosis and surgical treatment of necrotizing fasciitis. *Surg Gynecol Obstet* 1983;157:197–200.
5. Findlay GH, Hazelhurst JA, Franz RC: Gangrenous erysipelas and necrotizing fasciitis. *S Afr Med J* 1982;62:125–131.
6. Majeski JA, Alexander JW: Early diagnosis, nutritional support, and immediate extensive debridement improve survival in necrotizing fasciitis. *Am J Surg* 1983;145:784–787.
7. Brenner BE, Vitullo M, Simon RR: Necrotizing fasciitis. *Ann Emerg Med* 1982;11:384–386.
8. Daltrey DC, Rhodes B, Chattwood JG: Investigation into the microbial flora of healing and non-healing decubitus ulcers. *J Clin Pathol* 1981;34:701–705.
9. Kucan JO, Robson MC, Heggers JP, et al: Comparison of silver sulfadiazine, povidone-iodine and physiologic saline in the treatment of chronic pressure ulcers. *J Am Geriatr Soc* 1981;29:232–235.
10. Miller BJ, Perron WR: Myocutaneous flaps: the Saskatoon experience. *Can J Surg* 1980;23:569–572.
11. Hurwitz DJ, Swartz WM, Mathes SJ: The gluteal thigh flap: a reliable, sensate flap for the closure of buttock and perineal wounds. *Plast Reconstr Surg* 1981;68:521–530.
12. Raimer SS, Pursley TV: Office management of viral skin infections in the elderly. *Geriatrics* 1981;36:53–63.

18

Bone and Joint Infections

Richard H. Parker

Infection of bone and/or joints in the elderly is a devastating disease even if it is not a component of a fatal septic process. Bone and joint infections often result in prolonged loss of activity and hospitalization. Elderly patients bedridden because of bone or joint infections are now susceptible to other problems associated with inactivity, for example, thromboembolic disease, aspiration pneumonia. Even with recovery the patient may not be able to resume full activity either because of generalized weakness or loss of an extremity. Vertebral osteomyelitis may lead to spinal cord injury and its sequelae. Promptness in recognition and institution of therapy can prevent or decrease in magnitude some consequences of the infection.

Both bone and joint infections occur when microorganisms infect those structures either hematogenously, by direct inoculation (puncture wound), or by contiguous spread of infection from a focus of infection. Each of these three pathologic processes has a different clinical pattern.

The clinical presentation of bone and joint infection in the elderly is generally less acute than a similar infection seen in the younger patient. The bones infected in the elderly are much more varied than what occurs in the young person. Part of this is due to the fact that the microorganisms in the elderly often seek out bones that are susceptible to infection because of degenerative changes, vascular insufficiency, neoplasms, or other disease. Infection of a prosthetic joint in the elderly patient frequently results in subacute or even chronic symptomatology and is caused by a much wider variety of bacteria than is seen in septic arthritis in the young adult.

OSTEOMYELITIS

Hematogenous Osteomyelitis

Hematogenous osteomyelitis is usually an acute infection of long bones of children. Rarely do the elderly have a similar illness. However, bacteremia in the elderly does occasionally cause vertebral osteomyelitis. Over 50% of reported cases of vertebral osteomyelitis are in patients who are more than 50 years old and at least 20% are in patients older than 60.[1] Hematogenous infection of other bones does occur in the elderly, but this usually occurs only in the setting of pre-existing disease in the bone. Persistent fever in a patient with bony metastasis may be related to hematogenous osteomyelitis complicating the areas of metastases.

The sources of bacteremia leading to osteomyelitis and their estimated incidence are listed in Table 18-1. A common clinical picture is the onset of back pain weeks or months after a genitourinary (GU) tract infection; however, it is more common that the preceding factor that caused the bacteremia is not identified. Classic vertebral osteomyelitis is an insidious and vague disease that defies recognition. Most patients (90% of cases) have back or neck pain, with or without fever (50%). Less frequently the patient presents with pain that directs attention away from the spine. A major reason that infection is often not considered is the long duration of symptoms prior to the patient being hospitalized. At least 50% of patients have symptoms for more than 3 months and only 20% have symptoms for less than 3 weeks.

The microbiology of vertebral osteomyelitis is listed in Table 18-2. In approximately one third of cases the etiology is not established microbiologically. Multiple specimens and improved microbiologic technology may increase the number of positive cultures. Nearly 60% of all vertebral osteomyelitis in which the bacterial etiology is determined is caused by aerobic gram-postitive cocci. Over 80% of the gram-postitive cocci are *Staphylococcus aureus*, often secondary to a soft tissue infection. The

Table 18-1
Sources of Bacteremia Associated with Pyogenic Vertebral Osteomyelitis

Source	Estimated Incidence (%)
Genitourinary tract infections and/or procedures	30
Soft tissue infection	15
Respiratory tract infection	10
Intravenous device and drug abuse	5
Diarrhea	2
Endocarditis	1
Unidentified	37

Table 18-2
Bacteriology of Pyogenic Vertebral Osteomyelitis

Microorganism	Frequency of Cases (%)
Aerobes	
Gram-positive cocci	
Staphylococcus aureus	35
Staphylococcus, coagulase-negative	2
Streptococcus, nonenterococcal	5
Enterococcus	< 1
Total	< 45
Gram-negative bacilli	
Escherichia coli	7
Klebsiella or *Enterobacter*	3
Proteus	5
Pseudomonas	4
Other	< 2
Total	< 20
Anaerobes	
Bacteroides fragilis	< 1
Others	2
Total	2
Unknown	33

From Sapico and Montgomerie.[1]

most common aerobic gram-negative bacilli are *Escherichia coli* and *Proteus* species, which often originate from an antecedent urinary tract infection.

The complications of vertebral osteomyelitis include paralysis, paravertebral abscess, epidural abscess, retropharyngeal abscess, endocarditis, and death from sepsis.[2]

Osteomyelitis secondary to a contiguous focus of infections includes both postoperative infections and spread of infection to bone from soft tissue infections unrelated to surgery (Table 18-3).

Table 18-3
Factors Associated with Osteomyelitis Secondary to Contiguous Spread of Infection

Postoperative Infections	Nonsurgically Related Infections
Open reduction of fractures	Ulcers secondary to vascular insufficiency
Implantation surgery	Soft tissue infections
Disk surgery	Infected pressure sores
Craniotomies	Infected sinuses
Resection of malignant tumors	Infected teeth
	Burns

Diabetic Foot Infections

In elderly patients, vascular insufficiency with diabetes mellitus leading to infected cutaneous ulcers is a common clinical problem. It is stated that more patient hospital days are spent caring for diabetic foot infections than for any other complication of diabetes.[3] In addition, mismanagement of this common problem can result in unnecessary or premature amputation. The combination of peripheral neuropathy and vascular insufficiency result in the diabetic having a propensity for developing foot ulcers. This interruption of the skin barrier is the portal of entry for microorganisms to infect the underlying tissues.

Clinically, the development of the infected foot ulcer is rarely associated with systemic manifestations of an infectious disease; however, the patient may note increasing hyperglycemia. Elderly diabetics with diminished visual acuity and peripheral neuropathy may only recognize odor and drainage as manifestation of local infection. Specifically, the patients often do not experience pain or tenderness and do not observe redness. Only if drainage from an ulcer is obstructed by an eschar is the patient likely to become febrile and appear clinically septic. Early recognition of the extent of underlying bone infection requires utilization of a bone scan. Bone scans are probably necessary in evaluation of all diabetic foot ulcers except those that are clearly small superficial lesions. The major mistake made by many physicians managing patients with infected diabetic foot ulcers is failure to appreciate the severity of the problem. The microbiology of diabetic foot ulcer infections has been compromised by the difficulty of easily obtaining specimens not contaminated by surface (skin) microorganisms.

Sapico et al[4] compared quantitative aerobic and anaerobic cultures of deep tissue from infected lower limbs of diabetic patients with cultures of ulcer swabs, curettage of the ulcer base, and needle aspiration. Their study confirmed previous observations that swabs of the ulcer base rarely identify the causative microorganism of deep infections. Curettage and needle aspiration show better concordance with deep tissue culture results, but still may disagree 50% of the time. There are about 10^7 bacterial isolates per gram of deep tissue usually, with anaerobes 10 times more prevalent than aerobes. No single microorganism predominates, but specific bacteria frequently isolated include the aerobes *Staphylococcus aureus, Streptococcus* sp, Enterobacteriaceae (particularly *Escherichia coli* and *Proteus* sp), and *Pseudomonas* sp plus the anaerobic *Bacteroides, Peptococcus, Peptostreptococcus,* and *Clostridium* organisms. It should be emphasized that prior antimicrobial therapy does not invalidate results of deep tissue culture results.[4]

Pressure Sores

Osteomyelitis may occur beneath one third of pressure sores. The clinical evaluation is difficult, but there is little that differentiates the patients with bone infection from those that do not have infection. Swab cultures of decubiti are useless. Radionuclide scans must be done, but even when positive there may not be osteomyelitis.[5] Bone biopsy with histologic and microbiologic evaluation must be done. The microbiology of pressure sores is varied and similar to what is found in diabetic foot ulcers.

Postsurgical Osteomyelitis

Although severe open (compound) fractures that are classified as type III are seen most frequently in young adults, postoperative osteomyelitis in the elderly patient secondary to open reduction of fractures is not uncommon. Also, other surgical procedures on or near bone may be complicated by osteomyelitis. With the increasing amount of open-heart surgery, sternal osteomyelitis is seen more frequently and is a difficult therapeutic problem. Overall, the incidence of osteomyelitis following open fractures has been reduced by the combination of surgical techniques and antimicrobial prophylaxis to about 5% of cases.[6] In severe (type III) open fractures, infections may occur in over 20% of patients. Postoperative infections are often evident early (< 1 month after surgery). However, some infections are not apparent for months. The indolence of the late postoperative infections is usually related to the limited pathogenicity of the infecting microorganism, a low inoculum of microorganisms, and/or suppressive efforts of any antimicrobial agents that may have been administered postoperatively.

Clinical recognition of postoperative osteomyelitis is difficult. Often there is no fever, little or no inflammatory reaction, and no wound drainage. Continual pain or pain after days without pain should make one concerned about an infection. A persistent "superficial infection" should raise suspicion of a more serious problem and consideration given to bone scans. Roentgenographic studies are usually only helpful in 50% to 75% of cases. The more chronic the problem the more likely roentgenograms are to be helpful.

The microbiology of open fracture infections has changed during the "antibiotic era." Gram-positive bacteria, particularly *S aureus,* used to be the most frequent pathogens, but in recent years gram-negative bacilli are involved in over 75% of infections (Table 18-4). The specific gram-negative bacilli isolated from these infections include *E coli, Klebsiella pneumoniae, Enterobacter* sp, *Serratia marcescens, Morganella morganii,* and *Pseudomonas aeruginosa.* Because of the resistance of many of these

Table 18-4
Microbiology of Open Fracture Infections, Influence of Antibiotic Prophylaxis

	Percent of Cases		
Isolate	No Antibiotic Prophylaxis	Penicillin + Streptomycin	First-Generation Cephalosporin
Staphylococcus aureus	4	3	0
Streptococci, ß-hemolytic	1	1	0
Enterobacteriaceae	4	0	<1
Clostridium sp	3	0	0
Mixed gram-positive	1	2	0
Mixed gram-negative	1	3	3
Mixed gram-positive and -negative	0	1	<1
Total infected	14	10	4

Modified from Patzakis.[6]

organisms to multiple antimicrobial agents, it is essential to obtain good culture specimens so that the appropriate studies can be done.

Infections Following Implantation Surgery

An increasing number of elderly patients are having total joint surgery. Estimates indicate that currently approximately 100,000 total hip arthroplasties are done each year with about 50,000 total knee arthroplasties.[7] The average age of patients is over 60 years old. Infection rates have ranged from 1% to 4% for the initial operation and from 6% to 32% for revisional surgery.

Although the infections are often referred to as a "prosthetic joint infection," it is important to realize that these are actually infections of bone and adjacent soft tissues. Therefore the diagnosis is established by demonstrating inflammation and microorganisms in the soft tissue and bone. Infections associated with prosthetic joints occur either early (during the first postoperative year) or late (more than 1 year after implantation). The most common symptom in both types is pain.[7] Less than 50% of patients have fever, swelling, or drainage (Table 18-5). Leukocytosis is usually not present and the ESR can be normal at the time of infection. Radiographic studies of the joint are abnormal in approximately two thirds of late infections, but only one third of early infections. The causative microorganism of early infection is often a gram-positive coccus. In recent years *Staphylococcus epidermidis* has become the most common pathogen in many centers. Late infections are also predominately caused by gram-positive cocci, but there are increased numbers of infections due to aerobic gram-negative bacilli. Late

Table 18-5
Presenting Symptoms of Patients with Infection Associated with Prosthetic Joints

	Percent of Patients		
Symptom	Early	Late	Total
Pain	90	100	95
Fever	47	39	43
Swelling	43	33	38
Drainage	40	24	32

From Inman et al.[7]

infections are usually secondary to bacteremia and the early infections are often considered to be due to intraoperative wound contamination.

Sternoclavicular Osteomyelitis

Osteomyelitis of the clavicle has been observed as a complication of Swan-Ganz catheterization, a procedure widely used in the care of elderly patients. Patients with this problem usually have fever with pain and erythema in the clavicular area anywhere from days to weeks after catheter insertion. Clavicular roentgenograms are usually normal and either radionuclide bone scans and/or computed tomography (CT) are necessary to identify the involved area. The usual pathogens are *S aureus* or *P aeruginosa*.[8]

Sternal osteomyelitis associated with sternotomy wound infections is an infrequent complication of cardiac surgery, but does result in significant morbidity and mortality.[9] Usually, sternal wound infections are easily recognized because there will be a classic manifestation of erythema, induration, pain, and purulent drainage. However some sternal wound infections are more subacute and present as prolonged wound drainage (>2 weeks), with the drainage often being watery and associated with minimal erythema and tenderness. The difference in clinical presentation has in part been explained by the characteristics of the causative microorganism.[10] Pyogenic bacteria (eg, *S aureus*) usually result in an acute problem whereas nonpyogenic microorganisms such as *Mycobacterium* sp produce a more indolent process.

Osteomyelitis Secondary to Direct Inoculation

Osteomyelitis secondary to direct inoculation is classically represented by infection of the calcaneous secondary to stepping on a nail. Although it could occur in an elderly patient it is rarely reported. The presentation may be a simple one of persistent pain and the diagnosis requires surgical exploration. The most common pathogen is *P aeruginosa*.

SEPTIC ARTHRITIS

An increasing number of patients with nongonococcal septic arthritis are over 60 years of age.[11] Since the 1940s the percentage of cases of septic arthritis in patients over age 60 more than doubled at one institution.[12] In the elderly septic arthritis occurs in patients with pre-existing joint disease in about 75% of cases and there is an associated infection in about 50% of cases. The associated infection may be septicemia, endocarditis, urinary tract infections, or a contiguous soft tissue infection.

The most frequent joints involved are knee, wrist, hip, and shoulder. Multiple joint infections have been observed. If alert, most patients complain of pain and usually swelling; erythema and warmth are noted except when the infection involves the hip, sacroiliac, or shoulder joint. Ten percent of patients may be afebrile. On admission the elderly patient with septic arthritis is usually not toxic, which is similar to what is observed in other adult patients, but strikingly different from the toxicity often seen in children with septic arthritis.

Microbiologically, 50% of cases are caused by *S aureus*. The remaining cases are caused by streptococci (20%) and gram-negative bacilli (30%), including *E coli*, *Klebsiella*, *Serratia*, and *Pseudomonas* spp. *Neisseria gonorrhoeae* is an infrequent cause of septic arthritis in elderly patients even though it is usually the most common cause of septic arthritis in young and middle-aged adults. *Haemophilus influenzae* is causing increasing infection in elderly adults and must be considered as a possible cause of septic arthritis in this age group, as it is in children.[12,13]

LABORATORY TESTS

Radiologic studies. Standard roentgenographic studies should be obtained in all cases of suspected bone and joint infection. However, negative studies do not rule out the presence of infection, particularly in cases where there is recent onset (<2 weeks) of symptomatology.

Bone scans. Three-phase bone scanning currently is the most sensitive and specific noninvasive technique for identifying early osteomyelitis. Focal arterial hyperemia combined with focal increased activity on blood pool and delayed (2- to 3-hour) scans indicates osteomyelitis. Scans showing only venous hyperemia suggest pathologic changes in soft tissue only. Prior antibiotic therapy and/or peripheral vascular disease do not adversely effect the usefulness of the three-phase scan in diagnosing osteomyelitis.

CT scans. Computed tomography has limited need in evaluation of bone and joint infections. It is of acknowledged value in the diagnosis of vertebral osteomyelitis. Here, as in selected other situations, it may be of value in evaluation of the articular surface of bone and periarticular soft tissues, definition of the extent of involvement, and identification of sequestra.[13]

Synovial fluid examination. Diagnosis of septic arthritis requires examination of synovial fluid. The findings in elderly patients are similar to those observed in younger patients with septic arthritis. It must be emphasized that although most patients have grossly purulent synovial fluid when first examined, over 5% of patients may have bacterial infection even though arthrocentesis reveals only "normal" or blood-tinged synovial fluid.

Microbiology. Determination of the cause of osteomyelitis requires cultures of deep tissue specimens obtained surgically or by needle biopsy and aspiration techniques. Anaerobic cultures must be obtained, particularly where there is a subacute to chronic clinical course. Swab culture of cutaneous lesions (diabetic foot ulcers or decubitus ulcers) should not be utilized to plan therapy of underlying osteomyelitis. Synovial fluid cultures must be obtained even if synovial fluid is not grossly purulent. Also, bloody synovial fluid should be cultured if the patient is febrile because a hemarthrosis does not rule out concomitant infection.

Erythrocyte sedimentation rate. This nonspecific test continues to be of value in identifying patients with possible bone infection and for monitoring therapeutic response. A normal ESR makes active bone infection very unlikely.

TREATMENT

Osteomyelitis

In adults with osteomyelitis the primary role of antimicrobial therapy is to control any sepsis, cellulitis, or other dissemination of bacteria. With the exception of vertebral osteomyelitis, antimicrobial therapy without appropriate surgical therapy infrequently, if ever, results in cure of osteomyelitis in the adult. This is in sharp contrast to the success of early antimicrobial therapy alone in curing acute hematogenous osteomyelitis in children. Because of the wide diversity of bacteria causing bone infection in adults the initial therapy must be "broad spectrum" and cultures must be obtained so that therapy can be quickly tailored to the drug(s) which offer the best efficacy, least toxicity, and least cost.

In addition to utilizing antimicrobial agents with the proper spectrum of activity, consideration must be directed to the ability of these drugs to achieve therapeutic concentration in bone. Numerous studies of the concentration of antimicrobial agents in both cortical and cancellous bone have been done. Unfortunately the variability of results has tended to cause confusion rather than clarification as to which are the superior drugs. This variability has been attributed to the effects of protein binding, tissue binding, metabolic alterations, technical problems, and differences in sampling times. However, it is now generally agreed that the serum concentration of an antimicrobial agent is actually the major determinant of the bone–interstitial space fluid concentration of drug. The actual bone concentration achieved is primarily dependent on capillary blood flow in bone; however, penetration of drug will in part be effected by molecular size, protein binding, fat solubility, and the partition coefficient. The latter four factors do not appear to have major clinical relevance. Since chronic osteomyelitis is often associated with a compromised vascular supply it is imperative to use high doses of antimicrobial agents and debride avascular tissue. The recommended drugs and doses for empiric and specific therapy are listed in Table 18-6.

Duration of therapy is poorly defined, but usually at least 4 weeks of antimicrobial therapy is needed and in selected cases therapy may continue for 3 to 6 months. Oral therapy is useful for prolonged, less costly treatment provided efforts are made to assure compliance.[14]

Vertebral osteomyelitis Antimicrobial therapy and bed rest are sufficient for successful therapy of vertebral osteomyelitis. Operative fusion of the spine is rarely necessary. The optimal choice of antimicrobial agent requires identification of the causative microorganism by either culture of bone aspirate or blood culture. If the patient has a well-defined primary infection, then the causative bacteria for this may be presumed to be the cause of the osteomyelitis (ie, a patient with *E coli* urinary tract infection is more likely to have *E coli* as the cause of the bone infection). Although useful the above should only be utilized in decision making when a tissue specimen cannot be obtained.

Initial antimicrobial therapy should utilize parenteral (intravenous) drugs. Empiric therapy before culture results should utilize an antimicrobial agent(s) which will be active against most *S aureus*, nonenterococcal streptococci, and aerobic gram-negative bacilli. Therapy should continue for at least 4 weeks. In order to reduce the cost of prolonged hospitalization outpatient therapy with either an oral drug or outpatient intravenous (IV) regimen should be used (Fig. 18-1).

Osteomyelitis secondary to contiguous infection Therapy of osteomyelitis secondary to diabetic foot ulcers and decubitus ulcers requires a combination of surgery and antimicrobial therapy. Even if deep cultures are obtained, which allows choice of specific drugs, antimicrobial therapy alone will not result in cures. In all cases debridement is essential and usually should be done within the first 24 hours of hospitalization. With osteomyelitis secondary to diabetic foot ulcers or associated with other causes of vascular insufficiency, cure is dependent on successful revascularization procedures and conservative amputations (Fig. 18-2). With osteomyelitis secondary to pressure sores, reconstructive surgery may be needed to protect the area from secondary infection.

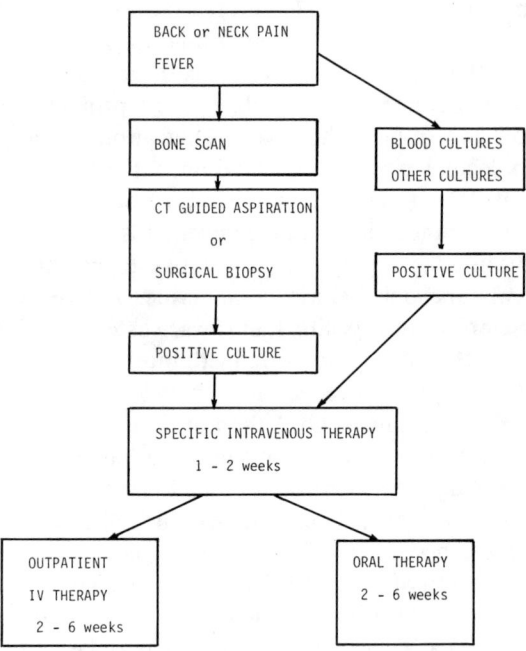

Figure 18-1 Management of patient with vertebral osteomyelitis.

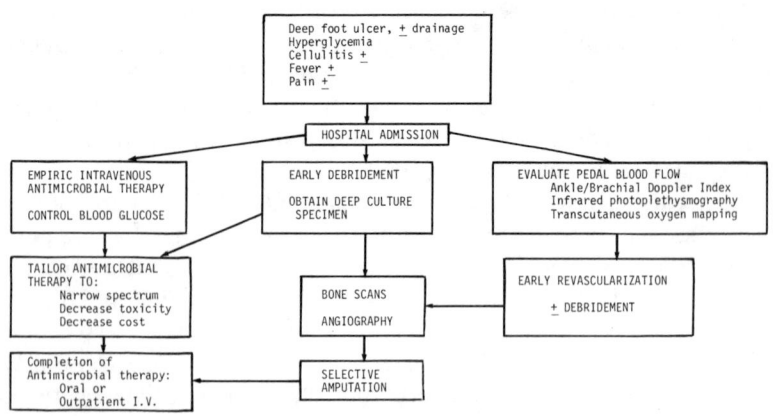

Figure 18-2 Management scheme for patient with osteomyelitis secondary to diabetic foot ulcer.

Table 18-6
Recommendations for Empiric Therapy of Osteomyelitis in Elderly Adults

Clinical Problem	Pathogens of Concern	Drug and Intravenous Dose*
Vertebral osteomyelitis		
Community-acquired		
No UTI	Staphylococcus aureus	Nafcillin sodium 2 g q6h
UTI	Escherichia coli Klebsiella Enterococci[†]	Cefazolin sodium 1 g q8h Ampicillin 2 g q6h plus gentamicin sulfate[‡] 1.0 mg/kg/q8h
Nosocomial		
No UTI	S aureus, MR, or S epidermidis	Vancomycin hydrochloride 0.5 g q12h
UTI	Enterobacteriaceae, betalactamase-positive[§]	Third-generation cephalosporin, eg, cefotaxime sodium 2 g q8h
	P. seudomonas aeruginosa	Ceftazidime 2 g q8h or ticarcillin 4 g q6h plus tobramycin, 1.0 mg/kg/8 h
Osteomyelitis secondary to contiguous infection		
Diabetic foot ulcer, first infection	S aureus E coli Anaerobes	Cefoxitin 2 g q6h or clindamycin 600 mg q8h plus tobramycin, 1.0 mg/kg/8h

Table 18-6 (con't)
Recommendations for Empiric Therapy of Osteomyelitis in Elderly Adults

Clinical Problem	Pathogens of Concern	Drug and Intravenous Dose*
Diabetic foot ulcer, prior therapy or nosocomial infection	S aureus Enterobacteriaceae, betalactamase-positive Bacteroides fragilis P aeruginosa plus above bacteria	Cefotaxime sodium 2 g q8h or ticarcillin plus clavulanic acid 3.1 g q6h Ceftazidime 2 g q8h or ticarcillin plus clavulanic acid
Decubitus ulcer	S aureus Enterobacteriaceae betalactamase-positive B fragilis	Cefotaxime 2 g q8h plus metronidazole 1 g q12h or ticarcillin plus clavulanic acid 3.1 g q4h
Post – open fracture or prosthetic joint	S aureus, MR S epidermidis Enterobacteriaceae betalactamase-positive P aeruginosa	Vancomycin hydrochloride 0.5 g q12h plus ceftazidime 2 g q8h

UTI = urinary tract infection or other known infection caused by gram-negative bacilli; MR = methicillin-resistant.
* Dosages are for elderly patients with serum creatinine < 1.5 mg/dL. Refer to chapter 15 for dosage adjustments for renal failure.
† Enterococci rarely cause vertebral osteomyelitis so empiric therapy is only justified if patient has had prior enterococcal UTI.
‡ Gentamicin must be used for empiric therapy of enterococcal infection because some enterococci are resistant to tobramycin.
§ Betalactamase-positive Enterobacteriaceae include E coli, Klebsiella, Enterobacter, Proteus, Providencia, Morganella and Serratia spp resistant to first-generation cephalosporins.

Empiric therapy with relatively high doses of parenteral antimicrobial agents must be initiated prior to the availability of the culture and susceptibility results. The following guidelines should be utilized to help select a specific regimen. The antimicrobial agent(s) should have good in vitro activity against *S aureus*, Enterobacteriaceae, and anaerobic bacteria. If patients have been hospitalized, are in a chronic care facility, or on antimicrobial therapy, then consideration has to be given to the risk of the infection being caused by methicillin-resistant *S aureus*, multidrug-resistant Enterobacteriaceae, and/or *Pseudomonas* sp. Specific examples of empiric therapy are included in Table 18-6. As soon as culture and susceptibility data are available, the empiric therapy should be tailored accordingly. Usually after 1 to 2 weeks, therapy can be continued out of the hospital with either oral regimens or outpatient IV therapy provided the causative bacteria are susceptible to drugs that can be administered by these routes.

Septic Arthritis

Therapy of septic arthritis requires antimicrobial therapy and drainage. Drainage may be accomplished by repeated arthrocentesis if the joint is accessible and the patient seen early (<4 days of symptoms) and provided that the synovial fluid is not already thick, viscous pus. Arthrocentesis to be effective must be repeated if fluid reaccumulates. If fluid continues to rapidly reaccumulate after three arthrocenteses or if arthrocentesis becomes technically difficult because of pain or viscosity of fluid, then it is best to establish surgical drainage. The reason for attempting drainage by repeated arthrocentesis is that if successful there is greater preservation of joint function and a decreased incidence of articular pain problem.[15]

At one time there was major concern regarding whether antimicrobial agents given systemically achieved therapeutic concentrations in synovial fluid. This has been resolved and provided sufficient dosage is given to obtain good serum levels, therapeutic levels of drug in synovial fluid will be obtained.[16] This obviates the need for any instillation of antibiotic into the joint — a practice which can result in synovitis unless low concentrations of drug are utilized. Suggested initial (empiric) therapy regimens based on results of microscopic examination of gram-stained smears of synovial fluid are listed in Table 18-7.

Table 18-7
Recommendations for Empiric Therapy of Septic Arthritis in the Elderly Adult Based on Microscopic Examination of Synovial Fluid*

Finding on Gram-Stained Smear	Pathogens of Concern	Antimicrobial Therapy
Gram-positive cocci:		
Chains	β-Hemolytic streptococci (groups A, B, F, G) Streptococcus pneumoniae	Penicillin G IV 2.5 million units q6h
Clusters, community-acquired	Staphylococcus aureus	Nafcillin sodium 2 g q6h
Clusters, hospital-acquired	S aureus, methicillin-resistant Staphylococcus epidermidis	Vancomycin hydrochloride 0.5 g q12h
Gram-negative coccobacilli	Haemophilus influenzae	Third-generation cephalosporins,[†] low-dose (eg, cefotaxime sodium 1 g q12h) or trimethoprim-sulfamethoxazole[‡] 2 ampules q8h
Gram-negative bacilli	Enterobacteriaceae	Third-generation cephalosporins, high-dose[§] (eg, cefotaxime sodium 2 g q8h)
No microorganisms seen	H influenzae Neisseria gonorrhoeae Neisseria meningitidis Enterobacteriaceae	Third-generation cephalosporin, high-dose

* All recommendations for initiating therapy are considered "aggressive" in that the drug and dosage is chosen to provide activity against the probable most resistant pathogen. Culture results should provide information for tailoring therapy to less toxic and less costly drugs.
† Third generation cephalosporins in low concentration are active against ampicillin-susceptible and ampicillin-resistant H influenzae.
‡ Trimethoprim-sulfamethoxazole should not be used if fluid restriction is necessary.
§ Although high doses of third-generation cephalosporins are recommended this should rarely be over 6 g/day of any one of them unless a need for high drug levels has been established by in vitro susceptibility data. The choice of third-generation cephalosporin should be based on local antibiogram, dosing habits, toxicity, and cost.

REFERENCES

1. Sapico FL, Montgomerie JZ: Pyogenic vertebral osteomyelitis: Report of nine cases and review of the literature. *Rev Infect Dis* 1979;1:754–776.
2. McHenry MC, Alfidi RJ, Wilde AH, et al: Hematogenous osteomyelitis. A changing disease. *Cleve Clin Q* 1975;42:125–153.
3. Gibbons GW, Eliopoulos GM: Infection of the diabetic foot, in Kozak (ed): *Management of Diabetic Foot Problems.* Philadelphia, WB Saunders Co, 1984, pp 97–102.
4. Sapico FL, Canawati HN, Witte JL, et al: Quantitative aerobic and anaerobic bacteriology of infected diabetic feet. *J Clin Microbiol* 1980;12:413–420.
5. Sugarman B, Hawes S, Musher DM, et al: Osteomyelitis beneath pressure sores. *Arch Intern Med* 1983;143:683–688.
6. Patzakis MJ: The use of antibiotics in open fractures. *Surg Clin North Am* 1975;55:1439–1444.
7. Inman RD, Gallegos KV, Brause BD, et al: Clinical and microbiological features of prosthetic joint infection. *Am J Med* 1984;77:47–53.
8. Hunter D, Moran JF, Venezio FR: Osteomyelitis of the clavicle after Swan-Ganz catheterization. *Arch Intern Med* 1983;143:153–154.
9. deSilva MI, Rissing JP: Postoperative wound infections following cardiac surgery: significance of contaminated cases performed in the preceding 48 hours. *Infect Control* 1984;5:371–377.
10. Gurevich I: Infectious complications after open heart surgery. *Heart Lung* 1984;13:472–481.
11. McGuire NM, Kauff CA: Septic arthritis in the elderly. *J Am Geriatr Soc* 1985;33:170–174.
12. Gilliland BC, Petersdorf RG: Infectious arthritis, in Braunwald E, Isselbacher K, Petersdorf RG, et al (eds): *Harrison's Principles of Internal Medicine*, ed 11. New York, McGraw-Hill Book Co, 1987, pp 1462–1464.
13. Borenstein DG, Simon GL: *Hemophilus influenzae* septic arthritis in adults. A report of four cases and a review of the literature. *Medicine* 1986;65:191–201.
14. Wilson KH, Kauffman CA: Oral antibiotic therapy for osteomyelitis of the foot in diabetic patients. *South Med J* 1985; 78:223–224.
15. Norden CW, Bryant R, Palmer D, et al: Chronic osteomyelitis caused by *Staphylococcus aureus*: controlled clinical trial of nafcillin therapy and nafcillin-rifampin therapy. *South Med J* 1986;79:947–951.
16. Parker RH, Schmid FR: Antibacterial activity of synovial fluid during therapy of septic arthritis. *Arthritis Rheum* 1971;14:96–104.

SECTION III
SPECIAL PROBLEMS

19

Fever of Unknown Origin

Michael J. Strampfer
Burke A. Cunha

The patient presenting with a fever of unknown origin always represents a diagnostic challenge to the clinician. A fever of unknown origin occurring in an elderly individual is even more of a diagnostic challenge than in the younger adult. Temperature elevations in the elderly need to be interpreted with caution. Many individuals aged 60 years and older have "subnormal" temperatures (35.6° to 36.7°C). When such patients become febrile, their temperature elevations may reach unimpressive values by the usual criteria, and infectious process may not be appreciated in view of the patients "low-grade" fever.[1-5]

A temperature elevation for three or more weeks, for which the etiology has not been determined by simple tests and initial hospital evaluation, is defined as a fever of unknown origin (FUO). The causes of FUO have changed in the adult and elderly population over the years. Certain diseases associated with FUO in the adult, ie, trichinosis, adult juvenile rheumatoid arthritis (Still's disease), atrial myxomas, and SLE, are infrequent in the elderly population. Conversely, other diseases such as giant cell arteritis and extrapulmonary tuberculosis are seen almost exclusively in the elderly. Over the years, the diseases responsible for FUO have also changed in both the adult and elderly populations. Endocarditis and collagen vascular diseases were important causes in FUO in past decades. At the present time, subacute bacterial endocarditis and collagen vascular diseases are unusual causes of unexplained, prolonged fevers. Diagnostic modalities are available today that make the diagnosis of these entities relatively easy. Infectious causes of FUO, traditionally, have been the most frequent single disease category responsible for FUO. However, at the present time neoplastic diseases are a more frequent cause of FUO than infections (Table 19-1).[6-8]

Of the infectious etiologies responsible for FUO in the elderly, intra-abdominal/renal abscesses are the most common. The diagnosis of a perinephric or subdiaphragmatic abscess in the elderly may be a difficult undertaking. Patients usually give a history of antecedent urinary tract disease in the case of nephric/perinephric abscesses or previous abdominal surgery in the case of subdiaphragmatic abscesses. Elderly patients with peritonitis frequently have few if any localizing signs suggesting peritoneal irritation. Peritoneal signs and a rigid abdomen are unusual in the elderly and frequently only abdominal tenderness suggests the underlying septic process. Frequently the diagnosis of intra-abdominal abscess is not considered because of the low-grade fever or because the antecedent surgical procedure is forgotten in the history.[9-10] Subacute endocarditis continues to be the cause of FUO primarily in situations where the organisms are difficult to culture or cannot be cultured at all, ie, "culture negative endocarditis." The majority of patients with so-called culture negative endocarditis represent in reality endocarditis due to slow-growing fastidious organisms. The most common organisms responsible for apparent

Table 19-1
Causes of FUO in the Elderly

Etiology of FUO	Frequency
Infection	~35%
Abscesses	
Abdominal; hepatic; nephric-perinephric	
Subacute endocarditis	
Extrapulmonary tuberculosis	
Renal/genitourinary tuberculosis; miliary tuberculosis	
Miscellaneous/other	
Malignancy	~50%
Lymphomas	
Carcinomas	
Hypernephromas; pancreatic, colon, lung; metastatic carcinoma	
Preleukemias	
Rheumatic diseases	~5%
Giant cell arteritis	
Periarteritis	
Vasculitis	
Other	~5%
Drug fever	
Multiple, recurrent pulmonary emboli	
Undiagnosed	~5%

Adapted from Larson et al,[2] Gleckman et al,[3] Esposito and Gleckman,[4] and Weinstein and Fields.[5]

culture negative endocarditis before the cultures become positive are hemophilus species. *Haemophilus influenzae*, *H parainfluenzae*, *H aphrophilus*, and *H paraphrophilus* all have been associated with slow growth in artificial media mimicking true culture negative endocarditis. Elderly patients with chronic obstructive lung disease or residents of chronic care facilities frequently have endocarditis due to one of the hemophilus species.[6,11,12]

Tuberculosis remains a common cause of FUO in all age groups. Tuberculosis presenting as an FUO is almost always extrapulmonary tuberculosis or miliary tuberculosis. The chest film is frequently negative in such patients, which results in clinicians failing to consider the diagnosis. Tuberculosis meningitis, genitourinary tuberculosis, and intra-abdominal tuberculosis are the most common forms presenting as FUO in the elderly. Miliary tuberculosis may be particularly difficult to diagnose because the miliary calcifications associated with this disorder may take weeks to develop and may be too small for detection by the conventional chest film.[13-15] A variety of other infectious diseases have been associated with FUO in some series. Brucellosis, Q fever, sidocosis, typhoid fever, malaria, and dental abscesses have been difficult for many clinicians to diagnose. Of these, dental abscesses from poor dentition are by far the most frequent, and are easily overlooked in the diagnostic workup. Such patients usually have nonspecific symptoms such as headache, fatigue, or bad taste in their mouths without pain referrable to the jaws or teeth. If the diagnosis is considered, such patients usually have point tenderness over the affected area, and a presumptive diagnosis is easily made.[4,16]

Unfortunately, malignancy is the most frequent cause of FUO in the elderly population. This parallels the increasing incidences of the malignancies that occur with aging. However, most neoplasms are readily detectable and only relatively few present as obscure FUO. Hodgkin's and nonHodgkin's lymphomas are increasingly common in elderly patients and are a common cause of FUO. When presenting as unexplained fever, these tumors are nearly always found in the retroperitoneal area, and are thus difficult to detect. Such patients usually have vague constitutional complaints and may only complain of night sweats, fatigue, or pruritis. Organ dysfunction due to compression by a retroperitoneal lymphoma, ie, hydronephrosis secondary to ureteral compression, is distinctively unusual. Mediastatic carcinoma to the liver frequently is associated with obscure fevers. It should be remembered that the Kupffer cells of the liver are one of the few cells in the body capable of elaborating the endogenous pyrogen mediator of fever. Alkaline phosphatase levels in patients with mediastatic carcinoma to the liver are usually elevated, but may be entirely normal. Occasionally carcinomas of the colon, pancreas, or lung cause unexplained prolonged fevers and present as an FUO. Second only to lymphomas as a cause of FUO in the elderly are hypernephromas (renal cell carcinomas). Hypernephromas have classically been recognized as internist tumor because of their varied presentations due to their early and widespread metastases. The only clue to the presence of hypernephroma may be a low-grade fever with or without hemituria. In all patients presenting with otherwise unexplained pyrexia that is sustained over a period of weeks, and certainly in elderly persons, hypernephroma should be considered. Patients with acute leukemia are usually afebrile unless there is superimposed opportunistic infection causing the temperature elevation. For this reason leukemias are not usually considered in the differential diagnosis of a patient with longstanding low-grade fevers. However, patients presenting with "preleukemia" that eventually go on to develop acute myelogenous leukemia (AML) commonly present as FUOs. Many elderly patients have received chemotherapy or radiation therapy and these therapeutic modalities may eventuate in AML. Certain diseases such as chronic myelogenous leukemia may progress to a blast crisis and AML. Prior to their dramatic presentation during the blast crisis phase, all of these factors are increased possibilities for elderly patients presenting with FUO during the preleukemic period. Unfortunately most of the neoplastic causes of FUO are ultimately fatal disorders. Since the most frequent cause of FUO in the elderly are neoplasms, an elderly patient presenting with a prolonged fever of unexplained etiology commonly has an ultimately fatal illness.[12,17,18]

The rheumatic diseases are uncommon causes of FUO in the elderly with the exception of polymyalgia rheumatica/giant cell arteritis (GCA). Giant cell arteritis is a disease of aging and may be extremely difficult to diagnose. Patients usually complain of unimpressive symptoms such as headache or fatigue. Visual symptoms and temporal tenderness over the distribution of the temporal arteries is uncommon. Not infrequently GCA is a diagnosis made serendipitously from an unusual laboratory finding (unexplained increased alkaline phosphatase) or the unpredicted result of a biopsy specimen (bone marrow). Vasculitis due to a variety of causes affects all age groups. Periarteritis nodosa is a readily recognizable multisystem disease characterized by renal involvement, hypertension, multisystem involvement, and peripheral eosinophilia. Patients presenting with specific vasculitis may have high titers of IgM rheumatoid factors which may suggest the diagnosis. Together, the rheumatic diseases are a treatable but relatively rare cause of FUO.[3,4,8]

Recurrent pulmonary emboli may be difficult to diagnose in any age group, but are particularly clinically deceptive in the elderly. Increasing shortness of breath with or without unimpressive chest pain may be the only findings. Many elderly patients are inactive and are predisposed to phlebothrombosis and subsequent pulmonary emboli. Large pulmonary emboli are readily clinically recognizable by a variety of diagnostic techniques. However, recurrent pulmonary emboli are difficult to detect and their presence may only be suggested by unexplained elevations in fibrin split products. The clinician should be alert to this diagnosis in patients where the predisposing factors for the formation of pulmonary emboli are presented.[12]

Fever may be the sole manifestation of a hypersensitive response to a medication in a patient. Drug fevers are becoming increasingly appreciated as a cause of temperature elevation in hospitalized patients in both young adults and the elderly. The older patient is particularly likely to have a prolonged fever on the basis of drug reaction because the elderly person is usually on a variety of medications for one or more medical conditions. Polypharmacy increases the possibilities of an allergic reaction to one or more of the patient's medications. Virtually any medication may be sensitizing to certain individuals and only relatively few medications have been infrequently, if at all, associated with hypersensitivity reactions of the drug-fever variety. Nonantibiotic medications that are not usually associated with drug fever include digoxin, benadryl, steroids, and multivitamin preparations. Antibiotics not usually associated with drug fever are erythromycin, tetracycline, clindamycin, vancomycin, and chloramphenicol. With variable frequency, all other medications may be incriminated as the cause of drug fever in patients. Particularly treacherous are stool softeners containing sulfa moieties which may be unappreciated by the clinician as the drug responsible for the FUO presentation. Thiazides and sleep medications are other causes of drug fevers which are frequently overlooked when reviewing the patient's drug history. Great care is necessary in all patients with FUO to rule out a prolonged temperature elevation on the basis of drug hypersensitivity.[19-20] Lastly, after all causes have been considered and a thorough history taken, a small number of patients will remain undiagnosed. Not infrequently, patients who have received an initial workup and are released without a diagnosis will benefit from subsequent readmission. In many situations the passage of time permits the disease process to advance and become more readily recognizable. A lymphoma that is inapparent by gallium CT scan becomes large enough in time to be detected. Similarly, the preleukemic patient's condition eventually progresses so that the diagnosis is apparent. The diagnostic approach should take into account the relative frequencies of the different causes of FUO and should include a careful search for and evaluation of clues from the history, physical examination, and laboratory data.[1,5,8]

DIAGNOSTIC APPROACH

Historical Clues to FUO

A careful history, physical examination, and selected laboratory tests usually narrow diagnostic possibilities in the elderly patient with FUO. In most cases, there are findings in the history of physical examination that direct the course of diagnostic testing. As a general rule, the longer the patient has remained febrile without explanation, the more likely the process is neoplastic and not infectious. Repeated and prolonged observations, sometimes including readmission to the hospital and extensive retesting, will eventually reveal the cause of the most obscure, prolonged fevers.[2,12]

A history of mental confusion in the elderly patient with FUO may suggest a chronic meningitis (cryptococcal meningitis, tuberculosis, etc), metastatic carcinoma, brucellosis, Legionnaires' disease, or an encephalopathic presentation of acquired immune deficiency syndrome (AIDS). In the elderly patient, mental confusion may be unrelated to the febrile process and may represent cerebral hypoxia secondary to cardiopulmonary disease. Careful attention must be paid to eliminating the treatable infectious causes of mental confusion.[6,8]

The presence of headaches in combination with myalgias in the older individual strongly suggests the presence of GCA until proven otherwise. Alternately, dental abscesses are common in the elderly, and deserve careful consideration. Other unusual diseases may be associated with these historical clues, ie, the common zoonoses (psittacosis, Q fever, brucellosis, leptospirosis). Legionnaires' disease is recognized with increasing frequency in the elderly, and may infrequently present as an FUO. The combination of mental confusion and headache with unexplained diarrhea should suggest this diagnostic possibility.[1,7]

Myalgias alone are difficult to evaluate in the elderly because they are due to many causes. High on the list of diagnostic possibilities is the atypical presentation of rheumatoid arthritis; again, GCA commonly presents in this manner. Endocarditis may infrequently present with predominantly neuromuscular symptoms.[7,8]

Similarly, fatigue is difficult to evaluate because it is nonspecific. Neoplasms are the most frequent cause of fatigue as part of the presenting FUO complex in the elderly. Once again, GCA and dental abscess should be considered in all patients presenting with fatigue without localizing signs or symptoms. Occasionally, other diseases may present as an FUO, with fatigue as the prominent presenting syndrome (Table 19-2).

Jaw pain should immediately suggest the presence of an occult dental abscess or GCA. Back pain is characteristic of brucellosis, endocarditis, and if localized, suggests metastatic carcinoma. A chronic nonproductive cough associated with low-grade fever may suggest bronchogenic carcinoma or pulmonary fibrosis, as well as a variety of infectious diseases affecting the lung. The possibility of a drug fever should be considered in all patients with an undiagnosed prolonged febrile illness, if they are taking one or more medications on a chronic basis.[8,20]

Table 19-2
Historical Clues to Diagnosis of FUO

Mental Confusion —
  metastatic carcinoma, chronic cryptococcal meningitis/tuberculosis, brucellosis, typhoid fever, Legionnaires' disease, acquired immune deficiency syndrome, endocarditis
Myalgias —
  trichinosis, endocarditis, adult juvenile rheumatoid arthritis, toxoplasmosis, systemic lupus erythematosus, periarteritis nodosa, rheumatoid arthritis, giant cell arteritis
Sensitizing Medication —
  drug fever
Back Pain —
  brucellosis, endocarditis, metastatic carcinoma, tuberculosis
Jaw Pain —
  giant cell arteritis, dental abscess
Headache/Myalgias —
  giant cell arteritis, psittacosis, Q fever, brucellosis, leptospirosis, Legionnaires' disease, dental abscess
Nonproductive Cough —
  bronchogenic carcinoma, tuberculosis, Q fever, typhoid fever, Legionnaires' disease, pulmonary fibrosis
Fatigue —
  giant cell arteritis, carcinoma, lymphoma, dental abscess, anicteric hepatitis, cytomegalovirus, infectious mononucleosis, typhoid fever, systemic lupus erythematosus, rheumatoid arthritis, endocarditis

Physical Examination

Fever patterns are occasionally helpful in diagnosing FUOs. Low-grade continuous fevers are the most common, and suggest carcinoma, lymphoma, or GCA. Factitious fever is rarely, if ever, seen in the elderly but may be suggested by the unexpected finding of relative tachycardia. Relative bradycardia is a much more significant diagnostic finding than is relative tachycardia, and in the FUO patient, suggests typhoid fever, Legionnaires' disease, psittacosis, leptospirosis, or drug fever. Additionally, lymphomas may present as periodic fevers, with or without relative bradycardia. A double-quoditian fever is defined as two fever spikes within a 24-hour period not induced by antipyretic medications. A double-quotidian fever may be the clue to miliary tuberculosis or Still's disease. The reversal of the diurnal temperature rhythm with temperature spikes in the morning rather than the afternoon should suggest the possibility of periarteritis nodosa or extrapulmonary tuberculosis (Table 19-3).[1,8,15]

A physical examination should pay careful attention to the eyes, a mirror of systemic disease. Examination of the fundi may suggest endocarditis, systemic lupus erythematosus (SLE), or miliary tuberculosis. Dry eyes suggest rheumatoid arthritis as well as other diseases. A subtle conjunctival hemorrhage may be the only clue to endocarditis. Conjunctival hemorrhages are prominent in the early stages of trichinosis but may be absent by the time the disease presents as an FUO. Uveal tract

Table 19-3
Fever Patterns in FUO

Periodic fever — lymphoma Double quotidian fever — miliary tuberculosis, adult juvenile rheumatoid arthritis, psittacosis, Legionnaires' disease Reversal of diurnal rhythm — tuberculosis, periarteritis nodosa	Relative bradycardia — typhoid fever, Legionnaires' disease, psittacosis, leptospirosis, drug fever, lymphomas, 1°/2° CNS neoplasms, factitious fever Low-grade continuous fever — carcinoma, lymphoma, giant cell arteritis

involvement should suggest miliary tuberculosis, Still's disease, toxoplasmosis, regional enteritis, or SLE.[7,8]

The presence of splenomegaly and associated generalized localized adenopathy is frequently helpful in directing the diagnostic workup in the adult patient. Lymph node involvement suggests a variety of malignant diseases as well as tuberculosis, infectious mononucleosis, AIDS, galovirus, or toxoplasmosis. AIDS is being seen with increasing frequency in the elderly population. In the older patient, AIDS is usually acquired by blood transfusion or by contact with intimate secretions with a male/female partner. The diagnosis of Waldenström's macroglobulinemia may be suggested by fever and generalized adenopathy in association with multisystem involvement. Splenomegaly suggests the same sort of diseases causing generalized adenopathy, but particularly suggests endocarditis in the elderly FUO patient. Enlargement of the liver suggests lymphomatous involvement, metastatic carcinoma, or alcoholic liver disease. Careful auscultation of the heart is important in ruling out endocarditis. Atrial myxomas are common in younger patients, but are rarely, if ever, the cause of FUO in the elderly adult. Left upper quadrant pain suggests splenic abscess in the FUO patient. Splenic abscesses are usually associated with endocarditis, but are not uncommonly associated with typhoid fever or brucellosis. Spinal tenderness suggests vertebral osteometastatic carcinoma, brucellosis, or enterococcal endocarditis. Sternal tenderness may be the only finding in myeloproliferative diseases, or leukemias involving the sternal bone marrow. Temporal tenderness, although infrequently present, should suggest giant cell arteritis in an older individual. Costovertebral angle tenderness points immediately to a perinephric or intrarenal infectious disease process, which should be investigated. Arthritis may be the presenting feature of extrapulmonary tuberculosis, or may indicate a collagen-vascular disease. Epididymo-orchitis usually presents as an acute problem, but in the setting of an FUO in an older individual, the clinician should consider genitourinary tuberculosis or a lymphoma (Table 19-4).[1,4,12]

Table 19-4
Physical Clues to Diagnosis of FUO

Fundi —
  subacute bacterial endocarditis (Roth spots), systemic lupus erythematosus (cytoid bodies), miliary tuberculosis (choroid tubercules)
Dry Eyes —
  rheumatoid arthritis, systemic lupus erythematosus, periarteritis nodosa
Subconjunctival Hemorrhage —
  endocarditis, trichinosis
Uveal Tract Involvement —
  regional enteritis, adult juvenile rheumatoid arthritis, toxoplasmosis, systemic lupus erythematosus
Adenopathy —
  lymphoma, acquired immune deficiency syndrome, Waldenström's macroglobulinemia, carcinoma, tuberculosis, metastatic carcinoma, infectious mononucleosis, cytomegalovirus, toxoplasmosis
Sternal Tenderness —
  myeloproliferative diseases, metastatic carcinoma, brucellosis, leukemia
Heart Murmur —
  endocarditis, atrial myxoma
Hepatomegaly —
  lymphoma, metastatic carcinoma, alcoholic liver disease
Splenomegaly —
  leukemia, lymphoma, tuberculosis, brucellosis, endocarditis, cytomegalovirus, infectious mononucleosis, toxoplasmosis, systemic lupus erythematosus, rheumatoid arthritis, psittacosis
Temporal Tenderness —
  giant cell arteritis
Left Upper Quadrant Pain/Splenic Abscess —
  endocarditis, typhoid fever, brucellosis
Epididymo-orchitis —
  tuberculosis, lymphoma, brucellosis, leptospirosis, periarteritis nodosa, infectious mononucleosis
Spinal Tenderness —
  vertebral osteomyelitis, enterococcal endocarditis, brucellosis, metastatic carcinoma
Costovertebral Angle Tenderness —
  perinephric abscess, chronic pyelonephritis
Arthritis —
  tuberculosis, rheumatoid arthritis, systemic lupus erythematosus
Jaw Tenderness —
  dental abscess, giant cell arteritis (GCA)

Laboratory Tests

Routine laboratory tests, including the hemogram, erythrocyte sedimentation rate (ESR), urinalysis, and liver function tests frequently will suggest the site of organ involvement. Because many patients that are elderly are anemic, for a variety of reasons this finding alone is not helpful. Similarly, the total WBC count, unless it is very highly elevated or depressed, is not helpful in suggesting a specific cause. Leukopenia suggests miliary tuberculosis, lymphoma, preleukemia, or AIDS in the elderly individual with prolonged, unexplained fevers. Much more helpful than the total WBC count is the differential cell count. Monocytosis strongly suggests tuberculosis or neoplasm. Eosinophilia suggests lymphoma, carcinoma, periarteritis nodosa, or drug fever. Basophilia is infrequent but a fairly specific indicator of serious underlying disease, ie, a lymphoma or carcinoma. Lymphocytosis also suggests tuberculosis. Atypical lymphocytes are not frequently helpful in the elderly patient with FUO, but may point to an obscure, anicteric viral hepatitis.[7, 21]

The elevated ESR is most useful when elevations are greater than 100 mm/hr. A very elevated ESR in this range suggests GCA, hypernephroma, endocarditis, carcinoma, lymphoma, or drug fever in the elderly patient with FUO. Increased IgM rheumatoid factors suggest vasculitis, or chronic active liver disease. An increase in fibrinous blood products may suggest occult recurrent small pulmonary emboli.[1,22]

The most useful serum tests, unrelated to the hemogram, in the FUO workup are liver function tests and an elevated alkaline phosphatase suggests a bone or liver source. However, an isolated unexplained elevation of alkaline phosphatase may suggest miliary tuberculosis, lymphoma, subacute thyroiditis, GCA, hypernephroma, or periarteritis nodosa. Extrabiliary sepsis may also be responsible for isolated elevations of the

Table 19-5
Diagnostic Clues to FUO from Laboratory Findings

Monocytosis —
  cytomegalovirus, tuberculosis, brucellosis, endocarditis, lymphoma, carcinoma
Eosinophilia —
  trichinosis, lymphoma, carcinoma, drug fever, periarteritis nodosa
Leukopenia —
  miliary tuberculosis, brucellosis, systemic lupus erythematosus, lymphoma, leukemia, acquired immune deficiency syndrome
Basophilia —
  carcinoma, lymphoma
Sterile Pyuria —
  tuberculosis, brucellosis, leptospirosis
Atypical Lymphocytes —
  infectious mononucleosis, cytomegalovirus, toxoplasmosis, viral hepatitis
Increased Rheumatoid Factors —
  subacute bacterial endocarditis, chronic active hepatitis, rheumatoid arthritis, vasculitis
Increased Fibrin Split Products —
  recurrent pulmonary embolism
Lymphocytosis —
  tuberculosis, cytomegalovirus
Elevated Erythrocyte Sedimentation Rate —
  adult juvenile rheumatoid arthritis, giant cell arteritis, hypernephroma, endocarditis, drug fever, familial Mediterranean fever, carcinoma, lymphoma
Elevated Alkaline Phosphatase —
  metastatic carcinoma to bone, miliary tuberculosis, lymphoma, drug fever, mononucleosis, cytomegalovirus, adult juvenile rheumatoid arthritis, subacute thyroiditis, giant cell arteritis, cholangitis, infiltrative/alcoholic liver disease hypernephroma, periarteritis nodosa, extra-biliary sepsis
Elevated Serum Transaminases —
  infectious mononucleosis, cytomegalovirus, Q fever, psittacosis, leptospirosis, toxoplasmosis, brucellosis, Legionnaires' disease, drug fever

alkaline phosphatase. Serum transaminases suggest hepatocellular injury and are most frequently associated with Q fever, Legionnaires' disease or drug fever in the FUO setting (Table 19-5).[2,4,12]

DIAGNOSTIC PROCEDURES

A variety of noninvasive radiologic techniques are available to assist in the diagnostic workup of the FUO patient. Sonogram of the abdomen and pelvis may reveal occult abscesses or neoplasms. M-mode or 2-D echocardiograms of the heart are useful in visualizing vegetations or detecting myxomas. Gallium scanning may be useful in selected cases in detecting an occult neoplasm or infectious process. However, gallium scans have a high incidence of false negative/false positive results, making interpretation of findings difficult. Computed tomography and MRI scans have revolutionized the approach to the FUO patient suspected of having an intra-abdominal or pelvic source of fever. These techniques are particularly useful for detecting occult abscesses or retroperitoneal neoplasms. Chest films, skull films, barium examinations, or bone scans are rarely helpful in determining the source of fever in elderly patients.[23-27]

Invasive Diagnostic Procedures

In spite of noninvasive diagnostic methods, many patients will require an invasive diagnostic procedure. Lung biopsy may occasionally be helpful in confirming the presence of obscure lymphomas, or unusual infections associated with AIDS. However, liver biopsy or bone marrow biopsy are the two procedures most likely to provide the most useful diagnostic information. Liver biopsy would clearly be of use in confirming the presence of hepatoma, metastatic carcinoma, chronic active hepatitis, alcoholic liver disease, granulomatous hepatitis, cholangitis, brucellosis, toxoplasmosis, and most importantly, miliary tuberculosis. Biopsy of the bone marrow may reveal the preleukemic phase of AML, lymphoma or miliary tuberculosis. *Salmonella* or *Mycobacterium avium-intracellulare* in the bone should immediately suggest the possibility of AIDS in a patient with prolonged unexplained fevers.[28]

Only rarely has exploratory laparotomy been necessary with the combination of the newer noninvasive diagnostic procedures and liver and/or bone marrow biopsy. Exploratory laparotomy is most likely to provide diagnostic information if there are signs, symptoms, or laboratory tests pointing to an intra-abdominal explanation. Exploratory laparotomy for an FUO most frequently reveals an occult intra-abdominal abscess not visualized on sonogram or CT scan, lymphomas, periarteritis nodosa, or intestinal tuberculosis (Table 19-6). Temporal

Table 19-6
Clues to FUO Disclosed by Invasive Diagnostic Procedures

Liver Biopsy — hepatoma, metastatic carcinoma, chronic active hepatitis, alcoholic liver disease, miliary tuberculosis, granulomatous hepatitis, brucellosis, toxoplasmosis, cholangitis Lung Biopsy — acquired immune deficiency syndrome (eg, *P carinii* etc), lymphoma, metastatic carcinoma, bronchogenic carcinoma Temporal Artery Biopsy — giant cell arteritis	Bone Marrow Biopsy — lymphoma, leukemia (preleukemia, AML), histoplasmosis, miliary tuberculosis, brucellosis, endocarditis, toxoplasmosis, acquired immune deficiency syndrome (eg, *M avium intracellulare*, Salmonella) Exploratory Laparotomy — lymphoma, polyarteritis nodosa, tuberculosis, intra-abdominal abscess

artery biopsy is mandatory in an elderly patient with prolonged unexplained fevers with symptoms suggesting GCA. Since the arteritis is segmental, multiple sections should be obtained. Although not invasive in the usual sense, AFB smears of gastric washings are second only to liver or bone marrow biopsy in diagnosing miliary tuberculosis without pulmonary findings.[4,8,28,29]

SUMMARY

The great majority of patients presenting with perplexing pyrexia of undetermined origin will be found to have an ultimately fatal neoplastic disease. The diagnostic workup should be directed accordingly. Careful attention should be paid to the second most common cause of obscure fevers, infectious disease processes. A diligent search should be made for an infectious explanation, because these diseases are usually treatable. In the elderly patient, the clinician must be ever wary of the atypical presentations of GCA, vasculitis, miliary tuberculosis and dental abscesses. Intra-abdominal abscesses and retroperitoneal lymphomas may be particularly difficult to diagnose in the older individual. The diagnostic workup should be directed by clues obtained from the history, physical examination, and initial laboratory studies. If noninvasive visualizing techniques fail to suggest the source of the fever, then liver biopsy or bone marrow biopsy will usually make the diagnosis. Exploratory laparotomy is rarely required because of the accuracy of today's noninvasive radiologic techniques.[4,12,28]

REFERENCES

1. Cunha BA: Fever of unknown origin in the elderly. *Geriatrics* 1982;37:30-44.
2. Larson EB, Featherstone HJ, Petersdorf RG: Fever of undetermined origin: Diagnosis and follow-up of 105 cases, 1970-1980. *Medicine* 1982;61:269-292.
3. Gleckman R, Crowley M, Esposito A: Fever of unknown origin: a view from the community hospital. *Am J Med Sci* 1977;274:21-25.
4. Esposito AL, Gleckman RA: Fever of unknown origin in the elderly. *J Am Geriatr Soc* 1978;26:498-505.
5. Weinstein L, Fields BN: Fever of obscure origin, in Weinstein L, Fields BN (eds): *Seminars in Infectious Disease*. New York, Stratton International Medical Book Corp, 1978, pp 1-33.
6. Mandell GL, Douglas RG Jr, Bennett JE (eds): *Principles and Practice of Infectious Diseases,* ed 2. New York, Stratton International
7. Reese RE, Douglas RG Jr (eds): *A Practical Approach to Infectious Diseases*, ed 2. Boston, Little Brown & Co, 1986.
8. Braunwald E, Isselbacher KJ, Petersdorf RG, et al (eds): *Harrison's Principles of Internal Medicine.* ed 11. New York, McGraw-Hill, 1986.
9. Altemeier WA, Culbertson WR, Fullen WD, Shook CD: Intra-abdominal abscesses. *Am J Surg* 1973;125:70-79.
10. Hoverman IV, Gentry LO, Jones DW, Guerriero WG: Intrarenal abscess: report of 14 cases. *Arch Intern Med* 1980;140:914-916.
11. Weinstein L: "Modern" infective endocarditis. *JAMA* 1975;233:260-263.
12. Molavi A, Weinstein L: Persistent perplexing pyrexia: some comments on etiology and diagnosis. *Med Clin North Am* 1970;54:379-397.
13. Christensen WI: Genitourinary tuberculosis. *Medicine* 1974; 53:377-390.
14. Barza M, Weinstein L: Uncommon presentations of pulmonary tuberculosis in adults. *Postgrad Med* 1972;51:143-148.
15. Bottiger LE, Nordenstam HH, Webster PO: Disseminated tuberculosis as a cause of fever of obscure origin. *Lancet* 1962;1:19-20.
16. Young EJ: Human brucellosis. *Rev Inf Dis* 1983;821-842.
17. Browder AA, Huff JW, Petersdorf RG: The significance of fever in neoplastic disease. *Ann Intern Med* 1961;55:932-942.
18. Weinstein EC, Geraci JE, Green LF: Hypernephroma presenting as fever of obscure origin. *Proc Mayo Clin* 1961;36:12-19.
19. Cluff LE, Johnson JE III: Drug fever. *Prog Allergy* 1964;8: 149-194.
20. Cunha BA: Drug fever. *Postgrad Med* 1986;80:123-129.
21. Horwitz CA, Henle W, Henle G, et al: Clinical and laboratory evaluation of elderly patients with heterophil-antibody positive infectious mononucleosis. *Am J Med* 1976;61:333-339.
22. Bottiger LE, Molin L: Fever and elevated erythrocyte sedimentation rate. *Acta Med Scand* 1964;176:639-648.
23. Tisdale WA, Klatskin G: The fever of Laennec's cirrhosis. *Yale J Biol Med* 1960;33:93-106.
24. Fisher HC, White MJ Jr: Biliary tract disease in the aged. *Arch Surg* 1951;63:536-544.
25. Simon HB, Wolff SM: Granulomatous hepatitis and prolonged fever of unknown origin: a study of 13 patients. *Medicine* 1973;52:1-21.
26. Fauci AS, Wolff SM: Granulomatous hepatitis. *Prog Liver Dis* 1976;5:609-621.
27. McNeil BJ, Sanders R, Alderson PO, et al: A prospective study of

computed tomography, ultrasound, and gallium imaging in patients with fever. *Radiology* 1981;139:647-653.
28. Cunha BA: Fever of unknown origin, in Samiy AH, Barondess J, Douglas RG (eds): *Diagnostic Internal Medicine*. Philadelphia, Lea & Febiger, 1986.
29. Geraci JE, Week LA, Nichols DR: Fever of obscure origin: The value of abdominal exploration in diagnosis. *JAMA* 1959;169:1306-1315.
30. Mitchel DP, Hanes TE, Hoyumpa AM, et al: Fever of unknown origin. *Arch Intern Med* 1977;137:1001-1004.

20

Infections in the Nursing Home Patient

Dennis H. Sullivan
Richard P. Wenzel

The term *nosocomial infection*, which is used primarily in reference to an infection that is contracted within a hospital, may also be applied to an infection that is acquired within a nursing home. Although little research has focused on infections in long-term care institutions, the available evidence suggests that, as in acute care hospitals, nosocomial infections represent a major problem in nursing homes.[1] The purpose of this chapter is to present the available information on infection rates, discuss the medical and social factors which predispose the elderly to infections, and highlight infections of the urinary tract.

Infection control activities, which have always been a major priority for nursing homes, are today assuming an even greater significance. The phenomenal growth of the population at the upper end of the age spectrum[2,3] is generating increased numbers of elderly who are in need of extended medical care, often at a level which at present cannot be provided in the community due to underdeveloped home care services. Concomitantly, because of the perceived need to control rapidly rising health care costs, measures are being devised to limit the use of costly acute care inpatient hospital services. Stricter admission criteria are being enforced, and a greater reliance on outpatient care is being encouraged. Financial incentives are also being developed to meet the goals of the federally mandated prospective payment system to encourage physicians to discharge patients from the hospital as soon as possible. The result is placing a greater emphasis on other resources outside the acute care hospital to provide an increasingly larger proportion of the convalescent, rehabilitative, and maintenance care needed by many of the elderly. Frequently, few alternatives are available to provide this type of care to debilitated geriatric patients, particularly those who do not have the family and financial resources to stay at home. Consequently, an increasing number of elderly patients are seeking admission to nursing homes, and many in the unique environment of long-term care facilities are at high risk of developing infectious complications because of their advanced age and debilitated condition.

THE SIGNIFICANCE OF NURSING HOMES IN THE HEALTH CARE SYSTEM

Nursing homes today represent an extremely important and rapidly expanding component of the health care system in the United States. Over the last 15 years the growth in the number of nursing home beds has been dramatic. This fact is especially apparent when compared with the change in the number of acute care hospital beds during the same period. Between 1969 and 1984, the number of nursing home beds increased from a total of 881,000 to over 1.4 million, whereas acute care hospitals experienced a decline in the number of beds to less than 1.3 million.[4]

The ratio of nursing home to acute care hospital beds is projected to increase. Hospital beds are being closed down, reflecting the plateau of hospital utilization reached in the 1980s. In contrast, the demand for nursing home beds continues to increase, paralleling the growth of the elderly population. The proportion of the population in the United States that is elderly is increasing steadily, with the most dramatic growth at the upper end of the age spectrum.[2,3,5] Persons over the age of 85 represent not only the fastest growing segment of society, but also the group at highest risk of nursing home placement.[6] By the turn of the century it is estimated that, unless alternatives are found, 3.5 million nursing home beds will be needed.[7]

The important position that nursing homes have attained in our society is emphasized by several impressive statistics. Although only 5% of the elderly are in nursing homes at any one time, 15% to 20% of those over the age of 85 years are institutionalized.[6] Even greater numbers of the elderly spend at least part of their lives in a nursing home. Individuals over the age of 55 have, prior to their deaths, a 39% probability of being admitted one or more times to a nursing home and a 14% probability of staying more than 6 months. Individuals who reach the age of 85 have a 68% chance of being admitted to a nursing home sometime in their remaining lives and a 30% chance that they will stay longer than 6 months.[8]

The average length of stay for nursing home residents is 19 months,[6] although a more meaningful statistic reflects the bimodal distribution of this population depending on length of stay. Short-stay residents, who make up 58% of admissions and have an average length of stay of 1.8

months, are much more likely to be admitted from an acute care hospital and eventually to return to the community. In contrast, the long-stay group, which constitutes 91% of the nursing home residents at any point in time, has an average length of stay of 2.5 years. Over 50% of the residents from both groups ultimately die without ever returning to the community.[9]

PREVALENCE OF NURSING HOME–ASSOCIATED INFECTIONS

Infection control problems in nursing homes, although only recently attracting the attention of the academic community, have been known for many years. In 1964, Lester published the results of an interesting study in which public health nurses surveyed 101 chronic care facilities in Mississippi and observed both the resident and the staff for evidence of infection.[10] Even though these facilities were not classified according to current definitions, the study was significant for demonstrating a high prevalence of infections. Of the 2147 patients and the 896 personnel examined, 14% of the former and 6% of the latter were found to be infected. The infections were present in 50% of the residents and 40% of the staff prior to their entering the nursing homes. In both groups, skin and subcutaneous tissues represented the most common sites infected.

The difficulty of obtaining reliable nosocomial infection prevalence data was highlighted by a study Cohen et al conducted in 1976.[11] In a one-day survey of 18 skilled nursing homes in Connecticut, the authors focused attention on only three potential sites of infection: the urinary tract, the skin or subcutaneous tissues, and the respiratory tract. The overall prevalence of nosocomial infections at the three sites was 2.7%. Urinary tract infections, including asymptomatic bacteriuria, were the most common of the three categories, being present in 1.2% of the residents. The prevalence rates, which were recognized to be relatively low compared with the findings of previous studies, possibly reflected the limitations of the groups' survey techniques. The mechanism of case finding consisted only of a review of each patient's nursing home chart and the laboratory results. There was no direct patient observation. Although the epidemiologic methods employed by Cohen et al are standard in acute care hospitals, they are probably inadequate for use in nursing homes because in these facilities neither the patient charts nor the laboratory data are reliable sources of evidence for infection.

A study by Garibaldi et al in 1981,[12] which consisted of a series of one-day surveys in seven skilled nursing homes, identified a 16% prevalence rate of infections among the total group of 532 residents. Casefinding techniques included reviewing the nursing home medical records, asssessing the need for antibiotics, interviewing staff nurses, and performing limited physical examinations on selected patients. Although the study did not attempt to differentiate between infections that were present prior to the patients' nursing home admissions from those that developed subsequently, it did highlight several important findings. The most frequent sites of infections were decubitus ulcers (33%), eye (conjunctivitis 19%), urinary tract (symptomatic infections 8%), and gastrointestinal (Gl) tract (diarrhea 7%). An apparent association between certain types of infections and specific underlying conditions was identified. Patients who were nonambulatory, fecally incontinent, or diabetic had higher rates of skin infections, whereas patients who were prescribed sedatives or tranquilizers had a slightly higher risk of developing lower respiratory tract infections. Clusters of infections, especially conjunctivitis, diarrhea, and respiratory tract infections, were frequently observed and accounted for over 20% of all infections identified. Of the 600 patients with indwelling bladder catheters, 85% had asymptomatic bacteriuria, and most had multiple resistant organisms, which were endemic in their particular home. Interestingly, there was no association between the prevalence of infection and the age of the patients.

Several infectious disease prevalence surveys have been done in chronic care facilities associated with Veterans Administration hospitals. Nicolle et al[13] at the University of Manitoba prospectively followed 68 elderly men who were permanently residing on two chronic care wards of a VA hospital. Infections were identified by an infection control nurse who conferred several times a week with the ward staff and reviewed patient charts, microbiology reports, and antimicrobial therapy records. During the 12-month study period, 37 infectious episodes were identified in 50 (74%) residents. Lower respiratory tract infections (35 cases in 26 patients), febrile episodes without an identified source (25 episodes in 18 patients), skin and soft tissue infections (21 episodes in 15 patients), and gastroenteritis (19 episodes in 15 patients) were the most frequent categories identified. Although asymptomatic bacteriuria was a frequent finding, symptomatic urinary tract infections occurred in only three patients. Of the 19 residents who died during the study, infections were the primary cause of death in seven (37%) and contributed to death in two other cases. The crude mortality rate from infections was 10.3/100 residents per year.

Lower respiratory tract infections represented the most frequent infectious cause of death. No conclusions could be drawn about the efficacy of preventive health measures since pneumococcal vaccine was not administered and influenza vaccine was given to fewer than half of the patients. Despite the availability of diagnostic facilities in the hospital, infecting organisms were only rarely identified by culture or gram stain. Residents with ischemic heart disease had the greatest likelihood of developing any infections, and incontinence of bowel and bladder correlated with an increased risk of infection of the lower respiratory tract, skin, and soft tissues. Evidence of a potentially significant risk of cross-infection between residents and staff was suggested by the finding of a correlation between high rates of staff absenteeism due to short-term illness and high numbers of infectious episodes among residents.

In summary, despite the potential seriousness of the problem, very little information exists about rates of endemic infections in nursing homes. Various studies performed over relatively short periods of time with various survey techniques in a limited number of facilities have identified the prevalence rates for infectious diseases in these institutions to be between 3% and 18%.[11,14] Most of the studies, however, did not attempt to differentiate between infections that were present prior to nursing home admission from those that developed subsequently. Prospective studies are needed to identify the rates of nursing home–acquired infections precisely and the attributable morbidity and mortality. An attempt should also be made to assess the relationship between patients' underlying prognoses, the goals for their nursing home stays, and the rates of complications secondary to nosocomial infections.[15]

FACTORS PREDISPOSING TO A HIGH PREVALENCE OF INFECTIONS IN NURSING HOMES

Host Factors

Residents of nursing homes are at increased risk of developing nosocomial infections for a number of reasons. Age alone is a factor. Eighty-six percent of nursing home residents are over the age of 65 years, and 35% are above the age of 75. At this late stage in life, changes occur in multiple organ systems which contribute to the residents' increased risk of developing infections. Protective barriers to infection decline with age, producing potential portals of entry for invading organisms. The skin and subcutaneous tissues lose their elasticity and thickness,[16] and even minor trauma can result in an open wound. Furthermore, a delayed healing response aggravates the situation.[16] Decreased lacrimal and salivary gland production along with changes in the orbital structures and mouth predispose to an increased incidence of conjunctivitis and inflammatory disease of the gums.[17,18]

Age-related changes in the immune system are being studied with respect to the incidence of infection. Although it is known that antibody production in response to exogenous immune stimulation is attenuated[19] and the incidence of autoimmune antibody production is increased,[20] it is not yet certain whether these and other changes in the immune system, independent of malnutrition and chronic disease, are responsible for the elderly's accentuated risk of developing infections.

Nursing home populations consist predominantly of the very frail elderly who have multiple chronic medical problems. On average, each patient has 3.5 chronic diseases, the most common of which include various manifestations of arteriosclerosis (49%), heart disease (34%), and senility (35% – 70%).[21] Consequently, over 90% of the residents have significant functional impairments. Greater than 70% need assistance with bathing and dressing, 66% are unable to ambulate independently, and more than half are frequently incontinent of bowel and bladder or have an indwelling bladder catheter.[15]

The presence of chronic diseases and the resulting functional impairment predispose patients to infections through a variety of mechanisms. If not treated aggressively with active or passive physical therapy, the immobile patient, while steadily losing energy and muscle bulk, is at an ever-increasing risk of developing pulmonary atelectasis and pneumonia. The same individuals are also at high risk of developing decubitus ulcers which have the potential for becoming infected. Incontinence, which is a serious problem in over 50% of nursing home residents,[22] is associated with an increased occurrence of skin breakdown and cellulitis. Garibaldi et al observed that infected pressure ulcers were the leading site of infection among nursing home residents in their study and that this condition was significantly more common among patients who were nonambulatory, fecally incontinent, diabetic, or catheterized than among patients without these conditions.[12] Patients with indwelling bladder catheters frequently have urine colonized with antibiotic-resistant gram-negative bacilli and enterococci, all of which can lead to the development of systemic infections. Patients with severe peripheral vascular disease and diabetes are predisposed to ischemic ulcers, gangrene, and sepsis while individuals with reduced levels of consciousness resulting in diminished or absent gag and cough reflexes are at risk of developing pneumonia as a result of their predisposition for recurrent aspirations.[23] Advanced dementia or extensive CNS damage from vascular accidents are conditions commonly seen in the latter group.

Many of the medications prescribed for chronic conditions can have a detrimental effect on the patients' defense mechanisms against infection. Tranquilizers and sedatives may inhibit the cough and gag reflexes leaving the patients' airways relatively unprotected, while steroids and many chemotheraputic agents have the potential to suppress the immune system. Drugs with anticholinergic properties are likely to decrease lacrimal and salivary secretion, inhibit bladder contractions, and cause clouding of consciousness. Antibiotics, especially when administered indiscriminately, can produce changes in the normal flora of the skin and

GI tract and tend to select for resistant organisms. Medication-induced effects such as these, which attenuate the immune response or weaken the barriers to invading organisms, accentuate the patients' risk of developing infections. The subtle effects of the long-term administration of certain pharmaceutical agents on the patients' defense against infection have not yet been adequately evaluated.

Many additional factors come into play and compound the nursing home patients' risk of developing nosocomial infections. Oral hygiene is often not given high priority. Consequently, diseases of the teeth and related structures are prevalent health care problems in this population.[24] Dental caries and periodontal disease if left untreated can lead to more complicated conditions such as cellulitis, bacteremia, and osteomyelitis of the jaw.[25] In general, older patients have a higher frequency of acquiring gram-negative bacteria in the oropharynx,[26] and the percentage of elderly who carry these organisms is dependent on the level of institutional care they receive. Aspiration of oropharyngeal contents, the major mechanism leading to pneumonia, also increases with age and the presence of underlying disease. Recently, tuberculosis has been recognized as an important nosocomial infection in the elderly in nursing homes.[27-29]

Administrative and Physician Factors

Several interrelated factors within nursing homes create a condition favorable for the development of nosocomial infections. A large number of frail, elderly patients with weakened defenses against infection are closely congregated in an environment which harbors a reservoir of potential pathogens. Without appropriate preventive measures these organisms can be transmitted by various means to this susceptible host population.

An optimal policy of infection control is difficult to obtain in nursing homes. Seventy-seven percent of nursing homes are proprietary institutions (of which most are owned by large chains), 74% have fewer than 100 beds, and only a few are directly affiliated with academic institutions. Furthermore, economic incentives play a significant role in policy decisions. The profit motive coupled with the government's attempts to limit long-term health care spending has resulted in a concerted effort by nursing homes to keep costs low. These policies have kept wages to a minimum, making it difficult to attract top-quality professionals, resulting in a high percentage of nonprofessional staff, a relatively high patient-to-staff ratio, and a minimum of qualified supervisory personnel.

Evidence suggests that staff are often the vehicles for transmitting infectious agents to patients,[12] a problem which is made worse by inadequate training, poor supervision, and a work policy which penalizes employees for taking sick leave. Maintaining appropriate staff education programs designed to minimize problems of infection control is difficult in nursing homes because of a rapid turnover in the work force. As in acute care hospitals, it is difficult to enforce simple preventive measures such as proper handwashing between patient contacts.[14]

The design of nursing homes and the organization of activities within these facilities are special concerns for optimal infection control since a competing goal is the establishment of an ideal living environment for the residents, conducive to promoting socialization and functional maintenance or rehabilitation. Large group activities, communal dining, and liberal visitation policies create a sound social atmosphere but allow for the potential spread of infections. Only a well-organized program of infection control can minimize cross-infection. Regularly scheduled prevalence surveys to rapidly identify new cases of infection coupled with an aggressive immunization program for residents and staff are needed. Whenever residents are infectious, they need to be withdrawn from group activities and have appropriate medical treatment instituted. It is also necessary to restrict employees and visitors from entering the home when ill. Whether the attainment of such a goal is feasible in most nursing homes is a point of contention, particularly with the current economic forecast for long-term care institutions.

Many variables related to physicians' involvement in nursing homes have a bearing on the problems of nosocomial infection control. Physicians' visits to residents of nursing homes are cited as being inadequate by the staff of these facilities,[30] nursing home medical directors,[31] and physician reviewers.[32] The interval between visits is negatively influenced by federal reimbursement regulations which, although designed to set minimum standards of care and to control costs, have had the effect of deterring physicians from making rounds more frequently than the standard 30-, 60-, and 90-day requirements. The resulting long intervals between visits may lead to subtle and unrecognized signs of deterioration, with the development of an acute event necessitating the utilization of much more costly hospital and emergency services, which potentially increase overall long-term nursing home care costs.[33]

The lack of needed diagnostic support such as laboratory and x-ray facilities or even an ECG machine, in addition to the unfavorable reimbursement schemes, discourages physicians from making emergency nursing home visits. There is also a tendency for physicians to overprescribe antibiotics, a practice which may contribute to the emergence of resistant organisms. The high mortality rate resulting from the purposeful nontreatment of fevers and obvious infections in some patients[34] certainly suggests that infections can contribute to mortality in the institutionalized elderly.

The problem of establishing greater physician involvement in nursing homes may not be related entirely to economics. Some critics charge that the quality and the quantity of care rendered by physicians in nursing homes is insufficient and indifferent.[35] Physicians whose practice extends into nursing homes spend relatively little time with their institutionalized patients.[30] Furthermore, a substantial portion of care of nursing home patients is being rendered outside of these institutions.[36] In such instances, the unenlightened practitioner, who does not see the environment in which the patient lives or does not have the opportunity to assess the staff's ability to carry out his instructions, may unknowingly render less than optimal care.[36]

Some of the difficulties encountered in caring for the elderly nursing home patient reflect the lack of emphasis placed on geriatric medicine by physicians in general. Although the situation is steadily improving with the development of geriatric programs in many academic centers, the elderly still do not receive adequate care. Despite the greater prevalence of multiple diseases in the elderly and their need to take longer to give and receive information, the average length of encounters between physicians and patient declines with the patient's age.[37] Many treatable medical problems are left undiagnosed on patients discharged from acute care hospitals,[38] and multiple errors and omissions are found frequently in the diagnostic records of patients at admission to nursing homes.[39]

The problem has its roots in the earliest years of medical education. Medical students tend to have stereotyped negative images of elderly patients[40] which are often left unchallenged because of the lack of exposure to proper geriatric training. The provision of care in nursing homes is given very little, if any, attention by most medical school and residency training programs, and consequently there is no consensus by the graduates as to what the quality of care standards are for physicians in nursing homes. The point is that in addition to medical and economic factors predisposing to the development and subsequent recognition of infection in nursing home residents, there are also social and educational factors.

SPECIFIC INFECTIONS FREQUENTLY ENCOUNTERED IN THE NURSING HOME SETTING

Many of the specific types of infections, such as pneumonia, which are commonly encountered in the nursing home are dealt with in detail in other chapters. The remainder of this chapter concentrates on one of the most common sites of infection in this high-risk population — the urinary tract. An overview is presented and then the diagnostic considerations in the noncatheterized and catheterized patients are treated separately. Lastly, an approach to therapy is provided.

Urinary Tract Infections

Although various microorganisms can invade the urinary tract, bacteria are the most common agents to do so and are clinically the most significant in the elderly. Urinary tract contamination is an especially common condition among nursing home residents. However, in these individuals, it is often difficult to quantitate the level of bacteriuria accurately or to determine what constitutes a urinary tract infection. A resulting controversy exists as to which bacteriuric patients should be treated, what form of therapy should be initiated, and how long it should be prescribed. The latter issue is complicated by the fact that it is usually not possible to distinguish between upper and lower tract involvement.[41]

Diagnositic evaluation in the noncatheterized patient For years it was felt that a diagnosis of a urinary tract infection in either a symptomatic or asymptomatic person required the presence of at least 100,000 colony-forming units per milliliter of urine from a catheterized or clean-catch midstream specimen. It is now apparent that this definition is inadequate for some populations[42] and needs to be evaluated in the elderly. Studies have revealed that even a negative culture does not rule out the diagnosis of a urinary tract infection in young females since certain causative organisms cannot be isolated by routine culture techniques.[43] Currently it is uncertain if the same principles hold true for symptomatic elderly patients residing in chronic care institutions. Consequently, the clinician has to be aware that the failure to find high numbers of bacteria in the urine may not be sufficient to exclude a diagnosis of a urinary tract infection in these individuals.[43]

Elderly, noncatheterized patients with classic symptoms of dysuria and urgency, with or without accompanying fever and flank pain, need to be evaluated carefully. The urine culture is only one of several factors which should be used to guide treatment. Proper techniques must be used to obtain the urine specimen, which must reach the laboratory for culture quickly. In addition to the culture results, the diagnosis of a urinary tract infection should be based on the history and a carefully interpreted urinalysis and gram stain. Consideration also needs to be given to the possibility that the symptoms may be a manifestation of kraurosis vulvae or vaginitis and, when appropriate, a thorough physical examination should be performed to exclude these conditions.

As opposed to symptomatic patients, there is even more controversy as to the criteria used to define a urinary tract infection in the asymptomatic, noncatheterized elderly. It is known that the prevalence of bacteriuria increases with both advancing age and the functional disability of the patient population, reaching frequencies of 25% to 50% in the debilitated institutionalized elderly. The significance of these findings, however, is not well understood. The natural history of bacteriuria and its contribution, if any, to morbidity and mortality are unknown. Some studies suggest that deteriorating renal function is seen in association with chronic bacteriuria, although several other reports refute the relationship. There is an established correlation between chronic bacteriuria and increased mortality in the geriatric population. Elderly persons with chronic bacteriuria are reported to have a 30% to 50% reduction in survival compared with subjects of similar age living under identical conditions and with an equal prevalence of other risk factors. However, this association does not prove a cause-and-effect relationship, and data are still needed to prove that aggressive treatment of the bacteriuria will alter mortality rates.[44-46]

Short courses of antimicrobials, although not studied carefully, are probably ineffective in sterilizing the urine of bacteriuric patients for more than a brief period of time. Many bacteriuric institutionalized elderly patients have a spontaneous turnover of bacteria in their urine,[47] and up to 26% revert to negative cultures over a period of 1 year. However, 29% of patients with sterile urine and a history of previous bacteriuria will be reinfected by 6 months. This fact raises the question whether long-term antimicrobial therapy is useful. An excellent study by Nicolle et al[48] demonstrates that treatment with trimethoprimsulfamethoxazole for up to 3 months is usually unsuccessful in eradicating bacteriuria in institutionalized male patients and it does not alter the outcome in terms of attributable morbidity or mortality. Similar studies in other elderly populations are needed. It is known that the emergence of resistant organisms and the development of drug-related adverse effects are often a result of extended courses of antimicrobial therapy. Consequently, until evidence becomes available that such intervention is efficacious, long-term antimicrobial therapy of chronic asymptomatic bacteriuria cannot be recommended.[46, 48]

When considering the possibility that an individual has only asymptomatic bacteriuria, one must realize that the classic symptoms of a urinary tract infection are often absent in the elderly. Any type of infection can present in an uncharacteristic manner[49, 50] with signs and symptoms such as a subtle change of mental status, increased lethargy, or even a greater propensity to fall. Urinary tract infections in particular may lead to the development of urinary incontinence as the initial manifestation. The clinician therefore has to have a high index of suspicion that any form of deterioration in a frail nursing home patient may be the result of a urinary tract infection. In the absence of other causes of the individuals' decline, clinical judgment has to be exercised to determine if aggressive treatment for the bacteriuria should be instituted.

Evaluating the catheterized patient For the elderly person residing in long-term care facilities, the use of indwelling bladder catheters is the most important risk factor for the development of bacteriuria. Various studies of nursing home populations report prevalence rates for the use of indwelling urinary drainage catheters of 1.5%[51] to 55%.[22] This rate is significant given the fact that the risk of developing a urinary tract infection with just a simple in-and-out catheterization is approximately 2% to 6%.[28] Moreover, when an indwelling catheter is in place, even when the catheter is inserted using proper sterile technique and a closed drainage system is attached, the risk of developing bacteriuria increases by 5% to 10% per day.[52,53] Virtually all patients with long-term bladder catheters have bacteriuria, often with multiple organisms.[54]

Chronic catheterization and the resulting bacteriuria can lead to the development of multiple complications including fever, acute pylonephritis, urethritis, epididymitis, prostatitis, and, of greatest concern, bacteremia, and possibly death.[55] Although most of the data on this subject are derived from studies performed outside of long-term care institutions, some reports indicate that there is a significant incidence of such complications in the chronically catheterized nursing home population. Bjork et al followed ten chronically catheterized male nursing home residents over a period of 12 to 28 months, taking frequent urine cultures while monitoring for the development of symptoms.[56] During the study, four (20%) of 20 symptomatic urinary tract infections were associated with bacteremia. Three of the bacteremic episodes were produced by highly resistant organisms, and one resulted in death. Others have also reported a high incidence of complications resulting from the use of bladder catheters in nursing homes.[57]

There is insufficient evidence to prove that any form of treatment is effective in preventing infectious complications while a bacteriuric patient remains chronically catheterized. Several studies demonstrate that prophylactic antibiotics do not prevent colonization with bacteria, eliminate the bacteriuria for more than short periods of time once it develops, or decrease the incidence of fever.[28] Such a strategy usually results only in the acquisition of resistant organisms.[58] Current information suggests that the practice of administering antimicrobials for the treatment of asymptomatic bacteriuria in the clinically stable, chronically catheterized patient is not warranted. However, indirect evidence exists that certain procedures such as the use of antibiotics during narrowly defined times of risk may be beneficial.

It is known that the development of catheter-related urosepsis is often preceded within 72 hours by a traumatic event such as obstruction, manipulation, or removal of an inflated indwelling bladder catheter.[59] During a study designed to investigate the correlation between fevers and catheter obstruction, the authors noted that fever did not accompany any of 17 catheter obstructions in patients concurrently receiving antibiotics, whereas fever was associated with 12 (13%) of 90 catheter obstructions in patients not on antimicrobials.[60] Procedures designed to decrease the incidence of catheter obstruction, such as catheter changes or irrigation with normal saline, have also been studied to determine if they lessen the risk of fever. No conclusive results have been reported to date.

Although the treatment of asymptomatic bacteriuria is controversial, most physicians would agree that chronically catheterized patients who develop lower urinary tract symptoms or who demonstrate signs of acute clinical deterioration need to be evaluated carefully. If after considering other possibilities, the physician considers a urinary tract infection the most likely cause of the patient's decline, vigorous therapy is indicated. Working through the differential and establishing the correct diagnosis, however, can be exceedingly difficult. As mentioned previously, an invasive urinary tract infection, particularly in the severely debilitated nursing home resident, may not present with any of the classic symptoms of urgency, suprapubic pain, or even fever. Subtle changes such as a decline in mental status or the more dramatic consequences of sepsis, including hypotension and shock, may in these patients be the initial manifestation. A high index of suspicion is required in these situations in order to avoid erroneously ascribing the patient's situation to other causes. Conversely, in these very high-risk individuals, a fever can be the result of any number of infectious or noninfectious causes. Even a thorough physical examination and a laboratory assessment may not establish the diagnosis with certainty. The WBC count and the ESR are rarely helpful under these circumstances, and, in the presence of an indwelling catheter, the results of a urinalysis are less specific for infection than in the noncatheterized patient. Hematuria or pyuria, the finding of which usually favors a diagnosis of a urinary tract infection, may in these patients result solely from the irritation to the bladder and urethra caused by the catheter.

Treatment of urinary tract infections The treatment for urinary tract infections has to be tailored to the individual, particularly when dealing with the long-term care patient. Urinary tract infections of nursing home origin tend to be caused by organisms intermediate in virulence and antibiotic resistance to those organisms acquired from the community and hospitals. The most common isolates are species of *Proteus;* although *Enterococcus, Klebsiella,* and *Providencia* spp are found frequently.[12, 61] Several studies have shown that these organisms are often resistant to commonly administered oral antibiotics, particularly in institutions where antimicrobials are used for prophylaxis.[56] In such situations appropriate culture and sensitivity tests are crucial to guide treatment. Patients recently admitted from the community who become colonized prior to entering the nursing home are more likely to be infected with antibiotic-susceptible *Escherichia coli.* Of greatest concern are the patients who develop their urinary tract infections in an acute care hospital prior to nursing home transfer. Sherman et al report that of the 45 urinary tract infections that were documented during a 5-month study in a skilled nursing facility, 17 (38%) developed during a preceding stay in a general hospital.[62] Whereas proteus species were the most common organisms isolated, *Pseudomonas aeruginosa* strains were responsible for the of the hospital-acquired urinary tract infections.

The initial treatment for nursing home patients with symptomatic urinary tract infections has to be empiric, based on a knowledge of which organism is likely to be involved. Routine periodic surveillance cultures are of little help in choosing the appropriate antibiotics. As a study by Warren et al points out, the urinary microbial flora of nursing home patients with chronic indwelling bladder catheters often changes spontaneously, even in the absence of antibiotics.[54] The patients, whose urine cultures usually demonstrate the presence of multiple organisms, have a mean interval between new episodes of bacteriuria of approximately 1.8 weeks. A study of Alling et al reported the finding of a similar rapid turnover of organisms colonizing the urinary tract of both catheterized and uncatheterized nursing home residents.[61] The current data illustrate the necessity of culturing patients at the time they present with symptomatic urinary tract infections and not relying on previous susceptibility reports.

Even after the appropriate intervention is initiated, it can be difficult to establish an acceptable therapeutic end point. Most authorities would agree that aggressive treatment aimed at eliminating the responsible organisms from the urinary tract is warranted, even though it may be difficult to accomplish. Ideally, patients who are chronically catheterized should have the device removed and, if needed, prescribed a program of in-and-out catheterization until the infection clears. Noncatheterized patients, particularly women with structural abnormalities and men with prostatic disease, may require extended treatment of up to 6 weeks in order to eradicate the site of infection and prevent rapid relapse.[63]

Many questions remain regarding the proper evaluation and treatment of the bacteriuric patient. One of the most important is the issue of the appropriate uses of the indwelling bladder catheter. Today, catheters are used to monitor urine output, to provide bladder drainage in the presence of bladder outlet obstruction or detrusor failure, and for the treatment of urinary incontinence. The latter two indications are the most frequent reasons long-term indwelling catheters are used. Both are very controversial. A study by Marron demonstrates that the use of these devices can often be reduced to a minimum. In a 527-bed skilled nursing facility, they could limit the use of catheters to 1.5% of the resident population.[50] This report and others demonstrate that incontinence can usually be treated effectively without bladder catheters. The latter include toileting regimens and specialized pads. Further research is needed to determine how much urine residua can be tolerated before the risk of noncatheterization outweighs the benefits. Included in the benefit-risk analysis is the question of which patients would likely benefit from surgical procedures designed to alleviate outlet obstruction or to prevent incontinence. Sphincterotomy, for example, may benefit patients who cannot spontaneously void to completion secondary to outlet obstruction and who at present require and indwelling catheter. Even though the procedure, in relieving the outlet obstruction, often leads to another form of incontinence, the resultant constant leaking of urine may be better tolerated than a catheter. The physician and nurses in the nursing home need to make a conscious effort to avoid catheterization whenever possible. Educational efforts designed to update the staff on techniques of caring for the incontinent patient without using catheters can be a beneficial part of the infection control effort.

REFERENCES

1. Avorn J: Nursing home infections — the context. *N Engl J Med* 1981; 305:759.
2. *Prospective Trends in the Size and Structure of the Elderly Population, Impact of Mortality Trends, and Some Implications.* US Bureau of the Census, Current Population Reports, Special Studies, series P-23, No. 78. Government Printing Office, 1979.
3. *Demographic Aspects of Aging and the Older Population in the United States.* US Bureau of the Census, Current Population Reports, series P-23, No. 59 (rev). Government Printing Office, 1976.
4. *Statistical Abstract of the United States: 1984*, ed 104. Washington, US Bureau of the Census, 1983.
5. *Public Policy and the Frail Elderly. A Staff Report.* Federal Council on Aging. US Dept of Health and Human Services publication No. (OHDS) 79-20959. Government Printing Office, 1978.
6. *The Need for Long-Term Care: A Chart Book of the Federal Council on the Aging.* Federal Council on the Aging. US Dept of Health and Human Services publication No. (OHDS) 81-20704. Government Printing Office, 1982.
7. Beck JC, Benson DF, Scheibel AG, et al: Dementia in the elderly: The silent epidemic. *Ann Intern Med* 1981;97:231–241.
8. Vicente L, Wiley JA, Carrington RA: The risk of institutionalization before death. *Gerontologist* 1979;19:361.
9. Keeler EB, Kane RL, Soloman DH: Short- and long-term residents of nursing homes. *Med Care* 1981;19:363.
10. Lester MR: Looking inside 101 nursing homes. *Am J Nurs* 1964;64:111–116.
11. Cohen ED, Hierholzer WJ, Schilling CL, et al: Nosocomial infections in skilled nursing facilities: A preliminary survey. *Public Health Rep* 1979;94:162–166.
12. Garibaldi RA, Brodine S, Matsumiya S: Infections among patients in nursing homes: Policies, prevalence, and problems. *N Engl J Med* 1981;305:731–735.
13. Nicolle LE, McIntyre M, Zacharias H, et al: Twelve-month surveillance of infections in institutionalized elderly men. *J Am Geriatr Soc* 1984;32:513–519.

14. Magnussen MH, Robb SS: Nosocomial infections in a long-term care facility. *Am J Infect Control* 1980;8:12–17.
15. Franson TR, Duthie EH Jr, Cooper JE: Prevalence survey of infections and their predisposing factors at a hospital-based nursing home care unit. *J Am Geriatr Soc* 1986;34:95–100.
16. Tonnesen MG, Weston WH: Aging of skin, in Schrier RW (ed): *Clinical Internal Medicine in the Aged.* Philadelphia, WB Saunders Co, 1982; pp 296–304.
17. Kasper RL: Eye problems of the aged, in Reichel W (ed): *Clinical Aspects of Aging.* Baltimore, Williams & Wilkins Co, 1983; pp 479–488.
18. Hudis MM: Dentistry for the elderly, in Reichel W (ed): *Clinical Aspects of Aging.* Baltimore, Williams & Wilkins Co, 1983; pp 498–511.
19. Roberts-Thomas IC, Whittingham S, Youngchaiyad U, et al: Aging immune response and mortality. *Lancet* 1974;2:368–370.
20. Murasko DM, Nelson BJ, Sliver R: Immunologic response in an elderly population with a mean age of 85. *Am J Med* 1986; 81:612–618.
21. Ingram DK: *Profile of Chronic Illness in Nursing Homes, 1973–74.* US Dept of Health, Education, and Welfare publication (PHS) 78-1780, Vital and Health Statistics, series 13, No. 29. Hyattsville, Md: National Center for Health Statistics, 1977.
22. Ouslander JG, Kane RL, Abrass IB: Urinary incontinence in elderly nursing home patients. *JAMA* 1982;248:1194.
23. Huxley EJ, Viroslav J, Gray WR, et al: Pharyngeal aspiration in normal adults and patients with depressed consciousness. *AM J Med* 1978;64:564.
24. Kamen S: Oral care of the geriatric patient, in Steinberg FU (ed): *Care of the Geriatric Patient.* St Louis, CV Mosby Co, 1983, pp 388–405.
25. Chow AW, Roser SM, Brady FA: Orofacial odontogenic infections. *Ann Intern Med* 1978;88:392.
26. Valenti WM, Trudell RG, Bentley DW: Factors predisposing to oropharyngeal colonization with gram-negative bacilli in the aged. *N Engl J Med* 1978;298:1108–1111.
27. Stead WW, Lofgren JP, Warren E, et al: Tuberculosis as an endemic and nosocomial infection among the elderly in nursing homes. *N Engl J Med* 1985;312:1483–1487.
28. Toews GB: Determinants of bacterial clearance from the lower respiratory tract. *Semin Respir Infect* 1986;1:68–78.
29. Stead WW: Tuberculosis among elderly persons: An outbreak in a nursing home. *Ann Intern Med* 1981;94:606–610.
30. Solon JA, Greenawalt LF: Physician's participation in nursing homes. *Med Care* 1974;12:486–495.
31. Ballard RW: The trouble with nursing homes. *Postgrad Med* 1982;72:307.
32. Zimmer JG: Medical care evaluation studies in long-term care facilities. *J Am Geriatr Soc* 1979;27:62–72.
33. Willemain TR, Mark RB: The distribution of intervals between visits as a basis for assessing and regulating physician services in nursing homes. *Med Care* 1980;18:427.
34. Brown NK, Thompson DJ: Nontreatment of fever in ex-tended-care facilities. *N Engl J Med* 1979;300:1246.
35. *Doctors in Nursing Homes: the Shunned Responsibility. Nursing Home Care in the United States: Failure of Public Policy.* US Senate, Subcommittee on Long-Term Care of the Special Committee on Aging: Supporting Paper No. 3. Government Printing Office, 1975.
36. Kane RL, Hammer D, Byrnes N: Getting care to nursing home patients: A

problem and a proposal. *Med Care* 1977;15:174.
37. Kane R, Soloman D, Beck J, et al: The future need for geriatric manpower in the United States. *N Engl J Med* 1980;302:1327.
38. Rubenstein LZ, Agrass IB, Kane RL: Improved care for patients on a new geriatric evaluation unit. *J Am Geriatr Soc* 1981;29:531.
39. Miller MB, Elliott DF: Errors and omissions in diagnostic records on admission of patients to a nursing home. *J Am Geriatr Soc* 1976;24:108.
40. Perrotta P, Perkins D, Schimpfhauser F, et al: Medical student attitude toward geriatric medicine and patients. *J Med Educ* 1981;56:478.
41. Hawthorne NJ, Kurtz SB, Anhalt JP, et al: Accuracy of antibody-coated-bacteria test in recurrent urinary tract infections. *Mayo Clin Proc* 1978;153:651.
42. Stamm WE, Counts GW, Running KR, et al: Diagnosis of coliform infection in acutely dysuric women. *N Engl J Med* 1982;307:463.
43. Komaroff AL: Acute dysuria in women. *N Engl J Med* 1984;310:368.
44. Carty M, Brocklehurst JC, Carty J: Bacteriuria and its correlates in old age. *Gerontology* 1981;27:72.
45. Dontas AS, Kasuki-Charvati P, Papanayiotou PC, et al: Bacteriuria and survival in old age. *N Engl J Med* 1981;304:939.
46. Nordenstam GR, Brandberg CA, Oden AS, et al: Bacteriuria and mortality in an elderly population. *N Engl J Med* 1986;314:1152-1156.
47. Kasuki-Charvati P, Drolette-Kefakis B, Papanayiotou PC, et al: Turnover of bacteriuria in old age. *Age Ageing* 1982;11:169.
48. Nicolle LE, Bjornson J, Harding GKM, et al: Bacteriuria in elderly institutionalized men. *N Engl J Med* 1983;309:1420.
49. Finkelstein MS: Unusual features of infections in the aging. *Geriatrics* 1982;37:65.
50. Gleckman R, Hilbert D: Afebrile bacteremia: A geriatrics phenomenon. *JAMA* 1982;248:1478.
51. Marron KR, Fillit H, Peskowitz M, et al: The nonuse of urethral catheterization in the management of urinary incontinence in the teaching nursing home. *J Am Geriatr Soc* 1983;31:278.
52. Garibaldi RA, Burke JP, Dickman ML, et al: Factors predisposing to bacteriuria during indwelling uretheral catheterization. *N Engl J Med* 1974;291:215.
53. Warren JW, Platt R, Thomas RJ, et al: Antibiotic irrigation and catheter-associated urinary tract infections. *N Engl J Med* 1978;299:570.
54. Warren JW, Tenney JH, Hooper JM, et al: A prospective microbiologic study of bacteriuria in patients with chronic indwelling urethral catheters. *J Infect Dis* 1982;146:719.
55. Warren JW, Muncie HL, Bergguist EJ, et al: Sequelae and management of urinary infections in the patients requiring chronic catheterization. *J Urol* 1981;125:1.
56. Bjork DT, Pelletier LL, Tight RR: Urinary tract infections with antibiotic resistant organisms in catheterized nursing home patients. *Infect Control* 1984;5:173.
57. Gambert SR, Duthie EH, Priefer B, et al: Bacterial infections in a hospital-based nursing facility. *J Chronic Dis* 1982;35:781.
58. Warren JW, Anthony WC, Hoopes JM, et al: Cephalexin for susceptible bacteriuria in afebrile, long-term catheterized patients. *JAMA* 1982;248:454.
59. Gleckman R, Blogg N, Hibert D, et al: Catheter-related urosepsis in the elderly: A prospective study of community-derived infections. *J Am Geriatr Soc* 1982;30:255.

60. Roberts JA: Urinary tract infections: In-depth review. *Am J Kidney Dis* 1984;4:103–117.
61. Alling B, Brandbery A, Seeberg S, et al: Aerobic and anaerobic microbial flora in the urinary tract of geriatric patients during long-term care. *J Infect Dis* 1973;127:34.
62. Sherman FT, Tucci V, Libow LS, et al: Nosocomial urinary tract infections in a skilled nursing facility. *J Am Geriatr Soc* 1980;28:456.
63. Gleckman R, Crowley M, Natsios GA: Therapy of recurrent invasive urinary tract infections in men. *N Engl J Med* 1979; 301:878.

21

Tuberculosis

George A. Pankey
Gregory T. Valainis

Since the beginning of the twentieth century, the average life expectancy in the United States has increased more than 50% — from 49 to almost 75 years of age. The "graying of America" has emerged as medical care has made tremendous breakthroughs. One of the great medical conquests of this century has been the effective control of tuberculosis (TB) due to isolation of patients in sanatoriums and the pasteurization of milk, control of disease in cattle,[1] and antituberculous chemotherapy, each in part significantly decreasing the morbidity and mortality of this once dreaded disease. Data from the national survey in the United States reported to the US Public Health Service since 1953 confirm this decline which actually began in the early 1900s, prior to the advent of chemotherapy, for all age groups. Only the AIDS epidemic of the 1980s has reversed this trend.

Yet, despite the overall decline, TB in the 65 years and older age group did not decrease as rapidly as it did in the younger age groups. The percentage of total cases in patients over 65 increased from 13.8% in 1953 to 28.6% in 1979.[2] The 1982 data from the Centers for Disease Control reveal the case rate per 100,000 population to peak in the 65 years and older age group for all race-sex categories.[3] This increase in the percentage of cases is out of proportion to the increasing size of the geriatric population. Age groups are not broken down for the elderly; however, Stead and Lofgren[4] have shown that between 1971 and 1981 the age-specific case rate in Arkansas actually increased for those persons 80 years of age and older. This raises the issue that for certain elderly subgroups the case rate is actually increasing and more intensive surveillance is in order. Those 80 years old and over are part of the fastest growing age group in the United States.

Why is there a relatively slow decline in case rates among the elderly? The reasons are multifactorial. They have lived through the years when TB was more common and thus have a higher number of exposure years. The elderly, particularly males, in most cases acquired the infection early in life, and it has remained dormant, manifested only by a positive tuberculin skin test. Once infected, an individual can harbor the tubercle bacilli for the remainder of his or her life that is capable of causing disease when host defenses are inadequate. Is there an age-associated immunodeficiency in the aged? T cell lymphocyte function does decline with age as reflected in a diminished delayed hypersensitivity reaction to purified protein derivative (PPD). Despite these findings, it remains to be determined whether this immunologic decline is sufficient by itself to cause activation of tuberculosis in the aged. Other contributing factors are the chronic illnesses in the elderly that cause an increased risk for recrudescence. These illnesses include diabetes mellitus, achlorhydria, end-stage renal disease, alcohol abuse, malignancy, malnutrition, and glucocorticoid use.

A final consideration involves TB in the nursing home patient. Epidemics of TB in nursing homes can occasionally occur and as suggested by Stead,[5] new infections occur more frequently than is generally thought. He described an outbreak in which 47 (45%) of the 104 residents who were previously uninfected became infected from a single index case.[5] A later report, which looked at all nursing homes in Arkansas,[6] noted a low prevalence of infection on initial admission to the nursing home. However, the infection rate increased at an annual rate of about 3.5% to 5% suggesting exogenous reinfection, which may lead to progressive primary TB. What can be learned from this is that all residing and new patients entering a nursing home should have their tuberculin status clarified, and those who are positive should have a chest radiograph performed. Any patient with known positive reactivity who develops a new cough or fever of undetermined source should have sputum samples examined for tubercle bacilli.

As a disease gradually declines, caution must be observed because clinical awareness will also decline. This is especially true when referring to TB in the geriatric population. Another confounding factor in attempting to make the diagnosis is the protean nature of the disease which often manifests nonspecific signs and symptoms. Also, the elderly patient more than likely will also be suffering from another acute or chronic condition causing the physician to overlook the possibility of tuberculosis.

All of these reasons may result in the diagnosis being missed or not sought for, which can result in prolonged morbidity and death. A number of autopsy studies have confirmed this. Edlin[7] in 1978 reviewed 24 active cases of TB in a British hospital that came to autopsy from 1968 to 1975. Twelve (50%) of the 24 were not diagnosed premortem. The mean age of the undiagnosed cases was slightly over 65 years. Nine (75%) of the 12 died; the cause of their deaths was directly due to untreated TB. The author commented that despite the overall declining prevalence, the number of undiagnosed cases has not decreased. Bobrowitz in 1982[8] reported on 21 patients who expired from undiagnosed TB from 1955 to 1979. Eleven patients had pulmonary disease and the remaining ten had miliary TB. Fifteen (71%) of the patients were age 66 or older. Fever, seen in 20 of 21 (95%) of the patients, was the principal symptom premortem, followed in order of decreasing frequency by weakness, disorientation and confusion, anorexia, and cough, again exemplifying the nonspecific presentation of the disease.

As many as 80% or more of elderly patients have no symptoms and tend to seek a physician late in the course. Physicians who view a slow, indolent, wasting patient may attribute the findings to the aging process or to an occult malignancy. More than one physician has been "burned" by TB mimicking malignancy. The most common factors involved in the misdiagnosis are (1) the decreased prevalence, (2) the fact that it is an "unfashionable" disease, (3) the nonspecificity of signs and symptoms, (4) its masking by concomitant disease, and (5) the atypical roentgenographic findings. Two of the most common conditions that are confused with TB are bacterial pneumonia and lung malignancy.

Tuberculosis in the elderly patient has a myriad of presentations and only a few selected clinical syndromes will be mentioned.

PULMONARY TUBERCULOSIS

Far beyond the others, reactivation pulmonary tuberculosis (chronic postprimary) is the most common presentation in the elderly. Fever (usually low-grade) with anorexia and weight loss is frequently present; however, night sweats, cough, and hemoptysis are late manifestations that may not even occur. Chest radiograph findings may be so nonspecific and the disease so slow to progress that months to years elapse before a diagnosis is made. Other pulmonary presentations include pleurisy with effusion, which is becoming more common in the aged. Again, a slow indolent process may be seen. Primary infection, formerly a disease of children and adolescents, is being seen more in adults. In Stead's[5] report of a nursing home outbreak, eight (17%) of the 49 PPD converters developed progressive primary TB and of these one died. The patient may be asymptomatic, but a tuberculin skin test will usually be positive. If primary TB is undiagnosed, it can progress even to the development of the adult respiratory distress syndrome (ARDS).[9]

TUBERCULOUS MENINGITIS

Tuberculous meningitis has "aged" from formerly being an infection almost exclusively of infancy and childhood to one occurring in the elderly. The presentation is similar to that in younger age groups, and the sequelae can be disastrous. Hass et al[10] reviewed their hospital's experience with tuberculous meningitis and found 19 cases from 1966 to 1974. Three of the 19 were over 70 years of age; two died, and the third was left with seizures as a neurologic sequela. Kennedy and Fallon[11] reviewed 52 cases in Scotland between 1960 and 1976. Only five (10%) of the cases occurred in patients over the age of 50, but these five constituted 38% of the deaths. In all of these deaths, the patients had concomitant liver disease which masked their meningitis. The authors also stressed the role of empiric antituberculous chemotherapy while waiting for cultures in a suspicious case. Delayed diagnosis and treatment led to a poorer prognosis.[11]

In the majority of cases, the identification by appropriate stains and microscopy is negative. Cultures are slow, with isolation of the tubercle bacilli requiring a minimum of 3 weeks. More rapid methods for identification are currently undergoing evaluation. Thus the clinician is faced with treating a patient with antituberculous chemotherapy for as much as 6 to 10 weeks pending culture identification and susceptibility testing. It should be obvious that one should not treat an elderly patient without obtaining appropriate culture materials.

MILIARY TUBERCULOSIS

Produced from the hematogenous dissemination of tubercle bacilli, miliary TB is the most common form of the disease in the elderly that is not diagnosed until autopsy. Numerous reports confirm the presentation of this disease in a cryptic fashion[12] with nondistinctive signs and symptoms. The classic miliary pattern may be absent on chest films, and in as many as 50% of the patients only nonspecific chest findings are seen.[13] Unexplicable low-grade fever is almost always present. If fever is present in a gradually wasting patient with anemia, leukopenia, or pancytopenia, the diagnosis of miliary TB should be strongly entertained. Empiric therapy can be lifesaving but some patients are beyond recovery when they are first seen. Sputum, bone marrow, or liver specimens should be obtained for culture and stains.

As aptly stated by Stead and Dutt,[14] once the diagnosis of TB is considered, the evaluation is generally easy using the tuberculin skin test and acquiring smears and cultures for *Mycobacterium tuberculosis* from clinical materials. A high index of suspicion, however, remains the essential key to the diagnosis in the elderly. Two adjuncts that can be very helpful in the diagnosis are the intradermal (Mantoux) tuberculin skin test and the chest roentgenogram.

DIAGNOSTIC TESTS

Skin Testing

Skin testing with the intradermal skin test using 5 tuberculin units of purified protein derivative (IPPD) remains an excellent screening test and is the most accurate test available for detecting infection. Several caveats are in order when applying skin testing in the geriatric population.

Tuberculin reactivity tends to wane the longer it has been since the initial infection. In fact, a positive skin test may revert to negative. To overcome this, sequential testing is performed in order to recall (boost) a previously reactive skin test that has diminished with time. The boosting phenomenon occurs in all age groups but is more common in those between 55 and 75 years of age. Therefore, an IPPD should be performed 1 week after an initial negative or weakly positive one before excluding tuberculin reactivity (10 × 10 mm of induration). All new patients entering a nursing home should have skin testing performed by the sequential method to help diagnose future outbreaks.

Elderly patients are more likely to be receiving immunosuppressive drugs or will have concomitant disease such as a hematologic malignancy, sarcoidosis, or malnutrition and may be anergic. Further evaluation with a battery of skin tests may be indicated to confirm this.

Overwhelming TB such as miliary or extensive cavitary disease may be associated with a weakly positive or negative IPPD even after sequential testing.

Chest Roentgenograms

Besides skin testing, the only other important diagnostic adjunct is the chest roentgenogram. Nevertheless, radiographic findings may be missed or misdiagnosed, which delays the diagnosis. Availability of previous films for comparison can decrease the likelihood of misinterpretation. Atypical features such as nodules, lower lobe infiltrates, bronchopneumonia, and masslike lesions may be ascribed to other diagnoses. In the review by Khan et al[15] of the radiologic manifestations of 88 patients with newly diagnosed pulmonary TB, 20 were inpatients older than 60 years of age. Of the 20 patients, 7 (35%) had atypical roentgenographic manifestations such as isolated disease in the middle or lower lobe or pleural effusion. Thus it is important to still consider TB in the differential diagnosis even when the chest film does not reveal the typical posterior segment infiltrate of the upper lobes with or without cavitation. Again the emphasis returns back to the clinician to consider TB despite radiologic interpretation.

TREATMENT

Fortunately, in most cases a positive acid-fast smear or a biopsy sample revealing granulomatous disease will lead the clinician to initiate therapy. Two bactericidal drugs, isoniazid (INH) and rifampin, should be included in the initial regimen of any form of the disease if drug resistance is not known beforehand. For pulmonary TB, 9 months of isoniazid and rifampin daily has been uniformly successful in eradicating the rapid and slow-growing (persistent) *M tuberculosis* as well as preventing the development of drug-resistant mutants. Dutt et al[16] have shown that for outpatient treatment of pulmonary disease, short-course chemotherapy is effective, less expensive, and has fewer drug side effects, even in the elderly. It consists of INH (300 mg) and rifampin (600 mg) daily for 1 month followed by twice-weekly therapy for 8 months consisting of isoniazid (900 mg) and rifampin (600 mg). In the study of Dutt et al 608 (59%) of the patients were over the age of 60 and the regimen was well tolerated. Many of the successfully treated patients suffered from chronic diseases associated with increased risk for TB.[16]

Extrapulmonary TB treatment regimens are less clear. Many physicians feel extrapulmonary TB should be treated more intensively and for a longer period of time. The need for a more intensive approach versus standard two-drug therapy used in pulmonary disease is lacking. Streptomycin should be avoided in the elderly because of ototoxicity and nephrotoxicity.[17] Dutt et al[16] have data to suggest that using two drugs (isoniazid and rifampin) for 9 months is comparable to using more intensive regimens for extrapulmonary TB. Ethambutol usage has declined considerably due to its bacteriostatic activity and is now considered a second-line agent.

The percentage of adverse reactions, and in particular isoniazid hepatotoxicity, increases with age, but in general the elderly patient tolerates isoniazid and rifampin without difficulty. There remains considerable disagreement as to the use of routine monitoring of hepatic enzymes to preclude serious liver damage. It would seem prudent that in a reliable elderly patient, monitoring of signs and symptoms suggestive of hepatitis, such as dark urine, nausea, vomiting, and anorexia, by the patient and physician should suffice. In an unreliable patient such as one suffering from chronic dementia, pre-existing liver disease, or ethanol abuse, laboratory monitoring is in order. One should stop both the isoniazid and rifampin when hepatic transaminases are 3 to 5 times above pretreatment levels. This appears to be less of a problem with short-course chemotherapy than with daily drug therapy.[16] If the use of streptomycin outweighs the risks, serum levels should be closely monitored as renal function normally declines with aging. One should be aware of possible drug interactions because the elderly are more likely to be taking other concomitant medications. Table 21-1 lists some of the more common drug interactions in the elderly.

Primary drug-resistant tuberculosis is rare in elderly patients born in the United States as compared with younger patients. It is especially high in people of Asian and Hispanic descent, but the rate varies across the country. If resistance is a strong consideration, four drugs should initially be used (isoniazid, rifampin, pyrazinamide, and streptomycin) pending susceptibility testing.

The adverse reaction rate from chemoprophylaxis with isoniazid is higher in the 35 years old and over age group. Partly because of this, chemoprophylaxis is usually reserved for the elderly patient with a positive tuberculin skin test and with at least one other risk factor such as recent skin test conversion, pulmonary infiltrates, concomitant disease such as end-stage renal disease, silicosis, achlorhydria, diabetes mellitus, malignancy, or an immunocompromised state. Stead[5] makes a convincing argument in his description of a nursing home outbreak for chemoprophylaxis. Thirty-nine patients with an average age of 72 were given isoniazid for a positive skin test with only three (7.7%) patients unable to complete the therapy due to hepatitis. None of the 36 converters developed disease compared with two of five converters who inadvertently were not treated and subsequently developed disease. In a recent report on TB as a

Table 21-1
Antituberculous Drug Interactions in the Elderly

	Adverse Reaction
Isoniazid plus	
Antacids containing aluminum	Decreased isoniazid absorption
Warfarin sodium	Increased prothrombin time
Diazepam	Increased diazepam effect
Phenytoin	Increased phenytoin levels
Rifampin plus	
Warfarin sodium	Decreased prothrombin time
Diazepam	Decreased diazepam effect (overrides INH effect)
Barbiturates	Decreased barbiturate levels
ß-blockers	Decreased ß-blockade
Digoxin	Decreased digoxin level
Glucocorticoids	Decreased steroid effect
Hypoglycemics (oral)	Decreased glucose control
Quinidine	Decreased quinidine levels
Streptomycin plus	
Furosemide	Additive oto- and nephrotoxicity
Pyrazinamide plus	
Isoniazid and rifampin	Possible additive hepatotoxicity

nosocomial infection in nursing homes,[6] incomplete data on toxicity were given. However, 605 positive converters received isoniazid prophylaxis, and in no case did liver failure or death occur. Only one case of clinical disease developed.

SUMMARY

Although great strides have been made in the twentieth century in the control of TB for the younger age groups, the elderly patient remains, in the words of Medlar et al, the "disregarded seedbed of the tubercule bacillus."[18] As the population of the United States continues to age, continuing education of the practicing physician regarding tuberculosis must be emphasized. The index of suspicion must remain high in order to prevent needless deaths from a disease that is relatively easy to treat.

REFERENCES

1. Myer JA: Tapering off of tuberculosis among the elderly. *Am J Public Health* 1976;66:1101−1106.
2. Powell KE, Farer LS: The rising age of the tuberculosis patient: a sign of success and failure. *J Infect Dis* 1980;142: 946−948.
3. Centers for Disease Control: Annual summary 1982: Reported morbidity and mortality in the United States. *MMWR* 1983; 31: 88.
4. Stead WW, Lofgren JP: Does the risk of tuberculosis increase in old age? *J Infect Dis* 1983;147:951−955.
5. Stead WW: Tuberculosis among elderly persons: an outbreak in a nursing home. *Ann Intern Med* 1981;94:606−610.
6. Stead WW, Lofgren JP, Warrren E, et al: Tuberculosis as an epidemic and nosocomial infection among the elderly in nursing homes. *N Engl J Med* 1985;312:1483−1487.
7. Edlin GP: Active tuberculosis unrecognized until necropsy. *Lancet* 1978; 650−652.
8. Bobrowitz ID: Active tuberculosis undiagnosed until autopsy. *Am J Med* 1978;1:650−652.
9. Sahn SA, Skeff KM: Tuberculous pneumonia with the syndrome of inappropriate secretion of antidiuretic hormone. *Chest* 1977;72:678−680.
10. Haas EJ, Madhavan T, Quinn EL, et al: Tuberculous meningitis in an urban general hospital. *Arch Intern Med* 1977;137:1518−1521.
11. Kennedy DH, Fallon RJ: Tuberculous meningitis. *JAMA* 1979;241:264−268.
12. Proudfoot AT, Akhtar AJ, Douglas AC, et al: Miliary tuberculosis in adults. *Br Med J* 1969;1:273−276.
13. Sahn SA, Neff TA: Miliary tuberculosis. *Am J Med* 1974;56:495−505.
14. Stead WW, Dutt AK: What's new in tuberculosis? *Am J Med* 1981;71:1−4.
15. Khan MA, Kovnat DM, Bachus B, et al: Clinical and roentgenographic spectrum of pulmonary tuberculosis in the adult. *Am J Med* 1977;62: 31−38.

16. Dutt AH, Moers D, Stead WW: Short-course chemotherapy for tuberculosis with mainly twice-weekly isoniazid and rifampin. *Am J Med* 1984;77:233–242.
17. Dutt AH, Moers D, Stead WW: Short-course chemotherapy for extrapulmonary tuberculosis. *Ann Intern Med* 1986;104:7-12.
18. Medlar EM, Spain DM, Halliday RW: Disregarded seedbed of the tubercle bacillus. *Arch Intern Med* 1948;81:501–517.

22
Infections in the Diabetic Patient

Thomas T. Yoshikawa

Diabetes mellitus is an important clinical disorder in the geriatric population because of its high prevalence and its associated complications. Certainly, infection is one important cause of morbidity (and, in some instances, mortality) in the elderly diabetic. However, with the exception of select infectious diseases, there are no objective data to indicate that diabetics, regardless of age, are especially more prone to infections.[1] With the knowledge that the aged person even in the absence of diabetes mellitus is at great risk to infections,[2] it becomes even more difficult to demonstrate the impact of this metabolic disorder on the susceptibility to infections in the elderly diabetic.

In this chapter, we review the following topics: (1) defining diabetes mellitus in the geriatric population; (2) the demographic features and pathogenesis of diabetes mellitus in the elderly; (3) the impact of diabetes mellitus on host defenses of the elderly; and (4) the infections putatively associated with diabetes mellitus.

DEFINING DIABETES MELLITUS IN THE GERIATRIC POPULATION

The increased awareness of the importance of diabetes mellitus in the geriatric population, the inconsistent diagnostic criteria for defining this illness, and the greater knowledge of the clinical consequences of various forms of hyperglycemia led to the revision and standardization of the nomenclature, diagnostic criteria, and classification of this disorder. The National Diabetes Data Group has established specific criteria for the diagnosis of diabetes mellitus and the classification of various forms of glucose intolerance.[3]

Diagnosis of diabetes mellitus and other forms of glucose intolerance is based on (1) the classic symptoms of diabetes mellitus; (2) the fasting plasma glucose concentration; and (3) the plasma glucose concentration following an oral (75 g) glucose challenge. The specific criteria for classifying nonpregnant adults as having diabetes mellitus or impaired glucose tolerance are shown in Table 22-1. These would be the same criteria used to diagnose and classify diabetes mellitus or impaired glucose tolerance in the elderly. Although some investigators and clinicians suggest adding 10 mg/dL per decade after the age of 50 years for each of the diagnostic plasma glucose levels,[4,5] others argue that standard criteria for diagnosing diabetes mellitus be maintained regardless of age.[6,7]

Insulin-dependent diabetes mellitus (IDDM) or type I diabetes mellitus was previously termed juvenile diabetes, juvenile-onset diabetes, brittle diabetes, or ketosis-prone diabetes. The older terminology implied that the disorder occurred only in children. However, type I diabetes mellitus can occur in any age; many elderly diabetics require insulin for optimal management of their disease. Noninsulin-dependent diabetes mellitus (NIDDM) or type II diabetes mellitus occurs primarily after the age of 40 years and is the most common form seen in the elderly population. It was previously called adult-onset diabetes, maturity-onset diabetes, ketosis-resistant diabetes, or stable diabetes.

Impaired glucose tolerance should be called such and not asymptomatic diabetes, chemical diabetes, subclinical diabetes, borderline

Table 22-1
Classification and Criteria for Diagnosis of Diabetes Mellitus and Glucose Intolerance

Type	Criteria	Comment
Diabetes mellitus	1. Overt diabetic symptoms and unequivocal hyperglycemia; or 2. Fasting plasma glucose (FPG) ≥ 140 mg/dL; or 3. With FPG < 140 mg/dL, a plasma glucose (PG) following oral glucose tolerance test (OGTT) ≥ 200 mg/dL at 2 h and at some time between 0 and 2 h (0.5, 1.0, or 1.5 h)	1. Ex: polyuria, polydipsia, ketosis 2. Must occur on at least two occasions 3. Must occur on at least two occasions
Impaired glucose tolerance (Nonpregnant adults)	1. FPG < 140 mg/dL 2. Following OGTT, 2-hr PG ≥ 140 mg/dL and < 200 mg/dL, and 3. Following OGTT, one PG value ≥ 200 mg/dL at 0.5, 1.0, or 1.5 h	Criteria (1) and (2) sufficient for epidemiologic studies Criterion (3) necessary for clinical classification

diabetes, latent diabetes, or prediabetes. Only 1% to 5% of persons with impaired glucose tolerance develop overt clinical diabetes mellitus per year.[3] Many persons will return to a normal glucose tolerance status spontaneously, and others will remain unchanged for many years. Moreover, glucose intolerance in the elderly may be associated with other disorders, hormones, and drugs, and is not considered diabetes mellitus. Therefore, to avoid the psychologic stigma and potential socioeconomic impact of the term *diabetes*, these individuals should simply be labeled as having impaired glucose tolerance.

DEMOGRAPHY AND PATHOGENESIS OF DIABETES MELLITUS IN THE ELDERLY

The prevalence of diabetes mellitus will obviously depend on the criteria used to define this disease. Until the previously mentioned standardization for diagnosis of diabetes mellitus was established,[3] a variety of criteria and nomenclature (eg, clinical diabetes, latent diabetes) was used to define the frequency of this disorder. However, despite these inconsistencies, all studies have shown a consistent pattern of increased frequency of diabetes mellitus or glucose intolerance with advancing age.[5,8] A more recent study, using an oral 100-g glucose tolerance test and measuring only fasting and two-hour plasma concentrations, demonstrated in a population sample of 1009 persons, an age relationship with glucose intolerance.[7] A fasting plasma glucose exceeding 140 mg/dL was found in 3% of the population. However, fasting hyperglycemia occurred only in persons aged 50 years or older, with no difference in frequency between sexes. Similarly, two-hour postprandial glucose concentrations exceeding 200 mg/dL occurred only in individuals in the sixth decade or older (10%). The prevalence was age-related with a frequency in the sixth, seventh, eighth, and ninth decades of 8%, 12%, 16%, and 21%, respectively.

The glucose intolerance that is associated with aging has been ascribed to a number of different mechanisms or factors[4,5]: decreased physical activity, decreased lean body mass and increased fat tissue, increased glucagon blood levels, decreased and delayed insulin release, insulin antagonism, and peripheral insulin resistance. Despite these proposed pathogenetic mechanisms, most recent data suggest that carbohydrate intolerance in the elderly is related to loss of in vivo action of insulin.[9] This decreased peripheral insulin sensitivity is not due to a decreased number of insulin receptors or decreased insulin binding to receptors, but to a postreceptor defect.[10,11] This abnormality is not related to adiposity, and the severity of glucose intolerance in the elderly is correlated with the severity of the postreceptor defect.

IMPACT OF DIABETES MELLITUS ON HOST DEFENSES IN THE ELDERLY

The information currently available on the impact of diabetes mellitus on host defense mechanisms is at best confusing, contradictory, inconclusive and, often, seemingly clinically irrelevant. With this background of confusion, it is nearly impossible to interpret the effects of diabetes mellitus on the integrity of host defenses in the elderly, let alone find studies that investigate this problem. Moreover, since aging alone has an impact on host defense mechanisms,[12,13] the role of the concomitant presence of diabetes mellitus on susceptibility to infections becomes further unclear.

In this section, the published data (though incomplete and inconclusive) on the influence of diabetes mellitus on host defense mechanisms, as well as any available information on the role of aging, are briefly summarized.

Neutrophil Function

The functional integrity of neutrophils (polymorphonuclear leukocytes) has been studied by evaluating primarily four functions: adherence, chemotaxis, phagocytosis, and intracellular killing. Many of the investigations show divergent results and conclusions. These variations result from (1) differences in assay procedures; (2) variations in the state of the patient's diabetic control; (3) sampling type I and/or type II diabetics in the studies; (4) evaluating in vivo versus in vitro effects of hyperglycemia, acidosis, or ketosis; and (5) determining neutrophil function in infected versus noninfected patients.

There are limited studies on the impact of diabetes mellitus on *neutrophil adherence*. It appears that both poorly controlled type I or type II diabetes mellitus caused an impairment in neutrophil adherence which was reversed toward normal values with insulin or oral hypoglycemic agent therapy.[14,15] However, there is no information whether neutrophils from elderly diabetics perform differently than those from younger patients.

Neutrophil chemotaxis has been shown to be abnormally affected by diabetes mellitus.[16–18] The work of Molenaar et al suggested that the abnormal chemotaxis function was not related to insulin deficiency or hyperglycemia but to an inherent deficit in leukocyte function.[16] Increasing age did not appear to influence the data results. However, the mean age of the various study groups ranged between 40 to 49 years with the oldest patients being 71 years old. In contrast, Fikrig et al failed to demonstrate defective neutrophil chemotaxis in either type I or type II diabetics.[19] Moreover, sera from these diabetics were not different in their ability to generate chemotactic factors.

Impairments in *neutrophil phagocytosis* have been demonstrated using *Streptococcus pneumoniae* or *Staphylococcus aureus* as the test organisms.[20,21] Bagdade et al[20] studied eight noninfected patients who had poorly controlled, nonketotic, diabetes mellitus; two patients were insulin-dependent. Neutrophil phagocytosis of *S pneumoniae* was significantly reduced and this abnormality was dependent on the presence of hyperglycemia. Tan et al[21] using *S aureus* showed that phagocytic deficits are present in some diabetics but that the abnormality did not correlate with glucose concentration, history of recurrent infection, or patient's age. However, more careful analysis of the data suggests that the group with the phagocytic defects were somewhat older (mean age 57 years versus 50 years in diabetics with no phagocytic abnormalities). This might suggest that elderly diabetics have poorer neutrophil phagocytic function. Too few patients limit any meaningful conclusions. Alternatively, there are data showing the absence of defects in neutrophil phagocytosis in young and old diabetics. Crosby and Allison[22] examined neutrophil function in 19 diabetics (nine on insulin) ranging in age from 37 to 70 years with 15 patients over 50 years of age. No patient had ketoacidosis or infection. Using *S pneumoniae* as the test organism, neutrophil phagocytosis was similar to healthy controls. Moreover, when glucose concentration in the sera was increased up to 1040 mg/dL, phagocytosis was unaffected.

Intracellular killing (microbicidal capacity) is the final and most important step in the culmination of neutrophil function. Generally, the presence or absence of defects in intracellular killing of microbes by neutrophils in diabetics paralleled the presence or absence of phagocytic abnormalities. That is, studies showing neutrophil phagocytic impairment in diabetics could also demonstrate microbicidal deficits.[20,21] In contrast, Crosby and Allison[22] failed to demonstrate both phagocytic and microbicidal deficits in patients with diabetes mellitus. A more recent study by Repine et al[23] showed that poorly controlled uninfected diabetics had impaired neutrophil microbicidal activity. Additionally, this study found that untreated nondiabetics with acute bacterial infection had increased neutrophil killing, whereas neutrophils from diabetics failed to increase their microbicidal activity with infection (which was more pronounced with poorly controlled diabetics). Unfortunately, all the patients were young adults, and therefore the impact of age could not be determined.

Immune Function

The available data on the effects of diabetes on the immune system are also fraught with contradictory results. Furthermore, the impact of age on immune function is well recognized[13] and thus its (age) role in affecting the immune status in diabetics has not been clarified or elucidated.

Humoral immunity appears to be relatively unperturbed by diabetes mellitus.[24,25] In the study of Beam et al[25] using the pneumococcal vaccine in type I diabetics, antibody response was similar to nondiabetic controls. Moreover, age did not appear to be a factor in antibody response among the study population. However, in other studies of animal model diabetes mellitus and in patients, antibody formation was reduced.[26,27]

A number of investigations have demonstrated some type of abnormality in cell-mediated immune function in diabetics. However, since T lymphocyte function may be assessed by a variety of in vitro tests, the abnormalities found have varied considerably depending on the assays used. Abnormalities in sheep red blood cell rosette formation by T cells have been described in type I diabetics.[28] Lymphocyte response to mitogens such as phytohemagglutinin has been shown to be (1) depressed in poorly controlled type I diabetics but not in well-controlled patients[29]; (2) reduced greater in type I than in type II diabetics, which was related to severity of diabetes mellitus but not to age[30]; or (3) not significantly decreased in diabetics who are well controlled.[31] One study showed depressed T lymphocyte responses to *S aureus* antigen in diabetics compared with normal controls.[31] However, the median age for the diabetics appeared significantly older than the controls. Data on the responses by age in the diabetic group were not presented.

Other Factors

There are virtually no data on the relationship between diabetes mellitus and secretory immunity, natural killer cell activity, interferon, bacterial receptors and adherence, and complement. Moreover, such factors as microvascular disease, peripheral and autonomic neuropathy, minor trauma, complications of ketoacidosis or hypoglycemia, and aspiration are more likely contributors to infections in diabetics than any alteration in host defense mechanisms.

INFECTIONS PUTATIVELY ASSOCIATED WITH DIABETES MELLITUS

A number of reviews that discuss infections associated with diabetes mellitus have been published.[1,32-34] Although there are some differences of opinion, putative infections linked to diabetes mellitus include some forms of urinary tract infection, soft tissue infections, osteomyelitis, tuberculosis, malignant external otitis, and certain fungal infections. In many of these infections, elderly patients are more frequently affected.

Urinary Tract Infection

Whether diabetes mellitus itself or its associated complications, ie, repeated catheterization, bladder dysfunction (autonomic dysfunction), or microvascular disease, explains the apparent higher prevalence of urinary tract infections in diabetics has not been elucidated. Moreover, depending on whether the study sample included men, women, outpatients, inpatients, controlled or uncontrolled diabetics, or autopsies, the association of urinary tract infection and diabetes mellitus is quite variable.[32,35,36] Urinary tract infection has been shown to have a higher prevalence in diabetic women but no increase in diabetic men. Alternatively, young persons with well-controlled diabetes mellitus have been shown to have the same incidence of urinary tract infection in age-matched nondiabetic controls.[37,38] The frequency of urinary tract infection in elderly diabetics compared to elderly nondiabetics has not been investigated. Moreover, the prevalence of bacteriuria in the geriatric population is so high (as much as 50%) that it may be difficult to determine if diabetes mellitus could influence an elderly patient's risk to this infection.[39] The therapy of urinary tract infections in the elderly is complicated by (decreased excretory function) secondary to age as well as systemic diseases, for example, diabetes mellitus.[40]

Interestingly, more complicated forms of urinary tract infection appear to occur more frequently in older diabetics. Perinephric abscess cases reported by Thorley et al occurred more commonly in association with diabetes mellitus and older age when compared with patients with pyelonephritis only.[41] Emphysematous pyelonephritis has been described almost exclusively in diabetics. Moreover, of the 53 cases recently reported, 23 patients (43%) were 60 years or older (mean age 56 years).[42] Mortality from emphysematous pyelonephritis, including all forms of treatment, is 31%.[42] Surgical intervention, that is, incision and drainage or nephrectomy, is the definitive form of therapy.

Soft Tissue Infections

Skin and soft tissue infections are common in diabetics because of peripheral neuropathy, trauma, and peripheral vascular disease. Carriage or colonization with *S aureus* appears to be a function of diabetes mellitus[43,44] and may explain the higher frequency of staphylococcal skin infection in this population. The associated diminished peripheral circulation and resultant decreased oxygenation of tissue in diabetics predisposes them to serious anaerobic or mixed anaerobic-aerobic soft tissue infections including necrotizing fasciitis, synergistic necrotizing cellulitis, clostridial gangrene, and foot ulcers.[33,34,45,46] Many of these infections, especially foot ulcers and Fournier's gangrene (a form of synergistic necrotizing cellulitis involving the scrotum) occur more frequently in the elderly diabetic.[46,47] Not only is the frequency of some of these infections higher in older diabetics, the severity (and associated morbidity and mortality) is also greater. Therefore early diagnosis and treatment is paramount in the management of these patients.

Osteomyelitis

All forms of osteomyelitis, that is, hematogenous osteomyelitis, osteomyelitis secondary to contiguous foci of infection, and osteomyelitis associated with peripheral vascular disease, are more frequent in the middle-aged and elderly populations.[48] However, osteomyelitis secondary to peripheral vascular disease occurs predominantly in elderly diabetics[48] and involves the distal lower extremities. Moreover, these infections are frequently caused by anaerobic bacteria (or mixed aerobic and anaerobic organisms).[49,50] This results from adjacent soft tissue gangrene, ulceration, and infection associated with decreased tissue perfusion and oxygenation. Although conservative medical management with systemic antimicrobial therapy is preferred in these frail elderly diabetics, often surgical intervention including amputation may be required as lifesaving forms of treatment.

Tuberculosis

The concept that tuberculosis occurs with greater frequency in diabetics remains controversial.[32,34,51,52] Alternatively, cases of diabetics with atypical pulmonary involvement with tuberculosis have been described.[52] These four patients (out of 20 diabetics with pulmonary tuberculosis) had lower lobe involvement. The mean age of the 20 diabetics was 51 years but the ages of the lower lobe cases were not specified. This is an important consideration since (1) pulmonary tuberculosis increases in frequency with age (regardless of diabetes mellitus); and (2) middle and lower lobe involvement also occurs in nondiabetic elderly patients.[53] Therefore it remains to be demonstrated that tuberculosis and diabetes mellitus have a significant clinical or pathologic association.

Malignant External Otitis

Malignant external otitis is a life-threatening infection caused almost exclusively by *Pseudomonas aeruginosa*. Nearly all reported cases occur in diabetics and usually in persons over the age of 55 years.[54] The infection begins in the external auditory canal and then may spread to involve the periauricular tissues including the parotid gland, temporomandibular joint, and soft tissue of the base of the skull.[55] Further progression of the disease results in extension to the cranial nerves at the base of the skull or to the jugular vein causing thrombosis. Extension may also occur into the middle ear, mastoid cells, and brain structures. With such potential complications, it is not surprising that mortality with this infection exceeds 50%.[56] All patients suspected of malignant external otitis require immediate hospitalization, parenteral combination antimicrobial chemotherapy, that is, anti-*Pseudomonas* penicillin and aminoglycoside, and local surgical debridement.

Fungal Infections

Mucocutaneous candidiasis and possibly lower urinary tract infection with *Candida* occurs more frequently in persons with diabetes mellitus.[34,57] Moreover, vaginal candidiasis appears to be age-related, with the highest frequency occurring in women over 50 years old.[58]

Torulopsis glabrata urinary tract infection, especially pyelonephritis, occurs in an unusually high frequency in elderly diabetics.[59] Many of these patients also have coexisting gram-negative urosepsis and experience a high death rate.

Rhinocerebral zygomycosis (phycomycosis or mucormycosis) is classically associated with diabetes mellitus, especially in patients with ketoacidosis.[60,61] Although this infection does occur in all ages, there is a tendency for patients to be older than 45 years.[61] The fungus initiates its infection in the nasal mucosa and then spreads by local extension to the adjacent paranasal sinuses, cribiform plate, and CNS. Intravascular invasion also occurs resulting in thrombosis. Patients present clinically with facial or ocular pain; nasal discharge (blood-tinged or crusty); proptosis, ophthalmoplegia and visual loss; facial cellulitis; and neurologic changes including coma, seizures, or hemiplegia. Mortality is high despite antifungal (amphotericin B) therapy and aggressive surgical debridement, if meningitis or cerebritis occurs.[62]

REFERENCES

1. Greene DA: Acute and chronic complications of diabetes mellitus in older patients. *Am J Med* 1986;80:39–53.
2. Yoshikawa TT: Geriatric infectious diseases: an emerging problem. *J Am Geriatr Soc* 1983;31:34–39.
3. National Diabetes Data Group: Classification and diagnosis of diabetes mellitus and other categories of glucose intolerance. *Diabetes* 1979;28: 1039–1057.
4. Davidson MB: The effect of aging on carbohydrate metabolism: a review of the English literature and a practical approach to the diagnosis of diabetes mellitus in the elderly. *Metabolism* 1979;28:688–705.
5. Levin ME: Diabetes: the geriatric difference. *Geriatrics* 1982;37:41–45.

6. Sullivan JB, Mahan CM: Evaluation of age-adjusted criteria for potential diabetes. *Diabetes* 1971;20:811–815.
7. Mahler RJ, Romanoff NE, Dunbar A, et al: The dilemma of defining diabetes mellitus in the aging population. *West J Med* 1982;136:379–383.
8. Swerdloff RS, Pozefsky J, Tobin JD, et al: Influence of age on the intravenous tolbutamide response test. *Diabetes* 1967;16:161–170.
9. Rosenthal M, Doberne L, Greenfield M, et al: Effect of age on glucose tolerance, insulin secretion, and in vivo insulin action. *J Am Geriatr Soc* 1982;30:562–567.
10. Rowe JW, Minaker KL, Pallotta JA, et al: Characterization of the insulin resistance of aging. *J Clin Invest* 1983;71:1581–1587.
11. Fink RI, Kolterman OG, Griffin J, et al: Mechanisms of insulin resistance in aging. *J Clin Invest* 1983;71:1523–1535.
12. Yoshikawa TT: Aging and infectious diseases: state of the art. *Gerontology* 1984;30:275–278.
13. Makinodan T, James J, Inamizu T, et al: Immunologic basis for susceptibility to infection in the aged. *Gerontology* 1984;30:279–289.
14. Bagdade JD, Walters E: Impaired granulocyte adherence in mildly diabetic patients. *Diabetes* 1980;29:307–311.
15. Bagdade JD, Stewart M, Walters E: Impaired granulocyte adherence. *Diabetes* 1977;27:677–681.
16. Molenaar DM, Palumbo PJ, Wilson WR, et al: Leukocyte chemotaxis in diabetic patients and their nondiabetic first-degree relatives. *Diabetes* 1976;25(suppl):880–883.
17. Mowat A, Baum J: Chemotaxis of polymorphonuclear leukocytes from patients with diabetes mellitus. *N Engl J Med* 1971;284:621–627.
18. Miller ME, Baker L: Leukocyte functions in juvenile diabetes mellitus: humoral and cellular aspects. *J Pediatr* 1977;81:979–982.
19. Fikrig SM, Reddy CM, Orti E, et al: Diabetes and neutrophil chemotaxis. *Diabetes* 1977;26:466–468.
20. Bagdade JD, Root RK, Bulger RJ: Impaired leukocyte function in patients with poorly controlled diabetes. *Diabetes* 1974;23:9–15.
21. Tan JS, Anderson JL, Watanakunakorn C, et al: Neutrophil dysfunction in diabetes mellitus. *J Lab Clin Med* 1975;83:26–33.
22. Crosby B, Allison F Jr: Phagocytic and bactericidal capacity of polymorphonuclear leukocytes recovered from venous blood of human beings. *Proc Soc Exp Biol Med* 1966;123:660–664.
23. Repine JE, Clawson CC, Goetz FC: Bactericidal function of neutrophils from patients with acute bacterial infections and from diabetics. *J Infect Dis* 1980;142:869–875.
24. Lipscomb H, Dobson HL, Green JA: Humoral immunity in diabetes mellitus. *South Med J* 1959;52:16–23.
25. Beam TR Jr, Crigler ED, Goldman JK, et al: Antibody response to polyvalent pneumococcal polysaccharide vaccine in diabetics. *JAMA* 1980;244:2621–2624.
26. Ludwig H, Fife M, Schernthaner G, Erdu S, et al: Humoral immunodeficiency to bacterial antigens in patients with juvenile onset diabetes mellitus. *Diabetologia* 1976;12:259–262.
27. Ishibashi T, Kitahara Y, Harada Y, et al: Immunologic features of mice with streptozotocin-induced diabetes. *Diabetes* 1980;29:516–573.
28. Cattaneo R, Saibene V, Pozza G: Peripheral T-lymphocytes in juvenile-onset diabetics (JOD) and in maturity-onset diabetics (MOD). *Diabetes* 1976;25:223–226.

29. MacCuish AC, Urbaniak SJ, Campbell CJ, et al: Phytohemagglutinin transformation and circulating lymphocyte subpopulations in insulin-dependent diabetic patients. *Diabetes* 1974;23:708–712.
30. Delespesse G, Duchateau J, Bastenie PA, et al: Cell-mediated immunity in diabetes mellitus. *Clin Exp Immunol* 1974;18:461–467.
31. Casey JI, Heeter BJ, Klyshevich KA: Impaired response to lymphocytes of diabetic subjects to antigens of *Staphylococcus aureus*. *J Infect Dis* 1977;136: 495–501.
32. Thornton GF: Infections and diabetes. *Med Clin North Am* 1971;55:931–938.
33. Galpin JE: Nosocomial infections of the aged. *J Nosocomial Infect* 1985;1:2–7.
34. Sen P, Louria DB: Infectious complications in the elderly diabetic patient. *Geriatrics* 1983;38:63–72.
35. Puxty JAH, Fox RA: Diabetes mellitus and infection, in Fox RA (ed): *Immunology and Infection in the Elderly*. New York, Churchill Livingstone Inc, 1984, pp 179–201.
36. Gallagher PG, Watanakunakorn C: Group B streptococcal bacteremia in a community teaching hospital. *Am J Med* 1985;78:795–800.
37. Huvos A, Rocha H: Frequency of bacteriuria patients with diabetes mellitus. *N Engl J Med* 1959;261:1213–1216.
38. Pometto D, Rees SB, Younger D, et al: Asymptomatic bacteriuria in diabetes mellitus. *N Engl J Med* 1967;276:1118–1121.
39. Yoshikawa TT: Unique aspects of urinary tract infection in the geriatric population. *Gerontology* 1984;30:339–344.
40. Brown WW, Davis BB, Spry LA, et al: Aging and the kidney. *Arch Intern Med* 1986;146:1790–1795.
41. Thorley JD, Jones SR, Sanford JP: Perinephric abscess. *Medicine* 1974;53: 441–451.
42. Hawes S, Whigham T, Ehrmann S, et al: Emphysematous pyelonephritis. *Infect Surg* 1983;2:191–196.
43. Smith JA, O'Connor JJ, Willis AT: Nasal carriage of *Staphylococcus aureus* in diabetes mellitus. *Lancet* 1966;2:776–777.
44. Tuazon CA: Skin and skin structure infections in the patient at risk: Carrier state of *Staphylococcus aureus*. *Am J Med* 1984;76:166–171.
45. Bessman AN, Sapico FL, Tabatabai M, et al: Persistence of polymicrobial abscesses in the poorly controlled diabetic host. *Diabetes* 1986;35:448–453.
46. Louie T, Bartlett JG, Tally FP, et al: Aerobic and anaerobic bacteria in diabetic foot ulcers. *Ann Intern Med* 1976;85:461–463.
47. Riegels-Nielsen P, Hesselfeldt-Nielsen, Bang-Jensen E, et al: Fournier's gangrene: 5 patients treated with hyperbaric oxygen. *J Urol* 1984;122:918–919.
48. Waldvogel FA, Medoff G, Swartz MN: Osteomyelitis, a review of clinical features, therapeutic considerations and unusual aspects. *N Engl J Med* 1970;282:198–206,260–266,316–322.
49. Raff MJ, Melo J: Anaerobic osteomyelitis. *Medicine* 1978;57:83–103.
50. Ger R: Prevention of major amputations in the diabetic patient. *Arch Surg* 1985;120:1317–1320.
51. Mullen LM, Higgins GK: Incidence of undiscovered adult diabetes in a tuberculosis sanitorium. *Can Med Assoc J* 1963;88:424–451.
52. Weaver RA: Unusual radiographic presentation of pulmonary tuberculosis in diabetic patients. *Am Rev Respir Dis* 1974;109:162–163.
53. Nagami P, Yoshikawa TT: Aging and tuberculosis. *Gerontology* 1984;30: 308–315.

54. Zaky DA, Bentley DW, Lowy K, et al: Malignant external otitis: a severe form of otitis in diabetic patients. *Am J Med* 1976;61:298–302.
55. Caruso VG, Meyerhoff WL: Trauma and infections of the external ear, in Paparella MM, Shumrick DA (eds): *Otolaryngology*. Philadelphia, WB Saunders Co, 1980, vol 2, pp 1345–1353.
56. Casey JI: Host defense and infections in diabetes mellitus, in Ellenberg M, Rifkin H (eds): *Diabetes Mellitus. Theory and Practice*, ed 3. New Hyde Park, NY, Medical Examination Publishing Co, 1983, pp 667–678.
57. Wise G, Goldberg P, Kozinn PJ: Genitourinary candidiasis: diagnosis and treatment. *J Urol* 1976;116:778–780.
58. Nagesha CN, Ananthakrishna NC: Clinical and laboratory study of monilial vaginitis. *Am J Obstet Gynecol* 1970;107:1267–1268.
59. Kauffman CA, Tan JS: *Torulopsis glabrata* renal infection. *Am J Med* 1974;57:217–223.
60. Meyers BR, Wormser G, Hirschman SZ, et al: Rhinocerebral mucormycosis. Premortem diagnosis and therapy. *Arch Intern Med* 1979;139: 557–560.
61. Salaki JS, Louria DB, Chmel H: Fungal and yeast infection of the central nervous system: A clinical review. *Medicine* 1984;63:108–112.
62. Abramson E, Wilson D, Arkey RA: Rhinocerebral phycomycosis in association with diabetic ketoacidosis. A report of two cases and a review of clinical and experimental experience with amphotericin B therapy. *Ann Intern Med* 1967;66:735–742.

23

Immunizations

Peter A. Gross

Just as the prevention of measles, mumps, and rubella are the aim of preventive public health programs in the young, so should the prevention of influenza and pneumococcal disease be the target of public health efforts in the old. The impact of respiratory tract infections with influenza virus and *Streptococcus pneumoniae* in the young is relatively small compared with the impact of these infections in the elderly. Immune senescence, age-associated diseases, concomitant use of diagnostic and therapeutic modalities, and the normal physiologic and anatomical changes of aging all conspire to make influenza and pneumococcal infections significant in the elderly.

INFLUENZA VACCINE

Influenza virus is the only major human virus that is genetically unstable. This characteristic makes control of influenza difficult. As a result of genetic instability, the virus changes in minor ways (*antigenic drift*) frequently and in major ways infrequently (*antigenic shift*).

Antigenic drift occurs every 2 to 3 years for influenza A viruses and every 5 to 7 years for influenza B. Antigenic shift occurs at intervals of 10 or more years for influenza A and does not occur with influenza B. Antigenic shift is associated with local or regional epidemics while antigenic shift is characterized by worldwide pandemics.

The influenza vaccine is updated annually to take into account the changes in prevalent influenza strains. Because of these changes, annual immunization is necessary to protect against new strains. The vaccines in recent years have had two influenza A viruses (an H3N2 strain and an H1N1 strain) and one influenza B strain.

Epidemics of influenza virus infection have been associated with 10,000 or more deaths 15 times in the years between 1957 and 1982. All but one epidemic followed antigenic drift of an influenza A or B strain. Only one epidemic in 1968 was due to a major antigenic shift in the influenza A virus. Some 10,000 excess deaths occurred as recently as the winter of 1982–1983 and this one was due to antigenic drift, that is, a relatively minor change in the influenza A strain.[1]

When excess deaths due to influenza and pneumonia are studied it is apparent that mortality in those aged above 65 years is far in excess of that seen in younger persons.[2-4] Whether age is the key factor or, more likely, the underlying disease is not clear. But it is likely that chronic disorders associated with age such as chronic respiratory diseases, cardiovascular diseases, and diabetes are the significant risk factors.

Transmission of influenza virus in the hospital is a frequent finding during community outbreaks of influenza. Introduction by hospital personnel and visitors permit easy access of the virus to hospitalized patients. The elderly are particularly susceptible to influenza infection in this setting.[5]

The significant and frequent impact of influenza on the population therefore is readily apparent. What is also readily apparent but not widely appreciated is that influenza vaccine is clearly effective in reducing the morbidity and mortality from influenza virus infection. Several studies have documented a reduction in respiratory illness rates, hospitalization rates, and mortality in the elderly.[3-6] While these studies were not randomized, prospective, placebo-controlled clinical trials, conducting such idealized studies in the elderly probably will never be possible given the ethical dictates of our society.

The side effects of the influenza immunization are typically benign and short-lived. Local reactions such as pain and redness at the injection site occur in about one third of vaccinees and last for one to two days. Systemic reactions such as fever and myalgias occur in a few percent of vaccinees and last for one to two days.

Allergic reactions are extremely rare and are usually due to egg proteins. Therefore anyone who has had an anaphylactic reaction on eating eggs should not receive influenza vaccine.

Guillain-Barré syndrome was associated with the swine influenza vaccine given in 1976. The reasons for this association remain unclear. Subsequent influenza vaccines, however, have not been associated with an increased frequency of Guillain-Barré syndrome.[1]

The current vaccines are inactivated vaccines, not live attenuated virus vaccines. The vaccine is composed of either whole virus inactivated by formalin or detergent-treated virus vaccine (so-called split product or subunit vaccine) which is also formalin-inactivated.[7] The route of administration for vaccine is intramuscular. Smaller doses given intradermally may be immunogenic but this route has not been tested in vaccine efficacy studies and is therefore not recommended for routine use.

The target groups for immunization since 1963 have been the persons who are at high risk of lower respiratory tract complications and death following influenza virus infection. Currently, the elderly with chronic disorders of the cardiovascular or pulmonary systems, diabetes, renal disease, severe anemia, or compromised immune function are considered at greatest risk when their medical condition has required regular medical follow-up or hospitalization in the preceding year. Residents of nursing homes and other chronic care facilities are also in this high-risk group.

Medical personnel can transmit influenza to high-risk persons. So physicians, nurses, and other personnel who have close contact with the high-risk elderly patients should also be immunized.

After the immunization needs of these two groups have been met, then vaccine should be made available to otherwise healthy individuals over the age of 65 years as they are at moderately increased risk of serious illness compared with the general population.[1]

After influenza appears in the community, vaccination can still be given. For optimal protection, amantadine hydrochloride should be given for 2 weeks until vaccine-induced immunity develops. Giving amantadine hydrochloride for the entire influenza season, however, is not a cost-effective or safer alternative to vaccination.[1,8]

PNEUMOCOCCAL VACCINE

Pneumococcal pneumonia is still the most common community-acquired pneumonia. The incidence of pneumococcal pneumonia increases with age beginning at 40 years. Over 60 years, the incidence doubles. As a cause of hospital-acquired pneumonia, it is rare. Despite the widespread use of effective antibiotics, the mortality from pneumococcal bacteremia is as high as 40% in high-risk patients. The mortality associated with pneumococcal meningitis is even higher.[9]

The conditions likely to place a person at high risk of serious complications of pneumococcal pneumonia are sickle cell anemia, Hodgkin's disease, multiple myeloma, cirrhosis, alcoholism, nephrotic syndrome, renal failure, chronic pulmonary diseases, other causes of splenic dysfunction, and a history of splenectomy or organ transplant.

Other patient groups may also be at greater risk of acquiring pneumococcal infection or of developing severe complications of infection. The groups include those with diabetes mellitus, congestive heart failure, or immunosuppressive conditions. Patients with a cerebrospinal fluid leak from a skull fracture or neurosurgical procedure may develop recurrent meningitis due to the pneumococcus.

Pneumococcal vaccine has been a subject of investigation for many decades. Polysaccharide vaccines were tested as early as the 1930s. The current multivalent polysaccharide vaccines were licensed within the past 10 years. In 1977, a 14-valent vaccine was approved for use and in 1983, a 23-valent vaccine was licensed. The 23 bacterial types in the latest vaccine include 87% of the strains responsible for bacteremic pneumococcal disease in the United States. The 14-valent vaccine had covered 71% of the strains.[10]

While patients with these conditions are considered at high risk, the precise degree of risk has not been clearly defined. A large scale study was done in the elderly by Kaufman in the 1940s.[11] There were more than 5000 persons each in the vaccinated and unvaccinated groups. He demonstrated a 79% protective efficacy against types 1, 2, and 3. However, the incidence of the other types increased in the vaccinated group compared with the control group. And the vaccine was more effective in the first year following vaccination than it was in subsequent years.[11]

Multivalent vaccines have been recently tested in South African miners and in New Guinea where the incidence of pneumococcal disease is high.[12,13] While the vaccine efficacy was high, the relevance of these studies to vaccine efficacy in the elderly is unclear. In two recent studies conducted in the elderly, a low incidence of pneumococcal disease prevented an adequate test of vaccine efficacy.[14] In another study, vaccine efficacy was estimated to be 70% for all patients over 55 years of age.[15]

Vaccination is indicated in all those considered at high risk as described previously. In addition, it is now recommended in all adults over 65 years of age. Caution should be taken to administer vaccine to patients scheduled for splenectomy 2 weeks before the procedure. In addition, when vaccinating immunosuppressed patients, vaccine should be given so as to provide the longest interval possible between vaccination and initiation of immunosuppressive therapy.

Pneumococcal vaccine can be given at the same time as influenza vaccine without any adverse effect on immunogenicity of either vaccine.[16]

Consideration should be given to providing vaccine at the end of hospitalization for high-risk patients. Two thirds of persons who will develop serious pneumococcal disease are likely to be hospitalized within 5 years of that illness.[17,18] Consequently, a concerted effort to immunize patients at the time of discharge will be effective in most of the target population. Third-party payers will reimburse for pneumococcal vaccine.

Administration of pneumococcal vaccine is associated with local pain and redness at the injection site in about half of the vaccine recipients. Less than 1% of vaccinees will develop systemic symptoms of fever and myalgias. Allergic reactions are rare.

Revaccination is not currently recommended because Arthus reactions and systemic reactions are common following a second dose.[19]

Persons who have received the 14-valent vaccine should not be revaccinated with the newer 23-valent vaccine. The vaccine is not recommended for healthy pregnant women.

The duration of immunity is thought to be at least 5 years. Reactions to revaccination may be less as immunity wanes. This phenomenon is currently being investigated.

TETANUS TOXOID

Immunity to tetanus toxoid may be waning in many elderly persons. Either booster immunizations may not have been kept up to date or a complete primary series was never received. These reasons account in part for the above-average susceptibility to tetanus in the elderly.[20]

Immunization with adult Td (tetanus and diphtheria toxoids) should be done every 10 years in the primary care setting and at the time of penetrating trauma. If the history of prior immunization is questionable, human tetanus immune globulin should be administered in conjunction with tetanus toxoid.[21]

VACCINES FOR TRAVELERS

Many elderly persons are likely to spend time traveling in foreign countries. In most developing countries and many developed countries the childhood diseases (measles, rubella, mumps, diphtheria, and polio) are still common. Adequate protection against these diseases should be ensured if exposure is likely.

For polio, the killed or inactivated polio vaccine (IPV, Salk vaccine) given subcutaneously is preferred to the live attenuated oral polio vaccine (OPV, Sabin vaccine). The incidence of vaccine-associated polio, while small, is nevertheless increased in adults following OPV administration.[22]

The indications for vaccines against yellow fever, cholera, hepatitis B, meningococcal meningitis, typhoid, plague, Japanese encephalitis, and rabies should be reviewed for each individual and for each itinerary. Smallpox vaccine should no longer be administered.[23]

REFERENCES

1. Immunization Practices Advisory Committee: 1986–1987 update on vaccine and antiviral agent available for control of influenza. *MMWR* 1986;35:1–9.
2. Eickhoff TC, Sherman IL, Serfling RE: Observations on excess mortality associated with epidemic influenza. *JAMA* 1961;176:776–782.
3. Patriarca PA, Weber JA, Parker RA, et al: Efficacy of influenza vaccine in nursing homes. Reduction in illness and complications during an influenza A (H3N2) epidemic. *JAMA* 1985;253:1136–1139.

4. Barker WH, Mullooly JP: Pneumonia and influenza death during epidemics: implications for prevention. *Arch Intern Med* 1982;142:85–89.
5. Van Voris LP, Belshe RB, Shaffer JL: Nosocomial influenza B virus infection in the elderly. *Ann Intern Med* 1982;96:153.
6. Glezen WP, Six HR, Frank AL, et al: *Impact of Epidemics upon Communities and Families. Options for the Control of Influenza.* New York, Alan R Liss, 1986, pp 63–73.
7. Gross PA, Ennis FA: Influenza vaccine: split product versus whole virus types — how do they differ?, editorial. *N Engl J Med* 1977;296:567–568.
8. Horadam VW, Sharp JG, Smilack JD, et al: Pharmacokinetics of amantadine hydrochloride in subjects with normal and impaired renal function. *Ann Intern Med* 1981;94:454–458.
9. Austrian R: Pneumococcal pneumonia: Diagnostic, epidemiologic, therapeutic and prophylactic considerations. *Chest* 1986;90:738–743.
10. Broome CV, Facklam RR: Epidemiology of clinically significant isolates of *Streptococcus pneumoniae* in the United States. *Rev Infect Dis* 1981;3:277–281.
11. Kaufman P: Pneumonia in old age: Active immunization against pneumonia with pneumococcus polysaccharide; results of a six year study. *Arch Intern Med* 1947;79:518–531.
12. Austrian R, Douglas RM, Schiffman G, et al: Prevention of pneumococcal pneumonia by vaccination. *Trans Assoc Am Physicians* 1976;89:184–194.
13. Riley ID, Tarr PI, Andrews M, et al: Immunization with a polyvalent pneumococcal vaccine. Reduction of adult respiratory mortality in a New Guinea Highlands community. *Lancet* 1975;1:1338–1341.
14. Austrian R: *Surveillance of Pneumococcal Infection for Field Trials of Polyvalent Pneumococcal Vaccines*. Report DAB-VDP-12-84. Bethesda, Md, National Institutes of Health 1980.
15. Shapiro ED, Clemens JD: A controlled evaluation of the protective efficacy of pneumococcal vaccine for patients at high risk for serious pneumococcal infections. *Ann Intern Med* 1984;101:325–330.
16. DeStefano F, Goodman RA, Noble GR, et al: Simultaneous administration of influenza and pneumococcal vaccines. *JAMA* 1982;247:2551–2554.
17. Partriarca PA, Weber JA, Parker RA, et al: Risk factors for outbreaks of influenza in nursing home A case-control study. *Am J Epidemiol* 1986;124:114–119.
18. Barker WH: Influenza and nursing homes. *Am J Public Health* 1986;76:491–492.
19. Borgono JM, McLean AA, Vella PP, et al: Vaccination and revaccination with polyvalent pneumococcal polysaccharide vaccines in adults and infants. *Proc Soc Exp Biol Med* 1978;157:148–154.
20. Levine L, Wyman L: Survey of immunity of serologic methods: Results of three successive surveys of samples of the Massachusetts population for diphtheria and tetanus anti-toxin. *N Engl J Med* 1965;272:23–26.
21. Centers for Disease Control: *Toxoids. Adult Immunization: Recommendations of the Immunization Practices Advisory Committee*. *MMWR* 1984;33:10S–12S.
22. Centers for Disease Control: *Both Live-Virus and Inactivated-Virus Vaccines: Recommendations of the Immunization Practices Advisory Committee*. *MMWR* 33:20S–21S.
23. *Guide for Adult Immunization*, ed 1. Committee on Immunization, Council of Medical Societies, Philadelphia, American College of Physicians, 1985.

24

Antimicrobial Therapy

Burke A. Cunha

RENAL AND HEPATIC FUNCTION IN THE ELDERLY

Many age-related changes occur in the kidney as normal physiologic changes during the aging process. The normal renal mass of the kidneys decreases with age from approximately 250 g in the young adult to less than 200 g by age 70 years. The decrease in renal mass is primarily due to the loss of cortical mass. The total number of glomeruli are reduced by about 50% by age 70. Additionally, the number of nonfunctioning sclerotic glomeruli increase concurrently and may involve approximately 30% of the total nephron population. Renal vascular changes also occur with age and result in an altered renal blood flow pattern. Blood flow to the cortex selectively decreases and is preferentially directed to the medullary areas of the kidneys in the elderly. Furthermore, renal plasma flow decreases to less than 50% in patients over 70 years of age, which may be, in part, related to decreases in cardiac output associated with aging. Renal tubular function also decreases with age and parallels the decreases in renal blood flow. The reduction in renal tubular function is proportional to the remaining functioning nephron mass in the elderly patient. Elderly patients with these age-related renal changes also have difficulties with water conservation and have a salt-wasting tendency. Older adults appear to be more likely to develop syndrome of inappropriate secretion of antidiuretic hormone (SIADH) than young adults. In the geriatric patient, a proportional decrease in the length of the proximal convoluted tubule decreases proportionately with glomerular loss. Clinically, this results in a parallel decline in glomerular and tubular function with aging[1-3] (Table 24-1).

Table 24-1
Pharmacokinetic Age-Related Changes
in the Elderly

Pharmacokinetic Parameters	Age-Related Changes
Absorption	↓ Absorptive surface
(↓ gastrointestinal motility)	↑ Gastric pH
Distribution	↓ Total body water
(↓ body mass)	↑ Fat
Metabolism	↓ Liver blood flow
(↓ hepatic mass)	↑ Hepatic fibrosis
Excretion	↓ Glomerular filtration rate
(↓ renal mass)	↓ Tubular secretory function
	↓ Renal perfusion

SYSTEMIC DISEASES

It is important to emphasize that the normal physiologic process of aging and the obligatory decrease in renal function does not take into account the secondary factors which clearly affect renal function in the elderly. Elderly patients have a high incidence of systemic diseases which frequently cause or worsen the primary renal dysfunction associated with aging. Systemic diseases including arteriosclerosis, hypertension, congestive heart failure, diabetes mellitus, or malignancy are increased with advancing age. In the geriatric patient, the renal insufficiency is usually on a multifactorial basis and most frequently results from the combination of physiologic changes, superimposed systemic illnesses, etc, that affect the kidney. Other factors, such as urinary tract infections or nephrotoxic drugs, may also further decrease renal function on a transient basis. Multisystem disease more profoundly affects renal dysfunction in the already elderly compromised kidney than it does in the younger adult patient. Furthermore, renal diseases in the elderly tend to be more severe and prolonged than in the younger population. The most frequent renal diseases encountered in elderly patients include proliferative, cresentic, and membranous glomerulonephritis. The systemic diseases most frequently associated with renal involvement and insufficiency are vasculitis, amyloidosis and malignancy (multiple myeloma, lymphoma, etc). Interstitial nephritis and acute tubular necrosis as well as obstructive uropathy (secondary to prostatic enlargement or stone disease) is particularly frequent in the elderly [2-4] (Table 24-2).

RENAL FUNCTION TESTS

Renal function should not be estimated from the serum creatinine in elderly patients. The majority of elderly patients will have a greatly

Table 24-2
Renal Diseases in the Elderly

Renal Disease	Elderly Adults ($\geq$ 60 years)	Increased Incidence over Normal Adults ($\leq$ 60 years)
Crescentic glomerulonephritis	16.5%	4×
Membranous glomerulonephritis	13.0%	2.5×
Proliferative glomerulonephritis	4.0%	2×
Glomerulosclerosis	13.0%	1.5×
Vasculitis	5.0%	2×
Amyloidosis	4.0%	4×
Wegener's granulomatosis	3.0%	15×

Adapted from Samiy.[2]

reduced glomerular filtration rate (GFR) and yet maintain a normal serum creatinine. Creatinine excretion is related to muscle mass and is proportionally less in the elderly individual with decreased body mass. The decrease in renal function associated with aging is adequate to compensate for the decreased creatinine load, and therefore the serum creatinine remains at normal or near normal levels. Nomograms correcting for age are inaccurate and should not be routinely employed in predicting the serum creatinine. However, creatinine clearance may be approximated by a variety of calculations. A useful formula to estimate creatinine clearance is:

$$\text{Men} = \frac{(140 - \text{age}) \times \text{body weight (kg)}}{72 \times \text{serum creatinine level}}$$

$$\text{Women} = 0.85 \times \text{value for men}$$

Glomerular function is best assessed in the elderly patient by a 24-hour creatinine clearance. An eight-hour creatinine clearance may be adequate if it is not possible to obtain a 24-hour sample. Renal tubular function may be assessed by measuring the morning urine osmolarity after overnight fluid deprivation. As the result of the significant decrease in renal function in the elderly, drugs normally excreted via the renal route will have altered pharmacokinetics in elderly patients. Drugs with a "narrow" toxic-therapeutic ratio excreted via the kidney should not be given a full dose but rather should take into account the 30% to 40% decrease in GFR in the aged patient.[1,2]

LIVER FUNCTION TESTS

Traditionally, tests of liver function have not correlated well with hepatic function. Therefore abnormalities in serum transaminases, total bilirubin, or alkaline phosphatase are not proportional to decreases in hepatic inactivation and excretory function. Drugs that are primarily eliminated by hepatic metabolism may require dosage modification in patients with significant liver disease. Furthermore, abnormal liver function tests may be misleading since they are elevated in a variety of conditions. Specifically, alkaline phosphatase levels have been associated with extrahepatic biliary infection in the elderly. Nonhepatobiliary sepsis in elderly patients is not associated with increases in serum transaminase or bilirubin levels. The mechanism of alkaline phosphatase elevation in elderly patients is not known. Physiologically, both liver and bone alkaline phosphatase isoenzymes increase with age. As the kidney undergoes a decrease in functional capacity with age, it appears that similar age-related physiologic changes occur in the functional capacity of the liver. In elderly patients the most important diseases of the liver that have been shown to adversely affect liver function are cirrhosis and viral hepatitis. Unfortunately, relatively few antibiotics are excreted via the hepatic route and dosage modifications are not necessary with the majority of these agents with the exception of chloramphenicol and metronidazole in situations where liver function is known to be significantly impaired.[5-8]

ANTIBIOTIC DOSING CONSIDERATIONS

Antibiotics with "wide" toxic-therapeutic ratios that are eliminated via the renal route need little or no dosage adjustment in elderly patients with mild to moderate renal insufficiency. Drugs with a "narrow" toxic-therapeutic ratio usually need to be administered in reduced dose and/or decreased dosing frequency in elderly patients with even mild renal dysfunction. Commonly used antibiotics that are eliminated primarily via the renal route include the penicillins (except nafcillin), the first-, second-, and third-generation cephalosporins (except cefoperazone), trimethoprim-sulfamethoxazole (TMP-SMX), the aminoglycosides, the tetracyclines (except doxycycline), polymyxin B, pentamidine, and vancomycin. While dosing adjustments may be calculated on the basis of measured renal function, that is, 8- or 24-hour creatinine clearance determinations, renally eliminated drugs with a narrow toxic-therapeutic ratio should be avoided in patients with moderately severe renal insufficiency. In such situations, the use of an antibiotic primarily eliminated via nonrenal mechanisms, with an appropriate spectrum, would be preferable. Dosage modifications for hepatic insufficiency need to be considered only in patients with moderate to severe liver dysfunction. The serum albumin remains the best overall test of liver dysfunction; only chloramphenicol and metronidazole usually require dosage modification. Mild liver dysfunction probably implies a decrease of about 25% in the functional capacity of the liver. Moderately severe liver disease and severe liver disease signifies an approximately 50% to 75% decrease in hepatic function respectively. As with severe renal insufficiency, hepatically metabolized drugs should probably not be used in patients with severe reduction in liver function. In such situations, the use of an antibiotic, with an appropriate spectrum, excreted primarily by renal mechanisms, would be preferable.[9]

ANTIBIOTIC DOSING MODIFICATIONS

A variety of approaches (nomograms, formulas, computer programs, etc) have been used to estimate the correct dosage of antibiotics in patients with renal insufficiency. However, these estimation methods are cumbersome and complicated and have not been shown to be better than making an estimate based on the degree of renal impairment. A useful rule which applies to most renally eliminated antibiotics is as follows:

Formula for Renal Insufficiency

Moderate renal insufficiency (creatinine clearance ~50 mL/min):
Administer *half* the usual dose, but maintain the *usual* dosing interval.

Severe renal insufficiency (creatinine clearance ~10mL/min):
Administer *half* the usual dose and *double* the normal dosing interval.

Example: Cefazolin (first-generation cephalosporin)
Normal renal function (creatinine clearance ~100 mL/min):
Usual cefazolin sodium dose: 1 g IV q8h

Moderately severe renal insufficiency (creatinine ~50 mL/min):
Cefazolin sodium dose: 500 mg IV q8h

Severe renal insufficiency (creatinine clearance 10 mL/min):
Cefazolin sodium dose: 500 mg IV q16h

Utilizing this simple and easily remembered formula applied for the majority renally eliminated antibiotics, a reasonable estimation of the correct dose based on approximation of creatinine clearance.[9,10]

Formula for Hepatic insufficiency

In patients with hepatic insufficiency, proper dosing may be estimated from the degree of liver dysfunction.

Mild hepatic Insufficiency (25% reduction in functional capacity):

No dosage adjustment is usually necessary.

Moderately severe hepatic dysfunction (~10% reduction in functional capacity)
Administer *half* the usual dose.

Example: Chloramphenicol

Normal hepatic function:
Usual chloramphenicol dose (for patients without meningitis): 1g IV q6h

Moderate hepatic insufficiency (~50% reduction in functional capacity):
Chloramphenicol dose: 500 mg IV q6h

Severe hepatic dysfunction (10% reduction in functional capacity):
Chloramphenicol dose: 500 mg IV q12h

In the event of combined hepatic and renal insufficiency frequently seen in multisystem disease or trauma, complicated dosing calculations may be necessary, but no good guidelines exist. Therefore it would seem preferable to use drugs whose half-lives are not appreciably altered with significant hepatic or renal dysfunction. That is, doxycycline or cefoperazone. Both of these drugs may be used in full dosage in patients with significant hepatorenal dysfunction[9-11] (Table 24-3).

ANTIBIOTIC DOSING IN DIALYSIS PATIENTS

Because elderly patients are more frequently affected by renal disease than the younger adult population, progressive renal disease leading to renal failure is frequent. Chronic renal failure patients are usually managed by a variety of dialysis regimens; chronic ambulatory peritoneal dialysis (CAPD) and hemodialysis are the most commonly used techniques. Again, most clinicians caring for elderly dialysis patients need assistance with antibiotic dosing in this setting. General guidelines are usually better than complicated formulas since both approaches are only estimates, although both are fairly accurate.

Most antibiotics are removed to some degree by the dialysis process. In addition, metabolism (elimination) of the antibiotic continues during the dialysis period. Dosing estimates should take both of these factors into account.

Since most antibiotics are affected by dialysis, some modifications of dosage (see above) to account for the lack of renal function before and between dialysis treatments are usually necessary, and frequently a post-

Table 24-5
Common Infections in the Elderly: Antibiotic Selection

		Clinically Equivalent		Renal Function	
	Usual Pathogens	Usual *Pre*-Drug Selection	Most Cost-Effective Drug Selection	Normal to Mild Renal Insufficiency	Moderate to Severe Renal Insufficiency
Pneumonias					
Aspiration	Oral anaerobic flora	Penicillin	Cefonicid	Doxycycline or Clindamycin Cefonicid	Doxycycline or clindamycin
Community-acquired (normal ambulatory host)	Pneumococci Group A streptococci Staphylococcus aureus Klebsiella Haemophilus influenzae	Cefazolin	Cefonicid	Cefonicid or Cefuroxime	Ceftizoxime
Community-acquired (nursing home, chronic care facility, ETOH, diabetes mellitus)	Pneumococci H influenzae Klebsiella	Cefazolin TMP-SMX	Cefonicid	Cefuroxime or cefonicid	Ceftizoxime or chloramphenicol or ciprofloxacin
Nosocomial	Pseudomonas aeruginosa Gram-negative bacilli S aureus Pneumococci	Anti-*Pseudomonas* penicillin plus aminoglycoside or ceftazidime plus vancomycin	Cefoperazone (plus azthreonam only if *Pseudomonas* proved)	Cefoperazone (plus azthreonam only if *Pseudomonas* proved)	Cefoperazone (plus azthreonam only if *Pseudomonas* proved) Doxycycline
Atypical	Legionella pneumophila Legionella-like organisms (LLO's) Mycoplasma	Erythromycin	Doxycycline	Doxycycline	

Table 24-5 (con't)
Common Infections in the Elderly: Antibiotic Selection

		Clinically Equivalent		Renal Function	
	Usual Pathogens	Usual *Pre*-Drug Drug Selection	Most Cost-Effective Drug Selection	Normal to Mild Renal Insufficiency	Moderate to Severe Renal Insufficiency
Urinary Tract Infections					
Catheter-associated					
Low risk	*Escherichia coli*	Ampicillin	Nitrofurantoin	Nitrofurantoin	Erythromycin
High risk	Enterococci	TMP-SMX	Ciprofloxacin	Ciprofloxacin	Ciprofloxacin
Urosepsis	Gram-negative organisms Enterococci	Ampicillin or aminoglycoside or TMP-SMX	Ampicillin or aminoglycoside or TMP-SMX	Ampicillin or azthreonam or ceftizoxime	Ampicillin or azthreonam
Skin Infections					
Above waist	*S aureus* Group A streptococci	Antistaphylococcal penicillin	Cefonicid	Cefazolin	Nafcillin
Below waist	*S aureus* Group A streptococci *E coli* *Proteus mirabilis* *Klebsiella*	Cefazolin	Cefonicid	Cefazolin	Cefazolin
Decubitus ulcers	*S aureus* Group A streptococci *E coli* *P mirabilis* *Klebsiella* *Bacteroides fragilis*	Ceftizoxime Cefoxitin or Clindamycin plus aminoglycoside	Cefoperazone	Ceftizoxime	Cefoperazone

TMP-SMX = trimethoprim-sulfamethoxazole.

dialysis supplemental dose is required. With the exception of penicillin G, ampicillin, cefothxime, ceftriaxone, polymyxin B, amphotericin B, and vancomycin, renally eliminated antibiotics are dialyzable. Except for dosing modifications appropriate for the degree of renal insufficiency, additional changes in dose need to be made with antibiotics that are poorly dialyzed. Guidelines for dosing are presented in Table 24-4. In situations when data on dosing are unavailable or estimates are complicated or uncertain, then the use of antibiotics cleared by nonrenal mechanisms, with the appropriate spectrum, is preferable, for example, cefoperazone.[9-11]

COMMON INFECTIONS IN ELDERLY PATIENTS

The most common infections encountered in the geriatric population in the ambulatory and inpatient settings are bacterial pneumonias, urinary tract infections, and skin infections, for example, infected decubitus ulcers. The organisms responsible for pneumonias in the elderly are

Table 24-4
Practical Guide to Antimicrobial Therapy in Dialysis Patients

*Antibiotics Affected by Dialysis**
(dosage modification required)
  Hemodialysis
  1. Dose and dosing interval same as for severe renal insufficiency
  2. Postdialysis supplemental dose
     a. Antibiotics with wide toxic-therapeutic ratios: give *full* usual dose following dialysis
     b. Antibiotics with narrow toxic-therapeutic ratios: give *half* usual dose following dialysis
  Peritoneal Dialysis
  1. Dose and dosing interval same as for severe renal insufficiency
  2. Postdialysis supplemental dose
     a. Not usually required; if any doubt regarding serum concentrations, measure serum levels and
     b. Add antibiotic to dialysate fluid at serum concentrations
Antibiotics Unaffected by Dialysis
(no dosage modification required)
  Poorly dialyzed antibiotics

Penicillin G	Vancomycin
Ampicillin	Erythromycin
Cefatoxime	Metronidazole
Ceftriaxone	Clindamycin
Cefoperazone	Chloramphenicol
Polymyxin B	Doxycycline
Amphotericin B	

*Dosing by serum levels is always preferred.

the same as for the general adult population except there is an increased incidence of *Klebsiella* and *Haemophilus influenzae* in these patients, especially in nursing home patients. Legionnaires' disease and, to a lesser extent, mycoplasma pneumonia are being recognized with increasing frequency in elderly patients. Aspiration pneumonia due to oropharyngeal organisms of nosocomial origin is a frequent occurrence in this patient population with impaired gag reflexes. Elderly patients with urinary tract infections are of particular interest since renal dysfunction may be further compromised by a superimposed urinary tract infection. Obstructive uropathy due to stone disease or prostatic hypertrophy is common in the elderly and is a frequent cause of urosepsis in these patients. Many geriatric patients have indwelling Foley catheters which are readily colonized and may, in some patients, progress to upper tract disease or bacteremia.

Escherichia coli and aerobic gram-negative bacilli are the predominant pathogens in patients with obstructive uropathy or stone disease. *Escherichia coli* and group D streptococci (enterococci) are the most frequent pathogens in patients with indwelling Foley catheters. Skin infections in the elderly include cellulitis and pyoderma. In addition, the elderly skin is friable as a result of advancing age and these changes may be exacerbated by certain medications, for example, steroids. Elderly patients may have limited ability to turn themselves and are thus predisposed to skin breakdown with subsequent decubitus ulcer formation. Decubitus ulcers on the back and legs are quickly colonized by the skin flora below the waist (*Staphylococcus aureus*, group A streptococci, *E coli*, *Proteus mirabilis*, or *Klebsiella*). Deep infections of the soft tissues or bone may result from prolonged or penetrating infected decubitus ulcers. Elderly patients with diabetes and foot ulcers have all of the organisms mentioned above as potential pathogens, and, in addition, have *Bacteroides fragilis* as an important copathogen in this setting. Therefore coverage should be directed against aerobic gram-negative bacilli, *S aureus*, as well as *B fragilis*.

After appropriate diagnostic specimens are obtained, the early use of empiric antimicrobial therapy in elderly patients may be lifesaving. For non-life-threatening infections, drugs should be selected that are cost-effective, in the drug related group (DRG) sense, and are safe and easy to administer. As a general rule, "polypharmacy" should be avoided, if possible, in elderly patients. The average nursing home patient takes four to seven nonantibiotic medications per day, and a hospitalized patient takes ten to twelve nonantibiotic medications per day. In terms of a current cost-benefit analysis, it is preferable to use monotherapy versus combination therapy, and use drugs with long serum half-lives if possible. Appropriate spectra and the concern for potential toxicity remain the primary considerations in antibiotic selection. The anatomical location determines the appropriate empiric spectrum. For example, in the elderly patient with pneumonia, coverage should be directed against the pneumococcus, *Klebsiella*, and *H influenzae*. In the pre-DRG era, a first-generation cephalosporin, for example, cefonicid, would be a reason-initial empiric therapy. Currently, it is more cost-effective to use a long-acting second-generation cephalosporin, for example, cefonicid, which has good activity against the pneumococci and *Klebsiella*, better activity against *H influenzae* than cefazolin, and costs less to the institution than cefozalin on a daily basis. If an elderly patient with severe renal insufficiency presents with a pneumonia, and initial empiric therapy is required before culture results are obtainable, then the use of a hepatically metabolized drug without compromising the spectrum is advisable. Antibiotics such as chloramphenicol and cefoperazone would be particularly useful in this situation. Considering antimicrobial therapy in an elderly patient with pneumonia with severe hepatic disease, the use of a long-acting ond-generation cephalosporin, for example, cefonicid, would be a reasonable and cost-effective choice (Table 24-5).

If aspiration pneumonia is the working diagnosis and the patient is not penicillin-allergic, then penicillin may be given to elderly patients with all but the most extreme degrees of renal insufficiency. Again, in the current cost-conscious DRG era, a long-acting second-generation cephalosporin would be as effective and appropriate, and would be of less cost to the institution in treating such a patient. Patients that have been hospitalized for more than a week or that are residents of nursing homes are frequently colonized with *Pseudomonas aeruginosa*. When such patients aspirate and develop pneumonia, *Pseudomonas* becomes an important organism to cover in addition to the aspirated oropharyngeal flora. Cefoperazone is an ideal choice in the elderly patient with normal or abnormal renal or hepatic function since it provides the least expensive effective monotherapy in such patients. For elderly patients with suspected Legionnaires' disease, empiric therapy with erythromycin is appropriate if liver function is not severely compromised. In patients with suspected Legionnaires' disease or severe hepatic disease, doxycycline would be an appropriate and less costly anti-*Legionella* therapy.[12]

Patients that are not frankly septic from the urinary tract may be treated with a variety of orally administered urinary antiseptic agents. Patients with obstructive uropathy or stone disease will not be cured by antimicrobial therapy alone and require surgical correction of the lesion for resolution of the infectious process. Patients with catheter-associated bacteriuria usually do not require treatment since they are more commonly colonized than infected. However, if therapy is desired, then nitrofurantoin provides the best coverage against catheter-associated organisms, that is, *E coli* and group D streptococci. Nitrofurantoin should not be used in elderly patients with a creatinine clearance of less than 40 mL/min. Alternately, TMP-SMX may be given to patients with a

Table 24-3
Practical Guide to Antimicrobial Therapy in Hepatic and Renal Insufficiency in Adults

Antibiotic	Normal Dose	Route	Normal Dosing Interval	Renal Insufficiency			Hepatic Insufficiency	
				Mild	Moderate	Severe	Moderate	Severe
Penicillin G	2–4 μ	IV	q4h	No △	1–2 μ IV q4h	1–2 μ IV q8h	No △	No △
Ampicillin	1–2 g	IV	q4h	No △	0.5–1.0 g IV q4h	0.5–1.0 g IV q8h	No △	No △
Oxacillin	2 g	IV	q4h	No △	1 g IV q4h	1 g IV q8h	No △	No △
Nafcillin	2 g	IV	q4h	No △	No △	No △	1g Iv q4h	1g IV q8h
Anti-*Pseudomonas* penicillins (Ticarcillin, Azlocillin, Mezlocillin, Piperacillin sodium)	3 g	IV	q4h	No △	1.5 g IV q4h	1.5 g IV q8h	No △	No △
Sulbactam/Ampicillin	1.5 g	IV	q6h	No △	750 mg IV q6h	750 mg IV q12h	No △	No △
Erythromycin	1 g	IV	q6h	No △	No △	No △	500 mg IV q6h	500 mg IV q12h
Tetracycline	500 mg	IV	q6h	Avoid	Avoid	Avoid	Avoid	Avoid
Minocycline	100 mg	IV	q12h	No △	No △	50 mg IV q12h	No △	No △
Doxycycline	100 mg	IV	q12h	No △	No △	No △	No △	No △
Rifampin	600 mg	PO	q6h	No △	No △	No △	300 mg PO q6h	300 mg PO q12h
Gentamicin sulfate	80 mg	IV	q8h	40 mg IV q8h	40 mg IV q16h	Avoid*	No △	No △
Tobramycin	80 mg	IV	q8h	40 mg IV q8h	40 mg IV q16h	Avoid*	No △	No △
Amikacin	500 mg	IV	q12h	250 mg IV q12h	250 mg IV q24h	Avoid*	No △	No △
Aztreonam	2 g	IV	q8h	No △	1 g IV q8h	1 g IV q16h	No △	No △
Trimethoprim-sulfamethoxazole	10–20 mg/kg/d in 4 ÷ doses	IV	q6h	No △	5–10 mg/kg/d in 4 ÷ doses IV q6h	5–10 mg/kg/d in 4 ÷ doses IV q12h	No △	No △

Table 24-3 (con't)

Antibiotic	Normal Dose	Route	Normal Dosing Interval	Renal Insufficiency Mild	Moderate	Severe	Hepatic Insufficiency Moderate	Severe
Cephalexin	1 g	PO	q6h	No △	0.5 g PO q6h	0.5 g PO q12h	No △	No △
Cephalothin sodium	2 g	IV	q4h	No △	1 g IV q4h	1 g IV q8h	No △	No △
Cefazolin sodium	1 g	IV	q8h	No △	500 mg IV q8h	500 mg IV q16h	No △	No △
Cefuroxime	1.5 g	IV	q8h	No △	750 mg IV q8h	750 mg IV q16h	No △	No △
Cefonicid	2 g	IV	q24h	1 g IV q24h	1 g IV q48h	Avoid	No △	No △
Cefoxitin	2 g	IV	q6h	No △	1 g IV q6h	1 g IV q12h	No △	No △
Cefotaxime sodium	2 g	IV	q6h	No △	1 g IV q6h	1 g IV q12h	No △	No △
Cefotizoxime sodium	2 g	IV	q8h	No △	1 g IV q8h	1 g IV q16h	No △	No △
Ceftazidime	2 g	IV	q8h	No △	1 g IV q8h	1 g IV q16h	No △	No △
Ceftriaxone sodium	2 g	IV	q12h	1 g IV q12h	1 g IV q24h	Avoid	No △	No △
Cefoperazone sodium	2 g	IV	q12h	No △	No △	No △	No △	No △
Nitrofurantoin	100 mg	PO	q6h	100 mg PO q6h	Avoid	Avoid	No △	No △
Clindamycin	900 mg	IV	q8h	No △	No △	No △	500 mg IV q8h	500 mg IV q16h
Chloramphenicol	1–2 g	IV	q6h	No △	No △	No △	0.5–1.0 IV q6h	0.5–1.0 IV q12h
Vancomycin hydrochloride	500 mg	IV	q6h	250 mg IV q6h	250 mg IV q12h	500 mg IV q7d	No △	No △
Polymyxin B sulfate	10,000 u	IM	q12h	5000 u IM q12h	2500 u IM q12h	2500 u IM q24h	No △	No △
Metronidazole	500 mg	IV	q6h	No △	No △	No △	250 mg IV q6h	250 mg IV q12h
Amantadine hydrochloride	200 mg	PO	q24h	100 mg PO q24h	100 mg PO q48h	200 mg PO q7d	No △	No △
Acyclovir	500 mg	PO	q4h	No △	250 mg PO q4h	250 mg PO q8h	No △	No △
Imipenem	0.5–1.0 g	IV	q6h	250–500 mg IV q6h	250–500 mg IV q12h	Avoid	No △	No △
Ciprofloxacin	500 mg	PO	q12h	No △	250 mg PO q12h	250 mg PO q24h	No	No

* Dosing should be guided by serum levels.

creatinine clearance of less than 20 mL/min. Ampicillin should be used only if the organism is sensitive to the drug since widespread resistance to ampicillin exists. Ampicillin remains the preferred drug for known enterococcal urinary tract infections. Azthreonam in place of aminoglycosides should be used if possible in urosepsis in the elderly patient. In this situation, a third-generation cephalosporin with a high degree of activity against the common uropathogens (excluding group D streptococci) would be appropriate, for example, cefotaxime, or ceftizoxime. If significant renal insufficiency exists, then cefoperazone or ciprofloxacin may be used in such patients to provide both aerobic gram-negative and enterococcal coverage at the lowest possible cost.

Decubitus ulcers are usually colonized and ordinarily should be treated with local antiseptic solutions. Penetrating decubitus ulcers/bone involvement may be treated with a first-generation cephalosporin, for example, cefazolin (if methicillin-resistant *S aureus* is not a consideration). The dosage of cefazolin does not usually have to be modified in patients with mild renal insufficiency. Long-acting drugs such as cefonicid or ciprofloxacin are useful in the nursing home setting in patients with reasonable renal function. If renal insufficiency is a consideration, then cefoperazone would offer the least nephrotoxic approach to the problem. Patients with diabetic foot ulcers are usually treated with drugs like cefoxitin or alternately may be treated with clindamycin combinations (TMP-SMX or aminoglycosides). Cefoxitin or sulbactam ampicillin may be used in patients with mild to moderate degrees of renal insufficiency. In patients with advanced renal disease (ie, diabetic patients with nephrosclerosis) cefoperazone provides an appropriate spectrum, no nephrotoxic potential, and is cost-effective.

Elderly patients with hepatic or renal insufficiency may require dosing adjustments based on the decrease in organ function. Estimates may be made based on the degree of organ dysfunction. The preferred method for determining the serum concentration of various antibiotics in difficult dosing situations remains actual determination of peak serum levels by appropriate assay methods.[11,12]

SUMMARY

Elderly patients have a variety of common infectious diseases that may present atypically in their age group. Older individuals frequently have multisystem disease that usually includes significant renal insufficiency. The use of antibiotics in the elderly should take into account the most common diseases encountered in this age group, as well as the functional capacity of the liver and kidneys. Dosing modifications should be reflective of diminished hepatic and renal metabolism and the excretory capacity associated with aging and systemic diseases. Elderly patients with significant renal dysfunction should be given drugs excreted primarily by nonrenal mechanisms. Conversely, elderly patients with significant impairment of hepatic function optimally should be treated with antibiotics that are eliminated via renal mechanisms. Ever-increasing numbers of patients with end-stage renal disease are maintained by a variety of dialysis regimens. Careful attention to antibiotic selection and dosing in these patients is particularly important. Lastly, in today's DRG world of cost-conscious antibiotic prescribing, the clinician needs to efficiently treat elderly patients at home, in the nursing home or chronic care facility, or in the hospital, with the least expensive effective medications appropriate for the diseases of the elderly.

REFERENCES

1. Epstein M: Aging and the kidney: Clinical implications. *Am Fam Physician* 1985;31:123−137.
2. Samiy AH: Renal disease in the elderly. *Med Clin North Am* 1983;67:463−480.
3. Frocht A, Fillit H: Renal disease in the geriatric patient. *J Am Geriatr Soc* 1984;32:28−43.
4. Gambert RS, Csuka ME, Duthie EH, et al: Interpretation of laboratory results in the elderly. *Postgrad Med* 1982;72:147−152.
5. Hang MH, Ginsberg AL, Dobbins WO: Marked elevation in serum alkaline phosphatase activity as a manifestation of systemic infection. *Gastroenterology* 1980;78:592-597.
6. Kenny RAM, Hodkinson HM, Prendiville OF, et al: Abnormalities of liver function and the predictive value of liver function tests in infection and outcome of acutely ill elderly patients. *Age Ageing* 1984;13:224−229.
7. Chu CM, Liaw YF: High serum alkaline phosphatase in septicemic infection. *Gastroenterology* 1980;79:776.
8. Lubin JR, Millward BA, Coles JA, et al: Value of profiling liver function in the elderly. *Postgrad Med J* 1983;59:763−766.
9. Conte JE, Barriere SL: *Manual of Antibiotics and Infectious Diseases,* ed 6. Philadelphia, Lea & Febiger, 1988.
10. Lesar TS, Zaske DE: Modifying dosage regimens in renal and hepatic failure, in Ristuccia AM, Cunha BA (eds): *Antimicrobial Therapy.* New York. Raven Press, 1984, pp 95-112.
11. Cunha BA: *Antibiotic Selection and DRG's.* New York, Raven Press, 1986.
12. Cunha BA: Antibiotic dosing in renal insufficiency/dialysis patient. *Heart Lung* 1988 (in press).

INDEX

Abscess
  brain, 28–30
  diverticular, 207
  intra-abdominal, 207, 209, 210
  liver. *See* Pyogenic liver abscess
  periappendiceal, 206
  source of intra-abdominal abscess, 208
  spinal epidural, 29
  treatment of, 210–213
Acinetobacter calcoaceticus, 146
Acquired immune deficiency syndrome. *See* AIDS
Actinomyces israelii, 66
Acyclovir, 50, 64, 252
Adult respiratory distress syndrome, 100, 305
Age, as factor in infections, 289–291
AIDS, 9, 54, 276, 278, 303
Amantidine hydrochloride, 109
Aminoglycosides, 168, 212
Amputations, due to osteomyelitis, 263
Anemia, in liver abscess, 189
Anergy, 10
Antibody-coated bacteria (ACB), 226
Antigenic drift, and shift, 324–325
Antimicrobial therapy
  common infections, 338–343
  dosing considerations, 333–334
  dosing modifications, 334–335
  liver function tests, 332–333
  pharmacokinetic age-related changes, 331
  renal and hepatic function, 330, 331–332
  renal diseases, 332
  systemic diseases, 331
Aortic valve calcification, 160
Appendicitis, 205–206
Arborvirus, cause of encephalitis, 44
ARDS. *See* Adult respiratory distress syndrome

Arteriosclerotic changes in valves, 160
Arthritis, septic, 261
  recommendations for empiric therapy of 268
Arthrocentesis, 267
Aspergillus, 147
Atherosclerotic valvular or annualar disease, 2

Back pain, with fever, 276
Bacteremia, with vertebral osteomyelitis, 1, 255
Bacteriuria, 216, 219–221, 223, 224, 294–295
B fraglis group, 213
Bile. *See also* Biliary tract infections
  bacteria in (bactibilia), 173, 175
  thrombi, 196
Biliary tract infections
  abdominal radiography showing emphysematous cholecystitis, 178
  algorithm for evaluation of acute cholecystitis, 181
  bacterial findings in patients undergoing cholecystectomy, 174
  bacterial findings in cultures from bile in acute cholecystitis, 175
  clinical features of, 176–177
  diagnosis of, 177–180
  differential diagnoses, 181
  pathophysiologic features of, 174–176
  treatment of, 180–183
  ultrasonographic study of calculous cholecystitis, 179
Bilirubin levels, 182, 197
Bilroth II resection, 210
Biopsy
  bone, 258
  brain, 48
  laryngeal, 74

liver, 200, 281
lung, 151, 281
warts, 253
Bladder catheter, as cause of infection, 288
Bladder infection, with prostatitis, 235
Blood cultures, in endocarditis, 163
Boils, 244
Bone and joint infections
  laboratory tests with, 261-262
  treatment of, 262-263
Bone infections, 254-268
Bone marrow biopsy, 281
Brain abscess, 28-30
Branhamella catarrhalis, 131, 146
Bronchopneumonia, 122
Bronchoscopy, new method in, 124

Candida, 147
Candidiasis, 320
Cancer, liver, 196
Carcinomas, as cause of fever, 273-274
Catheter
  complications of, 296
  evaluating the patient, 295-297
  removal in treatment of infection, 298
  as source of infection, 288
  use of in bladder infections, 230-231
Catheterization, of bladder, 228
Cefoxitin, 212, 213
Cellulitis
  in foot of diabetic, 249
  fulminant, 245
Centers for Disease Control, 144, 303
Central nervous system infections
  antimicrobial agents in treatment, 39-40
  bacterial, 28-35
  bacterial meningitis, 30-34
  brain abscess, 28-30
  clinical manifestations of, 27-28
  complications of atypical pneumonia, 51
  with endocarditis, 162

  fungal and yeast, 35-36
  initial therapy of meningitis in various circumstances, 38
  management of, 37-39
  neurosyphilis, 34-35
  other infections, 36-37
  overview of, 25-26
  parameningeal focus, 28-30
  superinfecting pathogens in patients with specific underlying diseases, 27
Cervicofacial actinomycosis, 66
Chest roentgenogram, for diagnosis of tuberculosis, 307
Chlamydia pssittaci (psittacosis or ornithosis), 102, 103-104
Chlamydia trachomatis, 105, 240
Cholangiogram (IV), 177-178
Cholangitis, 186
Cholecystectomy, 174
Cholecystitis, statistics of, 173, 182, 186
  See also Biliary tract infections
Cholecystokinin (CCK), 180
Cholelithiasis, 173
Chronic diseases, as factor in infections, 290
Clostridium perfringens (or *tetani*), 248
Colitis (or bowel disease), 207
Colonization, 7
Common cold and influenza syndrome
  caused by, 67
  epidemiology, 67-68
  prevention and treatment of, 68-69
  symptoms of, 68
Community-acquired pneumonia, 116-133
  See also Nosocomial pneumonia; Pneumonia
  studies of civilian adults, 120-121
Compound fractures, 258
Conjunctival hemorrhages, 277
Counterimmunoelectrophoresis (CIE), of sputum, 124
Coxiella burnetii (Q fever), 102, 103

Creatinine clearance formula, 332
Creutzfeldt-Jakob disease, 27
Cryosurgery with liquid nitrogen, 253
Crytococcus neoformans, 35
Cutaneous ulcers. *See* Diabetic foot infections
Cystic duct, obstruction of, 177
Cystitis, 216
Cytomegalovirus, 194

Decubitus ulcers, 250–251, 343
Dehydration, in pneumonia, 123
Delta hepatitis virus (HDV), 200
Dementia, 27–28
Dental abscess, 276
Diabetes mellitus
  candidiasis in, 320
  classification and criteria for diagnosis of, 313
  criteria for diagnosis of, 312–313
  defined, 312–314
  demography and pathogenesis of, 314
  effect on immune system, 316–317
  emphysematous pyelonephritis in, 318
  foot infections, 248–250, 257
  fungal infections in, 320
  glucose, in urine, 219
  humoral immunity in, 317
  impact on host defenses, 315–317
  insulin-dependent (IDDM), or type I, 313
  malignant external otitis, 319
  neutrophil function in, 315–316
  noninsulin-dependent (NIDDM), or type II, 313
  osteomyelitis in, 319
  overview of, 12
  putative infections linked to, 317–320
  rhinocerebral zygomycosis in, 320
  soft tissue infections in, 318–319
  torulopsis glabrata in, 320
  tuberculosis in, 319
  urinary infections in, 318
Diabetic patient, infections in, 312–320

Diverticulosis, 206–207
Drugs, as cause of fever, 275

Ecthyma, 244
Elderly
  factors influencing clinical presentation of infections, 18–19
  infectious diseases in, 1–5
  numbers in nursing homes, 286
  special problems associated with pneumonia, 116
Emphysematous pyelonephritis, 318
Empyema, 152
Encephalitis
  herpes simplex, 47–50
  mycoplasma-associated, 51–53
  overview of, 44
  St. Louis, 45–47
  western equine, eastern equine, and California, 46
Endocarditis
  antibiotic regimens for treating, 164–166
  clinical features of, 161–163
  diagnosis of, 163–167
  increase in incidence of, 159
  infective, 36
  microbiology, 160–161
  predisposing factors in, 160
  prognosis, 167
  prophylaxis for, 170
  prosthetic valve, 169
  subacute infective, 2, 272
  treatment of, 167–170
  valve destroyed by, 168–169
Enterobacteraciae, 238
Enterococci, group D, 161
Enterococcus, 212–213
Enzyme-linked immunosorbant assay (ELISA), 197
Epiglottis. *See* Laryngitis and Epiglottis
Epstein-Barr virus (EBV), 70
Erysipelas, 65, 244
Erythematosis, systemic lupus (SLE), 277
Erythrocyte sedimentation rate (ESR), 262, 279–280

Escherichia coli, 339
Exthyma gangrenosum, 246

Fatty liver disease, 190
Fever, 19–21
  with abscesses, 272
  with back pain, 276
  bradycardia, relative, 277
  caused by stool softeners, 275
  clues to fever disclosed by invasive diagnostic procedures, 282
  diagnostic clues to fever from laboratory findings, 280
  diagnostic procedures
    invasive, 281–282
    noninvasive, 280
  as drug reaction, 275
  with endocarditis, 162
  headaches, 276
  historical clues to diagnosis of fever, 277
  in liver abscess, 188
  with liver enlargement, 278
  with mental confusion, 276
  with myaligias, 276
  in osteomyelitis, 255
  physical clues to diagnosis of fever, 279
  in rheumatic diseases, 274
Fever, of unknown origin (FUO), 271–282
  causes of, 272
  diagnostic approach, 275–282
  fever patterns, 278
  laboratory tests for, 279–280
  physical examination of patient, 277–278
Fiber, crude, reduction of, as related to diverticulitis, 206
Fiberoptic bronchoscopy (FOB), 150, 152
Fistula, 206
Foot ulcers, 318–319
Fournier's gangrene, 248, 318–319
Fractures, severe open (compound), 258
Francisella tularensis (tularemia), 102, 103
Fungal infections, 320
  and yeast, 35–36
FUO. *See* Fever, of unknown origin

Gallbladder, inflammation of, 176–177
  See also Biliary tract infections
Gallstones, 173, 174
Gangrene, 206
  gas, 248
  synergistic, 249
Genitourinary surgery, with prostatic infections, 241
Geriatric medicine, low emphasis placed on, 293
Giant cell arteritis (GCA), 274
GI tract obstruction, 207
Glucose, in urine, 219
Glucose intolerance, 313–314
Glucose tolerance test, described, 314
Gonococcus, 235
Gram's stain, 150
Green nail syndrome, 246
Guillain-Barré syndrome, 36, 109, 325

Haemophilus influenzae (HIO infections), 31, 146
Hemophilus influenza cellulitis, 67
Hemorrhages, conjunctival, 277
Hepatic insufficiency formula, 334–335
Hepatitis
  body fluid precautions with, 202–203
  clinical features of, 195–196
  cytomegalovirus as cause of, 194
  diagnosis of, 196–197
  fulminant, 196
  infectious period of, 198
  interpretation of hepatitis B serologic markers, 199
  laboratory tests for, 197–198
  leukopenia and lymphocytosis in, 197
  management of, 201–202
  non-A, non-B, 200–201
  prevention and prophylaxis of, 202–203
  relationship of liver enzyme elevation, stage of disease and antibody in hepatitis A, 197

relationship of serologic markers
of hepatitis B infection with
SGPT and course of disease, 198
Hepatitis A IGM, 198
Hepatitis B surface antigen
(HBsAG), 198
Herpes simplex, 251, 252-253
Herpes simplex encephalitis (HSV),
47-50
Herpes virus, 147
Herpes zoster (shingles), 1, 64-65,
251-252
Hodgkin's and non-Hodgkin's lymphomas, 273
Hospitals
number of beds *v* in nursing homes,
286
Host defenses, 6-14
alterations with age, 10-14, 118
defects and susceptibility to infection, 8
in diabetes, 315-317
Hypernephromas, 273-274
Hypertension, with bacteriuria,
223
Hypotension, masking gallbladder
infection, 176
Hypoxemia, 151-152

IDDM. *See* Diabetes mellitus
Immune globulin, for hepatitis, 202
Immune system
abnormalities of, 2
age-related changes, 289-290
Immunizations
influenza, 324-326
pneumococcal, 326-328
target groups for, 326
tetanus toxoid, 328
for travelers, 328
Implantation surgery, infections
following, 259
Infection control plans, 292
Infections
altered clinical responses to illness,
19
of biliary tract, 173-183
bladder, with prostatitis, 235
bladder catheters as cause, 288

bone and joint, 254-268
central nervous system, 25-40
cervicofacial
common, 62-63
uncommon, 65-67
changing patterns of illness, 19
of decubitus ulcers, 250-251
definition of, 7
diabetic foot, 248-250
due to poor oral hygiene, 291
factors that cause, 7-10
fungal, 35-36, 320
intra-abdominal, 205-213
intra-abdominal sepsis and pelvic
infections, comparative clinical
trials of antibiotic regimens, 211
of joints, 261
of kidneys, 217
liver, bacterial, 185-192
lowered immunity due to medications, 289-290
in nursing homes, 285-299
orofacial, odontogenic, and deep
cervical, 79-86
overview of, 1-5
postoperative, 258-259
of prosthetic joint, 254
prostatic, associated with genitourinary surgery, 241
Pseudomonas, 245-247
respiratory tract, 288-289
of skin and soft tissue, 243-253
skin, viral, 251-253
staphylococcal and streptococcal,
244-245
underreporting of illnesses, 18
upper respiratory tract, 61-86
urinary tract, 216-231, 294-299
Infectious diseases
as cause of fever, 273
in the elderly, an overview, 1-5
Infective endocarditis (IE), 36
Influenza, 106-109
complications of, 107, 108
epidemics, 118
incidence and mortality rates,
106-107
vaccine, annual immunization
recommended, 130

virus, 324-325
Insulin sensitivity, 314
Interferon and vidarabine (ara-A), 202
Interleukin, 8, 21
Intra-abdominal infections, 205-213
Iodine solutions, 251
Isoniazid, 308-309

Janeway's lesions, 163
Japanese encephalitis, 26
Jaundice
  in hepatitis, 197
  in sepsis, 182
Joint infections, 254-268
Joint disease, 262

Kidney infection, 217

Laboratories, need for in nursing homes, 292
Laparatomy, 281
Laryngitis and epiglottis
  diagnosis of, 74
  etiology, 72
  symptoms of, 73-74
  treatment of, 74-75
Legionella-like organisms (LLO), 99
Legionella micdadei, 99-100
Legionella pneumophila, 53-54, 56, 96-99, 147
Legionnaires' disease, 36, 53-57, 127-128, 277, 281, 340
  diagnostic features of, 96
  laboratory studies of, 98
  Pontiac fever, 97
  predisposing factors in, 97
  symptoms of, 98
  treatment of, 99
Leukemia, acute myelogenous (AML), 274
Life expectancy, 303
Listeria infections, 26
Liver, penetrating injuries to, 187
Liver biopsy, 281
Liver cancer, primary, 196
Liver disease, 278
  masking tuberculosis, 306
Liver function tests, 332-333

Liver infections. *See* Pyogenic liver abscess
Liver scan, 190
Lobar pneumonia, 122
Ludwig's angina, 83
Lung biopsy, 281
Lyme disease, 36-37
Lymphomas, as cause of fever, 273

Malignant otitis externa, 29
Mantoux skin test, 306
Mediastinitis, 86
Meningitis
  acute bacterial, 33
  enterococcal, 33
  tuberculous, 305-306
Mental confusion
  in central nervous system infections, 27
  related to fever, 276
Miliary tuberculosis. *See* Tuberculosis
Mitral valve prolapse, 160
Mononucleosis, infectious, 70
Murmurs, in endocarditis, 162
Musculoskeletal symptoms, with endocarditis, 162
Mycobacterium tuberculosis, culture for, 306
Mycoplasma-associated meningitis, 51-53
Mycoplasma pneumoniae, 1
Mycoplasma pneumonia, 100-102
National Diabetes Data Group, The, 312-313
National Nosocomial Infections Study (NNIS), 144
Necrotizing fasciitis, 247-248
Neisseria catarrhalis. See Branhamella catarrhalis
Neutrophil function, in diabetes
  adherence, 315
  chemotaxis, 315-316
  intracellular killing, 316
  phagocytosis, 316
NIDDM. *See* Diabetes mellitus
Nisseria meningtidis, 31
Nosocomial infection, 6-7, 285-299

Nosocomial pneumonia, 144-156
  See also Pneumonia
  altering host susceptibility,
    155-156
  cause of, 145-147
  control of pathogens, 154
  diagnosis of, 147-151
  limiting transmission of, 154-155
  management of, 153
  prevention of, 153-155
Nursing homes, 13
  average length of stay in, 286
  bacteriuria in, 220
  environment harboring pathogens,
    291-293
  factors causing infections, 289-293
  infection control plans in, 292
  prevalence of infections in,
    287-289
  significance of in elderly health
    care, 286-287
  tendency to infection of residents,
    285-299
Nutrition, in treatment of bed sores,
  251

Obstructive biliary tract disease, 186
Odontogenic infections
  anatomical and physiologic considerations, 80-81
  canine, buccal, and parotid space,
    82-83
  deep fascial compartment, 82
  dentoalveolar, gingival, and
    periodontal, 81-82
  etiology of, 79-80
  masticator space, 82
  retropharyngeal, danger, and
    prevertebral spaces, 83-84
  sublingual, submandibular, and
    lateral pharyngeal spaces, 83
  treatment of, 84
Oral hygiene, as source of infection,
  291
Orofacial, odontogenic, and deep
  cervical infections, 79-86
Osler's nodes, 163
Osteomyelitis, 254, 255-260
  amputations as a result of, 263
  bacteriology of pyogenic vertebral
    osteomyelitis, 256
  diabetic foot infections, 257
  duration of therapy, 263
  factors associated with
    osteomyelitis secondary to continuous spread of infection,
    256
  hematogenous, 255-256
  of jaws, 84-85
  laboratory tests for, 261-262
  management of patient with
    vertebral osteomyelitis, 264
  management scheme for patient
    with osteomyelitis secondary to
    diabetic foot ulcer, 264
  microbiology of open fracture infections, influence of antibiotic
    prophylaxis, 259
  postsurgical, 258-259
  presenting symptoms of patients
    with infection associated with
    prosthetic joints, 260
  pressure sores, 258
  recommendations for empiric
    therapy in, 265-266
  secondary to direct innoculation,
    260
  sources of bacteremia associated
    with pyogenic vertebral
    osteomyelitis, 255
  sternoclavicular, 260
  vertebral, 29, 255-256, 263
Otitis externa, 77-78, 246
Otitis media and mastoiditis, 78-79

Papilloma virus (warts), 251
Parotitis, acute bacterial, 62-63
Pasteurella multocida, 102
Percutaneous transhepatic
  cholangiography (PTC), 191
Periarteristis nodosa, 274
Peritonitis, 206
Petechiae, 163
Pharyngitis
  complications of, 71
  diphtheria and, 70-71
  infectious mononucleosis, 70
  overview of, 69

streptococcal, 70
  treatment of, 71–72
  viral, 70
Phlebothrombosis, 274–275
Physicians, need for care in nursing homes, 293
Pittsburgh pneumonia agent (PPA), 99–100
Plague
  bubonic, 104
  pneumonic, 104–105
Pneumococcal pneumonia
  high-risk conditions for, 326–327
  rates of occurrence, 119
Pneumonia, 2–4
  closed chest drainage of fluid, 152
  as complication of influenza, 107–108
  currently preferred antimicrobial drugs for initial presumptive therapy of community-acquired pneumonia, 132–133
  diagnosis and therapy of, 131
  epidemics of, 154
  Haemophilus influenzae, as cause of, 126–127
  historical evidence of, 116–117
  hypoxemia in, 151–152
  infection control program, 155
  mycoplasma, 100–102
  nonpneumococcal, 126–131
  nosocomial, 144–156
  outpatient treatment of, 119
  simultaneous viral and bacterial, 108–109
  sputum cultures, in diagnosis, 123
  viral, 105–110
  zoonotic, 102–105
Pneumonia, atypical
  differential features of typical and atypical pneumonias, 94
  empiric therapy, 95
Polio vaccine, Salk *v* Sabin, 328
Pontiac fever, 97
Posttransfusion hepatitis, 201
Primary influenza pneumonia, 108
Prostate gland, enlarged, 224

Prostatitis
  bacterial, 235–240
  nonbacterial, 240
Prostatodynia, 241
Prosthetic joint infection, 254
Prosthetic valve endocarditis, 169
Pseudomonas aeruginosa, 170, 238, 298, 319
Pseudomonas skin infection, 245–247
Pulmonary emboli, 274
Pulmonary function, diminished by aging, 118
Pulmonary tuberculosis, 305, 308
Pyelonephritis, acute, 217, 223, 227
Pyoderma, 246
Pyogenic liver abscess
  causes of, 186–187
  clinical manifestations of, 189
  drainage of, 191–192
  history and incidence of, 185–186
  isolates obtained on direct needle aspiration of, 188
  laboratory tests for, 189–191
  microbiology of, 187–188
  organisms isolated from, 187
  symptoms of, 188–189
  treatment of, 191–192

Radioactive gallium 67 scans, 209
Radioimmune assay (RAI), 197
Radionuclide scintigraphy, 178
Renal abscesses, as cause of fever, 272
Renal function tests, 331–332
Renal insufficiency formula, 334
Respiratory tract infections, 61–86
  as most frequent cause of death, 288–289
  predominant oral microbial flora, 63
Rheumatic diseases, as cause of fever, 274
Rheumatic heart disease, as factor in endocarditis, 160
Rhinocerebral phycomycosis, 76
Rhinocerebral zygomycosis (phycomycosis or mucormycosis), 320

Rhinoscleroma, 76
Rifampin, 308-309
Rimantidine, 110
Roth's spots, 163

Scalded skin syndrome, 245
Schlichter tests, 169. 170
Secondary bacterial pneumonia, 108
Septic arthritis, 261
Shingles. *See* Herpes zoster
Sialoadenitis, 63
Sinusitis
  etiology, 75
  symptoms and diagnosis of, 75-76
  treatment of, 76-77
Skin infections, viral, 251-253
Spinal epidural abscess, 29
Splinter hemorrhages, 163
Sputum screening system, 150
Staphylococcal and streptococcal infections, 244-245
Staphylococcus aureus, 146, 160, 161, 236
Sternoclavicular osteomyelitis, 260
Stevens-Johnson syndrome, 101
St Louis encephalitis, 45-47
Still's disease, 277
Streptococcal purpura fulminans, 245
Streptococcus bovis, 161
Streptococcus pneumoniae, 146
Study of the Efficacy of Nosocomial Infection Control (SENIC), 144
Swan-Ganz catheterization, 260
Swine influenza vaccine, 325
Syndrome of inappropriate secretion of antidiuretic hormone (SIADH), 330
Synovitis, 267

Technetium 99 brain scan, 29
Tetanus toxoid, 328
Tetracycline, 240
Thrombophlebitis, suppurative, jugular, and carotid artery erosion, 85
Thrombosis, septic, cavernous, sinus, 86

Thymus gland, 10
Thyroiditis, suppurative, 65-66
Tobramycin, 212
Toe web infection, 246
Torulopsis glabrata, 320
Toxic shock syndrome (TSS), 244-245
Transthoracic needle aspiration of the lung, 124
Transtracheal aspiration (TTA), 124, 146, 151
Transurethral resection, 240, 241
Trichinosis, 277
Tuberculin skin test, 304
Tuberculosis, 2-3, 303-310
  adult respiratory distress syndrome, as a complication of, 305
  adverse reactions to drug therapy, 308-309
  antituberculous drug interactions, 309
  as cause of fever, 273
  of central nervous system, 33
  diagnostic tests for, 307
  as disease of elderly, 7
  drug-resistant, 309
  epidemics of, in nursing homes, 304
  extrapulmonary, treatment of, 308
  frequency of, 303
  identification of, with stains and microscopy, 306
  liver disease and, 306
  meningitis in, 305-306
  miliary, 306
  nonspecificity of symptoms, 305
  positive skin test for, 304, 307
  pulmonary, 305, 308
  treatment of, 308-310
Tuberculous meningitis, 34, 305-306
Tumors, benign, virus-induced, 253
Typhoid fever, 277

Ultrasonography
  to diagnose cholecystitis, 179
  of intra-abdominal abscesses, 209

Ureaplasma urealyticum, 240
Urethra, 217
Urethritis, 216
Urinary drainage, in prostatitis, 236
Urinary tract infections. *See also*
  Infections
  bacteriuria, significance of,
    223–225
  catheter-associated, 230, 231
  clinical features of, 222–223
  closed drainage, 231
  comparison of mannose-sensitive
    Escherichia coli to uroephithelial
    cells, 218
  cumulative percentage of subjects
    with positive urine culture
    survey, 221
  diagnosis of, 225–227
  epidemiology, 219–221
  host defense mechanisms, 218
  microbiology, 221–222
  open drainage, with catheter, 230
  pathogenesis, 217–219
  prevalence of bacteriuria, 220
  radiologic evaluation of, 227
  relapse *v* reinfection, 217
  results of antibody-coated bacteria
    test (ACB) on urine specimens of
    subjects with bacteriuria, 227
  treatment of, 227–230
Urine specimens, clean-catch, 225–226
U.S. Public Health Service, 303

Vaccine
  inactivated *v* live attenuated,
    325–326, 328
  multivalent, testing of, 327
  for pneumococcal pneumonia,
    326–328
  polysaccharide, 327
  polyvalent pneumococcal, 125,
    155
  smallpox, 328
  polio, 328
  swine influenza, 325
  14-valent, 327
Valve replacement, 168–169
Varicella zoster virus, 64
Vertebral osteomyelitis, *See*
  Osteomyelitis
Virarabine (ara-A), 49, 50
Viral cholestatic disease, 196
Viral hepatitis, 194, 203
  See also Hepatitis
Viral pneumonia, 105–110
  See also Pneumonia
Viral skin infections, 251–253
Viridans streptococci, 160–161

Waldenström's macroglobulinemia,
  278
Warts. *See* Papilloma virus

Yeast infections. *See* Fungal
  infections
Yersinia pestis (plague), 102, 104

Zinc
  decreased level of, 238
  in treatment of decubitus ulcers,
    251
Zoonotic pneumonia, 102–105